YOU DON'T
NEED MEAT

Also by Peter Cox

Linda McCartney's Home Cooking

LifePoints

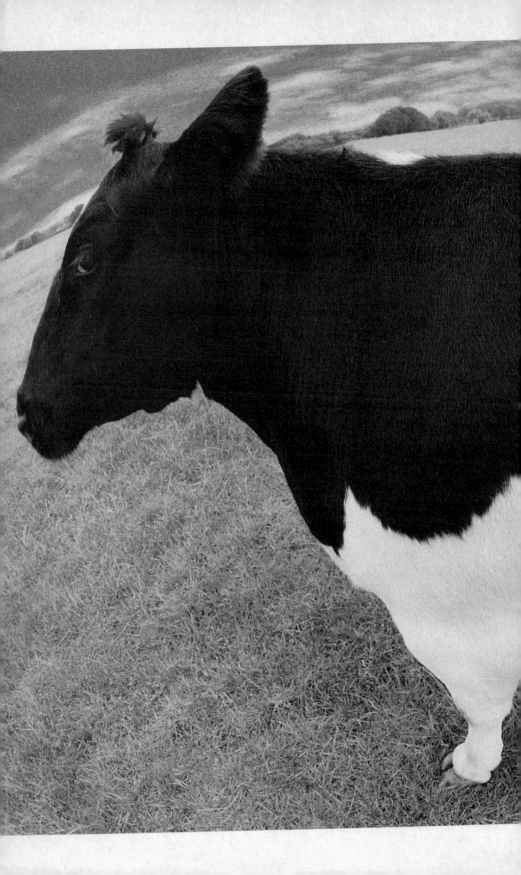

YOU DON'T NEED MEAT

PETER COX

THOMAS DUNNE BOOKS
ST. MARTIN'S GRIFFIN ⚯ NEW YORK

For Louise and Beau,
in the hope that your world will be
a nicer and kinder place
than ours was.

THOMAS DUNNE BOOKS.
An imprint of St. Martin's Press.

YOU DON'T NEED MEAT. Copyright © 2002 by Peter Cox. All rights reserved. Printed in the United States of America. No part of this book may be used or reproduced in any manner whatsoever without written permission except in the case of brief quotations embodied in critical articles or reviews. For information, address St. Martin's Press, 175 Fifth Avenue, New York, N.Y. 10010.

www.stmartins.com

Library of Congress Cataloging-in-Publication Data

Cox, Peter.
    You don't need meat / Peter Cox.—1st ed.
        p. cm.
    Includes bibliographical references (pp. 341–63).
    ISBN 0-312-27761-X (hc)
    ISBN 0-312-30338-6 (pbk)
    1. Vegetarianism. 2. Vegetarian cookery. 3. Meat—Health aspects.
    I. Title.

    RM236.C683 2002
    613.2'62—dc21   2001054814

First St. Martin's Griffin Edition: November 2003

10 9 8 7 6 5 4 3 2 1

CONTENTS

ACKNOWLEDGMENTS

Many people have helped me, in various ways, to write this book. I would like to express my sincere appreciation to the following people for most generously giving of their time and expertise:

Dr. Helen Grant, Colin and Lis Howlett, Barry and Sue Kew, Andrew Kimbrell of the Foundation on Economic Trends, Drs. G. and C. Langley, Dr. Alan Long, Philip L. Pick and the staff of the Jewish Vegetarian Society, Dr. David Ryde, Gregory Sams of the Realeat Company, Joyce D'Silva and Peter Stevenson of Compassion in World Farming, Sarah Starkey, Andrew Tyler, Michael Verney-Elliott, and the staff of the British Library, Science Reference and Information Service in London, the Sir Thomas Browne Library in Norwich, and the Addenbrookes Hospital Library in Cambridge. I would also like to express my gratitude to Tom Dunne and Marcia Markland for their publishing enthusiasm and editorial talent. My greatest debt, as always, is to Peggy for her encouragement and belief in the book.

FOREWORD

My friend Linda McCartney was kind enough to write a Foreword to the 1992 edition of this book, which is reproduced below. Her untimely death in 1998 from breast cancer robbed us of an important voice.

For many years now some of us have been saying "Stop eating animals" because we know that it is pointless and cruel. My friend Peter Cox is one of those who has been saying it loudest.

Unfortunately the majority of those who are steeped in the tradition of meat eating either closed their ears or said they didn't care about the moral arguments.

But now, in this remarkable book, Peter has researched arguments that the majority cannot ignore—not if they care for their health. Or their lives.

His conclusions are—for the meat eater—alarming. Those who believe that meat is somehow good for you should read the facts connecting it to heart disease, high blood pressure, and cancer before swallowing another mouthful.

This is a book that will change lives and save lives. I hope that yours is one of them.

Linda McCartney

PREFACE

This little book has had an interesting evolution. An instant bestseller when it was published in Britain all of fifteen years ago, it was less than half the size of the volume you now hold in your hands. From there, it went to Germany, Japan, Holland, and several other countries, arriving back in the U.K. again some five years later, where it was rewritten and greatly expanded. Then it went traveling all over again; back to Japan and Germany and other ports of call too numerous to mention. And so, eventually, it's arrived in America—rewritten once more and further expanded. Since Britain is guilty of unleashing such dubious delights as beef eating and Mad Cow Disease on the world, please consider this book as one Brit's way of saying "Sorry!"

Some people have said some very kind things about it along the way, and I blush to repeat them, but sometimes these things have to be done. Britain's most eminent food critic, Derek Cooper, scared me a great deal when he wrote, "I think from now on Peter Cox ought to lock his bedroom door at night; otherwise he might well be woken up by heavy breathing in the small hours and find two men in white coats trying to stun him with a bolt pistol prior to suspending him from a convenient meat hook . . . he just published the most forceful indictment of the meat industry I have yet seen; there must be large groups of men yearning for his blood in every cattle ring and slaughterhouse in the country. Since reading *You Don't Need Meat* I have crossed over the road every time I have approached a meat market."

Elle magazine said, "Cox's argument is riveting; his conclusions are utterly disturbing." I understand it takes quite a lot to disturb *Elle* magazine, so I guess that's a compliment. *The Financial Times*, however, was sure I was a modern-day Adolf Hitler. They wrote, "For Peter Cox, vegetarianism has all the appearance of a particularly austere religious order. . . . Austere men are often dangerous: Cromwell, Robespierre, Mussolini and Hitler, for example. . . . Cox and Hitler share a trait: they both believe the future belongs to vegetarians." Austere, *moi*? Surely they were jesting.

The *Nursing Times* reassured me a great deal when they concluded that I was not, in fact, severely delusional (and I think they are more of an authority on mental health than the *Financial Times* is): "Cox brings together in a readable form much recent research into nutrition and diet. This is a controversial and provocative book but, whatever one's ultimate conclusions concerning Cox's views, the arguments cannot be lightly dismissed; neither can they be relegated to the 'lunatic fringe' of food faddism."

Even the *Meat Trades Journal* concluded that "Peter Cox is a very convincing man," although they went on to say that I was probably the sort of person who, if I wasn't writing books, would probably be undertaking dastardly acts of despicable violence and terrorism.

This eruptive theme was continued by the *Birmingham Post*, who found the book "Explosive! If you've ever thought twice about the contents of the beef burger you're eating or felt unease when the latest meat-related disease hogs the headlines—then you should buy this book. . . . One of the most thought-provoking tomes you may read this year. . . . Do yourself a favor and buy this book now."

And even the conservative-minded *Daily Telegraph* welcomed the book "because it will rattle the cages, or perhaps crates, of people paid a lot of money to protect the interests of factory farming." Another national newspaper, *The Observer*, whined, "The trouble with Mr. Cox's book is that, having read it, it's all or nothing." Then they decided, I think, to come down on my side with the resigned, tight-lipped comment, "Pass me the tofu." *Raw* tofu? I think I'd prefer to eat Mussolini's hair shirt.

"Peter Cox's arguments are fascinating," said *The Lancet*, quite simply. ("Fascinating," I hope, because they're good arguments—not because they're fascinating examples of delusional psychosis.)

Today newspaper was more interested in my bank balance than anything else, writing, "Peter, who first spat out meat at the age of two, has sold more than half a million books—which must, at a conservative estimate, make him a millionaire." Now *that's* a good example of delusionary thinking.

The magazine *Vegetarian Living* more or less canonized me when they wrote: "Peter Cox is both energetic and amiable, with the kind of charm normally found in the diplomatic service. As he has become our foremost vegetarian ambassador perhaps this is not surprising."

But I was soon brought down to earth again by London's *Evening Standard*, who went for the jugular: "Peter Cox appears to have an identity problem, having at a young age confused himself with plant life." They didn't specify *which* plant, precisely, I had confused myself with, but it's true that I've always been weirdly attracted to carrots. Now I know why.

The *Sunday Times* also had their suspicions about me, although somewhat nicer ones: "Peter Cox looks like an off-duty TV presenter," wrote their reviewer, "And he's really not too loathsome at all. If, like him, you are taking on an £11 billion-a-year industry more or less single-handed, you need to be energetic, organised and brave. I suspect he may be some kind of genius." But what kind of genius, precisely? To my frustration, they didn't say. Since Hitler was an evil genius, I didn't find that comment necessarily reassuring.

At least the Sunday edition of *Independent* liked my clothes. "Peter Cox is a smartly turned-out former executive," they wrote, "with an impressive track record in advertising—an unlikely candidate to be an advocate of an alternative culture. But he is the meat industry's most effective foe. . . . If Mr. Cox's past campaigns are anything to go by, his latest assault on meat-eating will have the following consequences: his wife will receive warnings that he is about to be killed and be told how his corpse is about to be jointed; representatives of butchers and farmers will denounce him 'as an evangelist with few scruples'; and tens of thousands of people will become vegetarian."

Well, there you have it. Although it's startling to be compared to Hitler, and nice to be called a genius, I'm fortunate enough not to be troubled too much by either excessive praise or bloodcurdling threats. The only thing that really counts, for me, is *your* reaction to this book. After the first edition was published (in the days before e-mail— remember them?) it was my great pleasure to receive many hundreds of letters from readers with comments, thoughts, opinions, and information. For me, it was those letters, and sometimes the comments of members of the audience when I was giving a talk, that meant everything to me. Today, of course, we have e-mail, and if you feel like dropping me a line, I'd be truly delighted to receive it. The address is below.

Thank you for reading this book—I hope you enjoy it and find it useful.

To write to Peter Cox and to check for updates to this book, please visit www.yesitive.com/nomeat.

INTRODUCTION

Meat-eating. Never before has any part of the diet come under such scrutiny or been so hotly debated in circles spanning science, medicine, ethics, and environmentalism.

In medicine, it has certainly become an important consideration in treating patients. No matter what kind of issues we're dealing with, from high blood pressure to migraine headaches, good nutrition is essential to healing and prevention alike. In research studies at the Physicians Committee for Responsible Medicine (PCRM) in Washington, D.C., we've seen hundreds of people drop meat from their menus in favor of healthy plant foods. With this one simple change, we see body weight and blood pressure normalize, cholesterol levels drop, and immunity gain new strength.

Recently, we began a new focus on nutrition for cancer care, offering educational cooking classes for cancer survivors and their families. Led by our registered dietitians, participants roll up their sleeves and learn to prepare healthy, delicious meals packed with cancer-fighting nutrients. Not a single meal contains meat—or any animal product, for that matter. Invariably, these cancer survivors feel empowered with life-saving information that wasn't provided by the hospitals that treated their disease. Once they understand why meat is not part of the cancer-fighting menu, they no longer see it as an edible indulgence. Rather, they see it as the package of carcinogens it really is.

In the early 1990s, Dean Ornish, M.D., led a groundbreaking study to test whether a meat-free diet could improve the health of his patients with heart disease. By trading animal products for whole grain foods, vegetables, bean dishes, and fruits, along with moderate exercise and cessation of smoking, his patients began to recover. Not only did arterial blockages stop worsening, for most they began to dissolve away.

We have experienced similarly phenomenal results in our clinical research at PCRM. A study of women with menstrual pain found that simply eliminating hormone-boosting foods such as meat, dairy products, and eggs significantly reduced physical pain, tension, and irritability. The study also made medical history by showing the greatest cholesterol-lowering effect ever reported in women under fifty. And that's without medication or its troubling side effects.

In 1999, PCRM researchers studied whether a vegan diet, without the added benefit of exercise, could help people with Type 2 diabetes. The results were rapid. Without counting calories, subjects lost weight and saw their blood sugars drop dramatically. Kidney abnormalities improved, and many reduced or eliminated their diabetes medications. These are *powerful* findings that people anywhere can put to work in their daily lives.

Of course, if you told anyone in the general population that they "don't need meat," their surprise might be akin to hearing "you don't need air, water, or sunlight"—that is—until they give it a try. It's not that there is a lack of information available on all sorts of meat-eating-related topics. Epidemiologists are tracking heart disease and cancer rates among omnivorous and vegetarian populations, showing clear benefits for the latter group. Scientists are busy studying mad cow disease and its human variant Creutzfeld-Jakob disease. And anthropologists can brief you on the meat-eating habits of distant ancestors. (Did they or didn't they? The answers may surprise you.) Tragically, these telling studies reach the public at a dangerously slow rate, if at all. And that's where Peter Cox comes in.

You Don't Need Meat delves deeply into all aspects of our meat-eating culture, starting in the modern slaughterhouse, reviewing studies on diet-related disease epidemics, and questioning commercial influences on government food policies. You'll be shocked to learn how much information is convoluted through advertising and the leverage of businesses that profit from animal agriculture. This book unearths information that everyone should be taught, beginning with the first nutrition lesson in grade school. He translates complex scientific studies into language that we all can understand and immediately put to use. If you've ever considered getting away from meat, but didn't know where to begin, this book is the place. Peter has a gift for bringing humor and hope to even the bleakest aspects of animal agriculture. No matter what your notions about vegetarian diets, Peter's thoroughly researched volume will leave you questioning old beliefs and welcoming new ideas.

Beyond a deeply thought-provoking journey, readers of this book will gain invaluable information on staying healthy, even regaining health that may have been lost over the years. It is a wonderful contribution for doctors and their patients everywhere, and for anyone who would rather not become a patient at all.

Sometimes, patients tune out their doctors when we preach the virtues of exercise, a good diet, and other healthy lifestyle habits. *You Don't Need Meat* so thoroughly conveys the reality of what meat and other animal products are doing to industrialized human populations that we can't help but stop and listen. Take this opportunity to hear the whole story. What you learn just may save your life.

Neal Barnard, M.D.,
Physicians Committee for Responsible Medicine,
Washington, D.C.

A NOTE ON MEANINGS

As you will see, I detest pinning labels on people. However, we do need to be clear about the meaning of words used in this book; otherwise, we'll end up in an awful mess. So here are the words used to describe the different sorts of diets generally associated with or included within the term "vegetarian":

- **Vegetarian:** Someone who does not eat fish, flesh, or fowl.
- **Lacto-vegetarian:** Essentially the same as above, but a little more precise. Someone who does not eat fish, flesh, or fowl, but who consumes dairy produce. Usually encountered only in scientific or pedantic use.
- **Ovo-lacto-vegetarian:** Even more precise. Someone who does not eat fish, flesh, or fowl, but who consumes dairy produce and eggs. Again, not a term used in everyday speech. For most practical purposes, "vegetarian," "lacto-vegetarian," and "ovo-lacto-vegetarian" all mean the same thing.
- **Vegan:** Someone who doesn't consume or use any animal products. He or she avoids all fish, flesh, and fowl; eggs and dairy; and the use of animal products such as leather, silk and wool. Sometimes called "strict vegetarian," which is unnecessarily severe—a better description would be "pure vegetarian."

Inevitably, with the huge upsurge of interest in vegetarian living, various other terms have been used, often inaccurately. For example, it is incorrect to call someone who refrains from red meat, but who still eats chicken and fish, a vegetarian. Other terms, such as "semi-vegetarian" or "demivegetarian" are occasionally encountered, although they have very little practical meaning.

1

EVERYTHING YOU'RE
NOT SUPPOSED TO KNOW

I was twelve years old before I ever heard the word "vegetarian," and when I did, I didn't like it much. I grew up in a remote farming community of the British Isles, where there was no sewage system or electricity, and the water had to be pumped by hand from the well. I pretty much believed myself to be an isolated oddity of nature because I hadn't eaten meat since the age of two, and my parents firmly believed I was going to die, for the same reason. Many endless hours were spent sitting anxiously in the doctor's office.

"Is he eating meat yet?" the doctor would inquire.

"No!" my mother nervously replied, feeling guilty that she was failing in her duty to bring up a healthy boy child.

"Well, he doesn't look too bad, for the moment," the doctor would conclude. "Better bring him back again in six weeks."

And so it went on: more trips to the doctor, the death sentence postponed by another few weeks, more anxiety and anguish from my distracted parents, no sign of any dietary compromise from their fanatical son, and all the while, the doctor's pen poised and ready to make out the death certificate: *This child died from failure to eat meat.*

Except, it didn't happen.

Mostly, I was in pretty good physical shape—big enough to play second row in rugby, a rather brutal English game—and although my diet was somewhat restricted (my poor mother was driven to her wit's end trying to devise meals her finicky son would eat), there were no occurrences of rickets, anemia, edema, or plague. If anything, I seemed to be somewhat healthier than other kids my age.

Then, one day, someone told me what I was. "You're a vegetarian!" he exclaimed. My first instinct was to hit him as any right-minded boy would who'd just been insulted.

"What's that?" I scowled.

"Someone who doesn't eat meat! Like you!"

The truth slowly dawned. I wasn't entirely a freak of nature, then. There were others like me. How strange. Then I learned there was something called the Vegetarian Society. I wrote to them, got their newsletter, and was horrified. I had nothing in common with these people at all, other than the fact that we both excluded certain foods from our diet. They seemed middle-aged, obsessive, absurdly self-important, and fixated on something called nut cutlets. I happily went back to being a lone vegetarian.

The name struck me then, and still does, as being disagreeable; and rather than use the "V word," I preferred to say, "I'm sorry, but I don't eat meat," whenever it was offered. Note the apology.

If you like toast, you don't call yourself a "toastarian" (or if you did, most people would rightly think you'd taken leave of your senses). Similarly, if you appreciate an occasional dry martini, you wouldn't describe yourself as a "martinarian," unless you wished to cultivate a reputation for eccentricity. So why, then, should I be labeled after something I don't eat? It makes little sense to me, and in any case, I like to think of myself as something more than a set of dietary preferences. "Meet Peter Cox, the vegetarian" is about as illogical as "Meet Peter Cox, the free-hairian" (because I don't wear hats). Such is the blight of pinning labels on people.

Actually, it gets even worse, because as you'll see later in the book, I've moved on to veganism now. Can we let that one pass, just for the moment? I'll explain all in due course. Otherwise, we'll be on this page all day.

To conclude: Everything I'd learned about my deviant way of eating during the first three decades of my life can be summed up as follows:

1. It's dangerous, almost certainly life-threatening, and should only be attempted under strict doctor's supervision.
2. It has a name. Not a very nice one.
3. Other people do it, too, but they're even weirder than me.

And so I would have continued, but one day, my life took an unexpected turn, as lives invariably do.

EPIPHANY

I'd just turned thirty, and had recently left the advertising business. It's a great business to be in when you're young, and an even better business to leave when you're not. I was toying with a few other business ideas, but nothing seemed to pass the spreadsheet stage satisfactorily. Then one day, my wife said, "The Vegetarian Society is looking for a Chief Executive."

It seemed intriguing. Despite eating a vegetarian diet virtually all my life, I knew nothing about "vegetarianism," and the prospect of being a "professional vegetarian" initially seemed hilarious. However, they were an old, established nonprofit group apparently looking to update their image, and I was someone who could do that for them. Since the staff of some two dozen people was spread between a base in Manchester, England, and another in London, the first task was to make sure everyone was singing from the same song sheet.

The main challenge, however, was much more fundamental: what, precisely, were we supposed to be doing? Were we a pressure group? An animal rights group? A social tea party? There were many widely varying views, as indeed there had been since the founding of the society one and a half centuries earlier.

The first organized vegetarian movement in the West was born in a unique time of extraordinary religious, political, and social upheaval. We tend to think of our world today as being a chaotic place, but it can't hold a candle to the events of the midnineteenth century. Consider just a few taking place at that time. In 1848—the year after the Vegetarian Society was established—Marx and Engels produced *The Communist Manifesto*, and the first women's rights convention was held in Seneca Falls, New York. The horror of the Irish Famine was in full swing, killing a million or more people and generating extraordinary new levels of immigration to America. With increasing ferocity, the British Empire was struggling to retain its grip on its far-flung territories, such as India, China, and Canada, with war and revolution the inevitable backlash. In 1849, Thoreau published *On the Duty of Civil Disobedience*. Two years earlier, the Mormons sought religious freedom and founded Salt Lake City. Charles Darwin's on the *Origin of Species* would offer up a scientific challenge to the religious interpretation of man's place in the world in the next decade, and in 1861, America itself would be torn apart in the Civil War that set neighbor against neighbor, and brother against brother. Although Charles Dickens's novel *A Tale of Two Cities* (published in 1859) was ostensibly set at the time of the French Revolution some seventy years earlier, its sentiments, and indeed his opening words, perfectly captured the zeitgeist of this extraordinary period:

> It was the best of times, it was the worst of times, it was the age of wisdom, it was the age of foolishness, it was the epoch of belief, it was the epoch of incredulity, it was the season of Light, it was the season of Darkness, it was the spring of hope, it was the winter of despair . . .

From this fiery melting pot of great good and great evil belched forth many new movements and factions, and one of them was the Vegetarian Society. It is no coincidence that the society first took root in Manchester, England, cradle of the Industrial Revolution.

Manchester was the center of the new economy, the nineteenth century's equivalent of Silicon Valley, the most talked about and the most written about city in the Western Hemisphere. Extreme wealth and terrible poverty existed cheek by jowl, the one a consequence of the other, as the famous French social critic and writer Alexis de Tocqueville vividly describes:

> A sort of black smoke covers the city. The sun seen through it is a disc without rays. Under this half-daylight 300,000 human beings are ceaselessly at work. A thousand noises disturb this damp,

dark labyrinth, but they are not at all the ordinary sounds one hears in great cities. . . . From this foul drain the greatest stream of human industry flows out to fertilize the whole world. From this filthy sewer pure gold flows. Here humanity attains its most complete development and its most brutish; here civilisation works its miracles, and civilized man is turned back into a savage.[1]

So here, in Manchester—this cutting-edge city where the future was literally being forged—was where organized vegetarianism found fertile ground. It was a reform, protest, healthy-living, and religious movement all rolled into one. Yes, religious: many of the first vegetarians in Manchester were followers of the Swedish scientist, mystic, philosopher, and theologian Emanuel Swedenborg, who saw meat eating as "the most vivid symbol of our fall from grace and the source of all evil."[2]

Vegetarianism was therefore one of the earliest of all protest movements, and in its many elements, there could be found something for almost everyone. Its emphasis on consuming healthy, wholesome food (most manufactured foodstuffs of the time were scandalously adulterated) was a forerunner of today's consumer movement. Its denunciation of the appalling cruelties of the slaughterhouse, and endorsement of compassion and consideration to all living things, has clear parallels in today's environmental movement. Its assertion that animals—like women—might possibly have rights, brought it into direct conflict with the status quo, and has obvious political parallels today. In short, the early vegetarians of Manchester were dangerously free-thinking people. Indeed, some of them had to flee quickly across the Atlantic for their own safety, and from this grew the American vegetarian movement. Its chief proponent, Sylvester Graham, was one of the founders the American Vegetarian Convention in 1850. His immortality is assured, of course, by the flour and the crackers that still bear his name today.

The vegetarian movement acquired many and varied notable supporters, among them Gandhi, Tolstoy, and George Bernard Shaw, but the Vegetarian Society itself became something of a dying ember. It was more of a support group for its members than an active movement. That was the situation I inherited, and since there was insufficient support for a more proactive agenda, I decided I'd only be wasting my time to remain there; so I resigned.

Then something interesting happened. I'd been midway through negotiating an agreement with a publisher to put out a range of vegetarian books on behalf of the society. I phoned the publisher to say that I was leaving. "What will you do next?" he inquired. I said that I wasn't sure, but I'd probably start a business of some sort.

"Well, while you're planning that," he said, "why don't you write a book for us?"

"Sure," I replied, thinking nothing of it.

Ah, the naïveté of youth.

Aside from climbing Everest without oxygen, writing a book is possibly the most grueling torture yet devised by the human race. And a blank piece of paper (nowadays, a blank computer screen) is the most terrifying object yet created. After the first day, I went to bed early, exhausted with brain fatigue, and convinced I'd contracted a ghastly, debilitating disease. The second day, I managed to produce two hundred words. Then I stopped, because I'd said everything I could think of. That's what working in advertising does to you.

Then it came to me: research! That's what writers did, wasn't it? I clearly needed to do some research. So I went to a medical library, down a gloomy and far-flung corridor of a musty Victorian teaching hospital. It felt like a time trip into another era.

Big surprise.

I didn't expect to find much, if anything, and in truth I didn't even know what I was looking for. But I was desperate, in the way that authors and condemned men grow desperate when their time is running out. What I found was astonishing.

Going back to 1978, I unearthed an amazing piece of research (which I'll get to after a short digression) that was published in *The American Journal of Clinical Nutrition* and authored by Dr. Roland L. Phillips, one of America's most respected epidemiologists.[3] I had to check that word when I first encountered it. "Epidemiology" is defined as "the study of the relationships of the various factors determining the frequency and distribution of diseases in a human community."[4] To put it more simply, epidemiology is scientific detective-work.

The easiest way of comparing the health of meat eaters to vegetarians is just to watch them over a long period of time, and see who dies of what. Basically, it's not too difficult to do, although obviously it can takes years before you start to see any results. From the scientist's point of view, the main danger is that you'll die before the experiment has finished.

In some ways, epidemiology is a seriously overlooked discipline. It isn't as glamorous as the "wet" sciences, which make headlines with the latest high-tech brain transplant or potential cure for cancer. But because it concentrates on studying the way things actually are in the real world, it is capable of giving us extremely relevant insights into health and disease. You're going to see the results of some epidemiological studies now, and while you are considering them, please remember that the knowledge these studies give us has been obtained at a high cost—many millions of people have died to bring us the benefit of these findings.

Roland Phillips and his team were very interested in a subgroup of the American population called Seventh-Day Adventists. This group was particularly fascinating because their church advocates a very different diet and lifestyle than the typical meat-based American one. So the first thing Dr. Phillips did was to locate a large number of Seventh-Day Adventists. We're not talking about a few dozen, or even a few hundred people here. Dr. Phillips's sample size was massive—25,000 people, all of them residents of California. Obviously, the more people you study, the less likely it is that a few freak results are going to skew the analysis. In this case, the huge number of people involved makes the study very reliable, indeed.

Then the members of Dr. Phillips's team just waited. Every year, for six years, they would contact each one of those people, just to see if he or she was still alive. If the person had died, a death certificate was obtained, and the underlying cause of death was determined. Patience and tact are two key qualities for a good epidemiologist! At the end of the six-year period, the team had some highly significant results.

Compared to the average, meat-eating, Californian population, the risk of dying from coronary heart disease among Adventists was far, far lower. For every 100 ordinary Californians who died from heart disease, only 26 Adventists males had died—that's about one-quarter the risk. Among females, the risk was one-third. You can see this illustrated in Figure 1.1.

This is very forceful evidence. It isn't theoretical, or hypothetical, or a scientist's opinion or some other piece of cunning public relations. It is a straightforward, nonarguable, nonnegotiable fact. It is, quite simply, what happened. Counting dead bodies is pretty convincing, even for the most hardened skeptics.

Now the next question, of course, is why? Well, one reason must be the fact that most Seventh-Day Adventists do not smoke. "OK," say the skeptics, "it's nothing to do with eating meat, it simply proves that smoking isn't healthy. And we knew that already!" Unfortunately for the skeptics, that explanation doesn't hold up. You see, Dr. Phillips and his team had considered possibilities such as that, as, indeed, good epidemiologists should always do. So they next compared deaths from heart disease among Seventh-Day Adventists to deaths

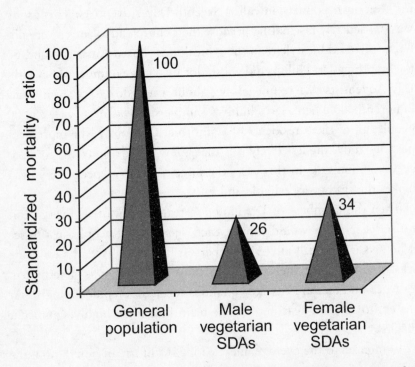

Figure 1.1. Deaths from heart disease. Seventh-Day Adventists compared to the general population.

from heart disease among a representative group of nonsmokers, as studied by the American Cancer Society. Clearly, if Adventists were healthier purely because they didn't smoke, then deaths rates in these two groups should be the same.

But they weren't—not by a long shot. The cold figures showed that Adventists had only half the risk of dying from heart disease, when compared to nonsmokers (actually, people identified by the American Cancer Society as "*never* having smoked"). So there was clearly something else very special about the Adventist lifestyle.

What could it be? Perhaps people with religious faith die less often from heart disease? Perhaps they have less stress in their lives? Perhaps they secretly take a magic potion that protects them? A determined opponent could throw up any number of possibilities to explain away these findings.

And that's where the sheer good science of Dr. Phillips's research really paid dividends. He thought that people might raise all kinds of possible explanations, such as these, and he accounted for them. Dr. Phillips realized that although the Adventist church advocated the vegetarian lifestyle, it wasn't compulsory. Some Adventists still ate meat. So he included this aspect in his research. He found that about 20 percent of them ate meat four or more times a week, about 35 percent ate it between one and three times a week, and the remaining 45 percent never ate it at all. To a bright mind, these facts created a unique scientific opportunity.

Why not simply compare the health of Adventists who never ate meat (i.e. vegetarians) to those Adventists who did eat it? In a flash, it would eliminate all other confounding factors. So that's what Dr. Phillips did.

You can see the result in Figure 1.2 on the following page. Among Adventist men who ate meat, the death rate from coronary heart disease was only 37 percent of the normal death rate for the average meat-eating population in California—impressive in itself, and certainly proof that the nonsmoking Adventist lifestyle is pretty healthy. But among those Adventists who were vegetarian, the death rate plummeted even further—right down to 12 percent of that of the normal population. Twelve percent!

Let me just put this another way, so that we're really, really certain

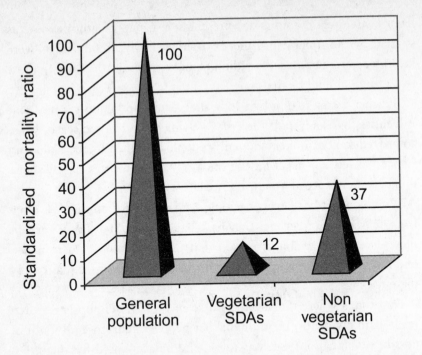

Figure 1.2. Deaths from heart disease. Seventh-Day Adventist vegetarians compared to Seventh-Day Adventist nonvegetarians.

that we understand each other. Vegetarian Seventh-Day Adventist men are about ten times less likely to contract coronary heart disease than a "normal" meat-eating person.

Now, one of the great things about large-scale studies such as this is the longer you are prepared to wait, the more interesting and more accurate the results become. So that's what happened next—they waited, and watched. For twenty years. Eventually, Dr. Phillips's team published the final results of the study, which had literally observed people growing old and dying over two decades.[5] This landmark project provided the first ever scientific proof that the more meat you eat, the more at risk you are of getting heart disease.

Look at Figures 1.3 and 1.4 (on pages 11 and 12) and you'll see a summary of the results. The relative risk of fatal heart disease closely correlates with the frequency of eating meat. Those Adventist males who consumed meat one or two times a week were 44 percent more likely to die from heart disease than Adventist vegetarians. Those who

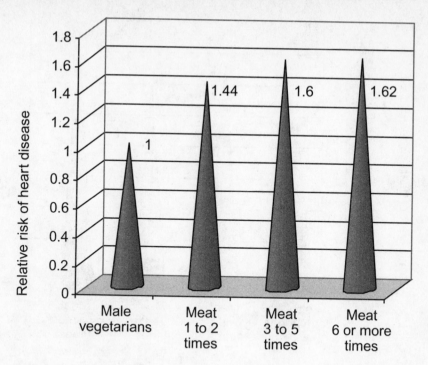

Figure 1.3. Weekly meat consumption correlated to risk of fatal heart disease, for males.

consumed it between three and five times per week were 60 percent more likely to die from heart disease. And for those who consumed it six or more times a week the rate rose to 62 percent. For females, the rates are 38, 25, and 58 percent, respectively. The significant finding is that even a small amount of meat—once or twice a week—greatly elevates the risk.

For men in one particular age group—forty-five to fifty-four—the stakes are particularly high. For these people, prime candidates for heart disease, the risk for meat eaters, when compared to vegetarians, is 400 percent greater!

Your head is probably spinning, and I apologize for that. I know mine was when I first came across this study. But quite clearly, it must be seriously flawed. I mean, if it was correct, your doctor would have told you, wouldn't he or she? And certainly, the government and its various agencies would surely by now have broadcast the message high and low: more meat means more heart disease, so go vegetarian!

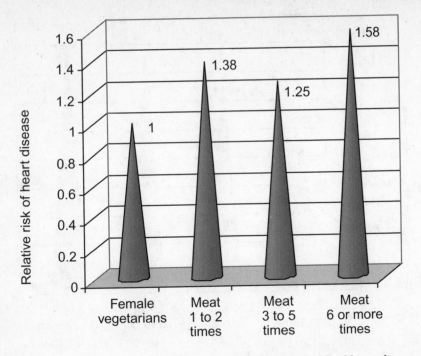

Figure 1.4. Weekly meat consumption correlated to risk of fatal heart disease, for females.

Any administration that had the interests of its citizens at heart (excuse the pun) would most certainly have publicized this extraordinary news without any delay. Unless I missed something, they didn't: so undoubtedly this study must be wrong. A freak, perhaps. Or a bizarre statistical quirk.

I continued researching.

The next thing I found was a study from Japan. Inspired by the insights gained from the American Seventh-Day Adventist studies, scientists from the National Cancer Center Research Institute, in Tokyo, embarked on a similar study.[6] Similar, that is, in concept—but even broader in scope. In this case, the Japanese decided to follow not a mere 25,000 people, but an astonishing 122,261 individuals, tracked over sixteen years. The logistics alone must have been daunting: each man (they only studied males in this survey) had to be interviewed at home, by specially trained public health nurses.

Because the size of the study was so large, it was possible to divide the participants into various subgroups according to their dietary and lifestyle preferences. After much hard work and computing time was expended in analysis, two lifestyles emerged as being very high risk and very low risk, respectively: The high-risk lifestyle included smoking, drinking, meat consumption, and no green vegetables.

The low-risk lifestyle was, not surprisingly, precisely the opposite. In Figure 1.5, you can see how the lifestyles compare. Deaths from all causes were elevated by 1.53 times greater among those who smoked, drank, ate meat, and didn't eat green vegetables. The risk of heart disease was 1.88 times higher in this group, and the risk of any kind of cancer was 2.49 times higher.

So far so good—and probably just what you were expecting to see. But the statistical power of this huge study was able to reveal, for the first time, some extraordinary relationships between meat consumption and ill health. Let me summarize:

- The Japanese found that simply adding one factor—meat—to an otherwise healthy lifestyle had a serious effect on mortality. The difference between the lowest risk group (no smoking, no

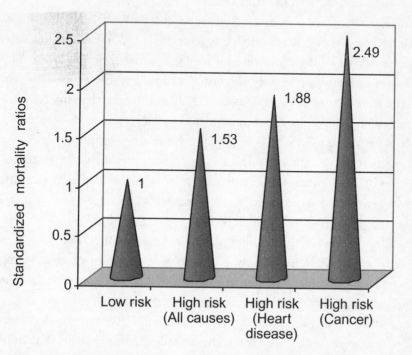

Figure 1.5. Risky lifestyles: how two opposite lifestyles compare.

drinking, no meat eating, and lots of green vegetables) and those people who led a similar lifestyle but ate meat was that the meat eaters boosted their risk of dying from heart disease by 30 percent.

- At the other end of the scale were the two most unhealthy groups. We generally think of smoking and drinking as unhealthy habits, and the study confirmed this—people who smoked and drank (but consumed green vegetables and didn't eat meat) were 39 percent more likely to die from any cause than the healthiest group. However, even more unhealthy were those people who smoked, drank, ate meat, and didn't consume green vegetables. These people increased their risk of dying from any cause by another 14 percent! In other words, the vegetarian lifestyle was conferring some protection, even on the smokers and drinkers!

Well, that's the Japanese, of course. Probably something funny in the water over there, which makes these statistics meaningless to Westerners. Then I found a study from Germany.

When the German Cancer Research Center advertised in *Der Vegetarier*, the German magazine for vegetarians, for participants in a similar tracking study, they were following a rather different angle. The scientists were particularly interested in the way the vegetarian diet seems able to protect against cancer. It is thought that nitrate consumption is linked to the development of cancer, and many vegetables contain nitrates. So why don't more vegetarians contract cancer? One possibility is that their overall diet contains other elements (vitamins A and C, for example) that protect them and lower their risk. This was one of the main areas the researchers were keen to investigate. Eventually, a total of 1,904 subjects were recruited.

After five years, the results began to emerge. Deaths from all causes were very low, indeed—only 37 percent of the average meat-eating population. All forms of cancer were slashed to 56 percent of the normal rate, and heart disease was down to 20 percent.[7]

Perhaps this was due to a lack of smoking? As in the two studies quoted previously, the researchers had already taken that into account. Even when vegetarian smokers were compared to nonvegetarian smokers, it was found that the vegetarians' rate of heart disease was still only 40 percent of the average population's. Clearly, the vegetarian diet was playing a significantly protective role.

I don't know. All this data was seriously spinning my head. And the results all seemed to be saying the vegetarian lifestyle is far, far healthier than the meat-eating one. Not at all what I'd been brought up to believe.

Then—please take a deep breath—I found a study from dear old Britain.

This one tracked the health of 4,671 British vegetarians (actually, it tracked their causes of death) for seven years and, knock me over with a feather, it reached very similar conclusions.[8] For male vegetarians, the death rate from all causes was 50 percent of the general population's; for females, 55 percent. Looking at heart disease alone, for the male vegetarian the death rate was only 44 percent of normal, and for female vegetarians, 41 percent.

The study also compared the vegetarians to a similar population group—customers of health food shops—and found that they were also at less risk for heart disease—60 percent of the average population. Presumably, this reflected health food shoppers' greater interest in their own health, and avoidance of smoking. However, when the two groups were compared, it was obvious that the vegetarians had reduced their risk of heart disease by a third when compared to the health food shoppers.

Finally (I think you'll be pleased to see me use that word), I found the great-granddaddy of them all. The China study. Hold on for a few more paragraphs, please, this is important.

If the Japanese study was impressive in terms of the number of participants, the China study is unprecedented in terms of the depth of information produced. So much so, in fact, that it made headline news in the *New York Times*.[9] Under the headline "Huge Study of Diet Indicts Fat and Meat," the report began:

Early findings from the most comprehensive large study ever undertaken of the relationship between diet and the risk of developing disease are challenging much of American dietary dogma. The study, being conducted in China, paints a bold portrait of a plant-based eating plan that is more likely to promote health than disease.

A "plant-based eating plan" . . . whatever could they mean? Surely not the "V word"?

Two major surveys were undertaken, one in 1983 and the other in 1989–90. In the 1983 survey, 367 items of information were collected on how people live and how they die in 138 rural Chinese villages; 6,500 adults and their families were surveyed. In the 1989–90 survey, more than 1,000 items of information were collected on 10,200 adults and their families in 170 villages in rural China and Taiwan.

"This is a very, very important study," commented Dr. Mark Hegsted, emeritus professor of nutrition at Harvard University and former administrator of human nutrition for the United States Department of Agriculture. "It is unique and well done. Even if you could pay for it, you couldn't do this study in the United States because the population is too homogeneous. You get a lot more meaningful data when the differences in diet and disease are as great as they are in the various parts of China."

Let me summarize some of the key findings of the China study to date:

- While 70 percent of the protein in average Western diets comes from animals, in China only 7 percent of the protein does. Although most Chinese suffer very little from the major killer diseases of the West, those affluent Chinese who consume similar amounts of animal protein to Westerners also have the highest rates of heart disease, cancer, and diabetes. Suspicious, or what?
- The Chinese consume 20 percent more calories than Westerners do. This should mean that they are fatter than Westerners, but the reality is that Westerners are 25 percent fatter than the Chinese! This is almost certainly due to the fact that the Chinese eat only a third as much fat as Westerners, but twice as many complex carbohydrates. That's another way of saying "plants."

- Current Western dietary guidelines suggest that we should reduce the fat in our diets to less than 30 percent of our calorie consumption. The Chinese study reveals that this is by no means enough to effectively prevent heart disease and cancer—it should be slashed to something closer to 10 to 15 percent.
- You don't need to drink milk to prevent osteoporosis. Most Chinese consume no dairy products and instead get all their calcium from vegetables. While the Chinese consume only half the calcium Westerners do, osteoporosis is uncommon in China, despite an average life expectancy of seventy years. "Osteoporosis tends to occur in countries where calcium intake is highest and most of it comes from protein-rich dairy products," says Dr. T. Colin Campbell, a nutritional biochemist from Cornell University and the American brains behind the study. "The Chinese data indicate that people need less calcium than we think and can get adequate amounts from vegetables."
- The study also reveals that meat-eating is not necessary to prevent iron-deficiency anemia. The average Chinese adult, who shows no evidence of anemia, consumes twice the iron an average American does, but the vast majority of it comes from plants.

The main nutritional conclusion from this study is the finding that the greater the consumption of a variety of good-quality, plant-based foods, the lower the risk of those diseases commonly found in Western countries (e.g., cancers, cardiovascular diseases, diabetes). Based on these and other data, the scientists behind the study predict that the majority of all such Western diseases could be prevented until we were about age ninety years old if we were prepared to cut out meat and basically go vegetarian.

Says Dr. Campbell: "We're basically a vegetarian species and should be eating a wide variety of plant foods and minimizing our intake of animal foods."

Well, all that gave me plenty of food for thought.

EXCUSE ME?

I don't know what you think of the preceding five studies I've mentioned, but I know what I thought. Either these studies are the result
of deranged and misguided minds run amok, or somebody's been
keeping the truth from me for decades. Remember, I'd been vegetarian all my life and had been conditioned to believe that it was an
unnatural and perilous thing to do. Now, suddenly, I had plain evidence in front of me that contradicted everything I'd been taught to
believe. It was like the frog all of a sudden learning that he was, in
fact, a prince (well, let's not stretch this analogy too far . . .).

So why hadn't I been told? Why hadn't *we* been told?

Imagine you have stock in a drug company. One day, the company
announces that it has a new product that will immediately slash heart
disease by 50 percent. No question about it. No side effects. No ifs or
buts. It works.

Now, do you think that would make headline news around the
world? Do you think you would be a very, very rich bunny, and a
very, very happy one, too? You bet you would.

So that's the problem I faced. If all this good news about the vegetarian diet is true, *why haven't we been told?*

The first group of people we turn to when we want health advice is
the medical profession. So that's where I turned, too. Surely, they
should know the truth? After all, the research results you've just seen
were published in medical and scientific journals, and you'd expect
that most doctors would keep up to date with these things.

Well, they try to. But the trouble is, an awful lot of other work gets
published in scientific journals, too. Dr. Vernon Coleman, a doctor
and medical writer, explains what happens to all this research:

There are so many medical journals in existence that a new scientific paper is published somewhere in the world every twenty-
eight seconds. . . . Because they know that they need to publish
research papers if they are to have successful careers, doctors
have become obsessed with research for its own sake. They have
forgotten that the original purpose of research is to help
patients. . . . Believe it or not, much of the research work that

has been done in the last twenty years has never been analyzed. Somewhere, hidden deep in an obscure part of a medical library, there may be a new penicillin. Or a cure for cancer. You don't have to go far to find the evidence proving that many scientific papers go unread: approximately twenty percent of all research is unintentionally duplicated because researchers haven't had the time to read all the published papers in their own specialized area.[10]

So the first reason more doctors don't know the truth about the benefits of the vegetarian lifestyle is, simply, because they just don't come across the evidence. But even if they did, there are two further problems: First, there's no one to sell it to them. This may sound rather cynical, but the truth is that doctors respond to the information they are fed, and most of it comes from one direction—the drug industry. Research has shown that by far the greatest influence over doctors' prescribing habits is the nonstop barrage of promotion that these companies produce.[11] By contrast, only 12 percent of their prescribing decisions are influenced by articles in professional journals. Second, doctors have traditionally focused on studying disease, rather than promoting health. As Dr. Joe Collier, a clinical pharmacologist who has studied and written about the drug industry, puts it:

"Doctors fail patients because they are preoccupied with, even obsessed by, disease. Right from their earliest days at medical school, training concentrates on the recognition and treatment of disease, rather than its prevention. . . . Disease is so much a part of a doctor's horizon that it may be difficult for a patient to escape the consulting room without an illness being diagnosed and at least one medicine being prescribed."[12]

Then we come up against the medical system itself. The sad truth is, information from major studies such as those described above are rarely used to offer advice that will improve people's lives. When medical science comes across studies that show that vegetarians have less heart disease than meat eaters, it doesn't respond by saying "Great! Let's advise all our patients to go vegetarian!" Instead, it asks itself,

"What is it about the meat eaters that makes them so unhealthy?" This then generates yet more research, as you will see.

Dr. T. Colin Campbell, the mastermind from Cornell University behind the China Study described above, explains this mode of thinking: "One line of investigation suggests that evidence is not sufficient for serious dietary recommendations until mechanisms are identified and understood. However, this logic is rather nihilistic. If this were necessary, then it should also be reasonable to require a full mechanistic accounting of the effect of the same food constituent upon other diseases as well. Such logic contradicts the true complexities of biology and discourages hope of public health progress ever being made."[13]

In other words, it isn't necessary to understand *every last detail* of the cause-and-effect relationship between meat eating and disease in order to start taking action now. Another expert, Dr. O. Turpeinen, of Helsinki, who himself has produced some fascinating work, which we will consider a little later, expressed it like this: "It is not always judicious to wait for the final results and the irrefutable proof before taking action. Many lives could be saved and much good done by starting a little earlier. Although we do not yet have an absolute proof for dietary prevention of Coronary Heart Disease, there is strong evidence for its effectiveness, and its safety."[14]

So studies such as the five mentioned above usually go unpublicized, and serve to generate more theories, which are then explored and tested, often by conducting animal experiments. You may be amazed to learn, as I was, that researchers have known for *decades* that feeding a naturally vegetarian species, such as rabbits, a meat diet will produce heart disease. And they've also known that in naturally carnivorous species, such as dogs, it is virtually impossible to produce clogging of the arteries, even when large amounts of cholesterol and saturated fat are fed to them.[15] Now for heaven's sake, doesn't this information tell us *something* about the sort of diet we humans should be eating?

What have they been doing all this time? Why haven't they given us this vital information?

What they've been doing is yet more research. Looking in ever closer detail at the mechanisms of disease. And, oh yes, producing wonderfully profitable new ranges of drugs and medications to avoid heart disease, treat heart disease, and fight cholesterol.

AN APPOINTMENT WITH THE DOCTOR

This is all rather depressing. It suggests that, although we already have a medicine that can prevent and treat heart disease and many other major problems of our time—it's called the vegetarian diet—it will never become widely recognized or prescribed. When I went to interview a hospital dietician, whose job it is to help people with high cholesterol levels reduce them by dietary means before drug treatment is prescribed, I was amazed to find her including meat and other animal products in the diet sheets she was giving out.

"Why aren't you encouraging people to go completely vegetarian?" I asked her. "Surely you're aware of the weight of evidence in favor of the vegetarian lifestyle?"

She replied dismissively, "Oh, people would never do that. There's no point giving people diets that you know they just won't follow."

It seemed to me that she was denying her patients potentially life-saving information, based on little more than her own prejudice. As a result, many of them could be condemned to a lifetime of taking cholesterol-lowering drugs.

Luckily, some doctors don't share this dismal attitude. Dr. Bruce Kinosian, an assistant professor of medicine at the University of Maryland in Baltimore, is one. "If you can lower cholesterol with diet, why use drugs?" he says. "There are clearly people who need drugs to lower their cholesterol, but there are other options out there that may be more cost-effective and are not being emphasized. There are a lot of people with high cholesterol levels in this country, and as a matter of social policy, you don't want to get in the habit of prescribing pills to everyone."

So there are a few glimmers of hope out there. In a free society, it is difficult to suppress the truth forever, particularly when it is something so eminently sensible as the vegetarian way of living.

In the course of my own research, I had heard about Dr. David

Ryde, a British family doctor, and I was curious to know if everything I'd heard was true, especially the revelation that he happened to be the lowest-prescribing general practitioner in Britain. Dr. Ryde is in every respect a conventionally trained and qualified doctor, but he has gradually acquired a reputation for preferring to treat his patients through dietary means. The vegan diet, to be precise. So I visited him in his office.

An athletic and vigorous man greeted me at the door with a big grin. I later learned that he is actually thirty years older than he looks. First, I asked him how he came to be vegetarian.

"The seeds were planted when I was walking home from school one day," he told me, "and I saw some pigs being beaten. That set me thinking. Was it really necessary to inflict so much cruelty just to have bacon for breakfast? Anyway, at the age of twelve, I stopped eating meat and fish, much to the horror of my parents. But they couldn't deny I was healthy enough—I was captain of athletics, rugby, and swimming at school, and I could easily cycle 100 miles or more in a weekend.

"When I went to medical school, we were taught nothing about nutrition. They simply said there were two types of protein—'first class' and 'second class.' It was only years later that I began to understand that plant protein could be entirely satisfactory for human needs. I was still keenly interested in sport, playing rugby for the county, and for the United Hospitals.

"Eventually, I began to become interested in the science of nutritional medicine, and I started to offer my patients nutritional advice. Some patients simply didn't want to know—they'd take the attitude that they didn't want a lecture, they just wanted me to write a prescription for some pills—that's what they regarded as 'proper' medicine. But other patients were more willing to try something new, and I started to get some extraordinary results.

My first was a patient with severe angina. His condition had been deteriorating for about five years, and he'd been into hospital, was taking all the medication, and so on. But his condition was, frankly, almost terminal.

It was a really pitiful sight to see him struggle to walk the few yards from the car to the surgery. Now a person in such a desperate state will listen, and they will try anything. So I suggested he try a strict veg-etarian diet, actually a vegan one.

"Just one month later, he could walk one mile, from his home to my surgery. Three months later he could walk four miles, while carry-ing shopping. 'It used to take him a quarter of an hour to climb three flights of steps,' his daughter told me. 'Now he's up in a few seconds!'

"That was my first success, and it encouraged me to try it with other patients. Another interesting case was a professor of medicine, actually the dean of a medical school. He had been taking antiulcer medication for four years, with little success. I suggested he try a vegan diet, and after three days, there was a remarkable improvement in pain reduction. A year later, he had lost about ten pounds of weight, and he looked a new man, light-hearted and happy.

"Another interesting case was a woman with severe headaches, and a blood pressure of 185/120. I suggested she try a vegan diet, and the pressure soon came down to 115/75. Now you'd never seen that kind of reduction using medication. And she felt fantastic! Which was another benefit, because antihypertensive medication often leaves patients feeling exhausted.

"I've seen results such as these in my patients too often to attribute them to coincidence. Really, this kind of treatment has no side-effects, and the benefits are so worthwhile, that there's no reason not to try it."

"What sort of reaction have you had from your colleagues?" I asked.

"In the early days, they used to warn me that I wasn't prescribing enough medication. When they charted the prescribing rates of GPs [general practitioners], I would always be right at the bottom, way off the graph. And I think that worried some people. But these days, I'm asked to give talks to colleagues and to administrators. Obviously, my methods are far less costly to the health service than usual.

"I also feel strongly that we doctors need to examine more closely what actually goes on in the consulting room. You know, the truth is that patients don't usually come and see us because they're ill; they come because they're *worried*. They're anxious about some aspect of their health. Now, if all we do is simply send them away with a bottle of pills, we have actually reinforced their anxiety, which can make a cure harder."

He paused, and smiled.

"Fundamentally, we must remember that we're not vending machines!"

Dr. Ryde isn't alone, but he is in a minority. Other caring members of the medical community have come to the same viewpoint as he has (that we are basically a "vegetarian species," as Dr. Colin Campbell calls it) and that we are today eating the wrong sort of food—with disastrous consequences. For example, I could mention

- Dr. Neal Barnard, president of the Washington, D.C.–based Physicians Committee for Responsible Medicine (PCRM), which encourages doctors to practice medicine based on nutritious vegetarian diets and other positive lifestyle changes, rather than reliance on, and the use of, drugs and surgery.[16]
- Dr. John A. McDougall. As a plantation physician in Hawaii, Dr. McDougall cared for 5,000 people, mostly of Chinese, Japanese, and Filipino ancestry. He observed that his first-generation patients, those who migrated to Hawaii from their native lands, were in excellent health and always trim. Their children and grandchildren became fatter and sicker. The only thing that changed was their diet. The older folks lived on a traditional diet, mostly rice and vegetables. Their offspring, raised in a modern society, learned to eat richer foods—meats, poultry, eggs, dairy products, and highly processed foods. He became fascinated by the effect of diet on health, wrote many bestselling books, and now runs a world-famous clinic. "The most powerful medicine ever imagined," he says, "is right there on your dinner plate."[17]
- Dr. Dean Ornish. Founder, president, and director of the nonprofit Preventive Medicine Research Institute in Sausalito, California, he is also a professor of clinical medicine at the University of California, San Francisco, and a founder of the Osher Center for Integrative Medicine there. For the past twenty-three years, Dr. Ornish has directed clinical research conclusively demonstrating that the meat-free diet and other lifestyle changes can reverse even severe coronary heart dis-

ease without the need for either drugs or surgery. He is the author of five bestselling books, including the *New York Times* bestseller *Dr. Dean Ornish's Program for Reversing Heart Disease*. We'll look at Dr. Ornish's work in detail later.[18]

- Dr. Michael Klaper. A surgeon, at the University of California Hospitals in San Francisco. Dr. Klaper began to realize that many of the diseases his patients brought to his office—clogged arteries (atherosclerosis), high blood pressure (hypertension), obesity, adult-onset diabetes, and even some forms of arthritis, asthma, and other significant illnesses—were made worse, or actually caused by the food they were eating. This prompted him to undertake a serious study of the link between diet and disease, eventually leading him to implement nutritionally based therapies in his practice. The results were dramatic. Nearly all of his patients who followed his vegan diet, exercise, and stress-reduction programs soon became leaner and more energetic, while their elevated blood pressure and cholesterol levels returned to safer values. (In twelve weeks on this same program, Dr. Klaper's own cholesterol dropped from 242 mg/dl to 140 mg/dl, while a twenty-two-pound "spare tire" of abdominal fat melted away—without dieting or restricting calories. He also observed that many of the chronic diseases mentioned above improved or resolved completely, often allowing his patients to reduce or discontinue their medication entirely. He is now director of the nonprofit Institute of Nutrition Education and Research, which seeks to educate physicians and other health professionals about the importance of nutrition in clinical practice, and is a member of the Nutrition Task Force of the American Medical Student Association.[19]

These and other doctors, such as Dr. William Harris,[20] Dr. Joel Fuhrman,[21] and Dr. Robert Kradjian[22] have all spoken out about the health impact of the meat-free way of living. And even though their voices are loud and clear, they are still very much in a minority. Why?

REDUCE ME TO TEARS

I think one of the answers to this perplexing question lies in the way much of modern scientific research operates. For a start, most research today is undertaken with a commercial aim: usually that of finding or creating a drug that can be sold to a profitable market niche. This is also the reason why many of the diseases that afflict Third World countries aren't given much attention by the pharmaceutical companies—they're simply not going to produce the return on investment that companies require. As far as dietary means of preventing or treating disease, well, where's the bottom line? If you can't patent it, package it, and sell it for a good markup, forget it.

As you'll see later, the vegetarian (and especially, the vegan) diet can work wonders for your cholesterol level. But that's not going to increase anyone's share price. "The ultimate wonder cure for a lousy lifestyle has arrived: the anti-cholesterol pill," reported a British newspaper. "Take one a day and you can go back to junk food, throw away the running shoes, and even take up smoking again and still escape a heart attack." Since Britain has one of the highest death rates from coronary heart disease in the world, the British market is certainly worth grabbing. Comments a stockbroker, "The drug companies want people to ignore dieting, even though it is much more effective than drugs for 90 per cent of people. Ideally the industry would like to prescribe anti-cholesterol drugs to everyone with a family history of heart disease—the market is enormous." And a doctor, who had just been whisked off to Rome for a lavish drugs company sales pitch adds, "Anti-cholesterols are the hottest property in the drug world and people are being hounded into their massive use even before some of the long-term trials are completed. In theory they allow people to live on hamburgers and sausages and yet have the blood cholesterol of a Chinese peasant who eats rice and soybeans."[23]

There's another reason, too, and it is well described by the term "reductionism." When studies are published that demonstrate the superiority of the vegetarian diet—in either a preventative or curative capacity—most doctors and scientists seem to respond (if they respond at all) by searching for the one "magic ingredient" that makes vegetarians healthier. Is it the lower animal fat in their diet? Or the larger amounts of vitamins A and C? Or the trace minerals? Or the amino acid pattern in the protein? If they could just put their fingers on it, then the problem would be solved. Meat eaters could make suitable adjustments—eat leaner meat, or take a few more vitamin pills—and then they'd be as healthy as vegetarians.

And that's the problem with reductionism: a classic case of not being able to see the wood for the trees. Reductionist science produces masses and masses of data. This is, in fact, a chronic problem with science today: too many people are providing too much information, yet too few people have time to read and digest it. I suspect that in some cases scientists are repeating the same work without knowing it. Too many people talking—too few people reading, digesting, analyzing, and synthesizing.

The aim of reductionist science is to find the single magic bullet . . . that one missing piece of the jigsaw . . . the ultimate answer . . . the quest for the Holy Grail. Hence most medical research today has as its aim the isolation of a pure form of a chemical compound with a clearly defined (stoichiometric) chemical formula, which can be administered in quantitative doses and shown in statistically designed clinical studies to significantly and reproducibly affect the outcome of the disease.

But what if it doesn't exist?

What if our belief in magic bullets is just that—magical, illusory, not based in reality? In that case, no amount of scientific research, and no amount of expenditure, will ever find it. A reductionist approach toward medical research also, sooner or later, runs into the law of diminishing returns, whereby we have to spend more and more economic resources in order to achieve less and less. That's why, for example, all the cancer charities you know seem to have an inexhaustible appetite for money—and many of them are the best-funded charities in existence. The only message we all seem to receive loud and clear is "Give us another billion or so, and give us another decade" and then, at last, we may finally have a cure that works. Yeah, right.

The straightforward reality is that *all* the ingredients of a healthy vegetarian diet work together to preserve health and combat disease. We know how some of them work, we think we know how others work, and we know nothing about how yet others might work. But that's not the point. The point is, it *does* work. So why aren't we all vegetarian by now?

MESSING WITH YOUR MIND

If you're of a cynical turn of mind (I'm sure you're not, but the next person who reads this book might be), you could be thinking right now, "I hear what you're saying, Cox, but give me a break—you know very well that, in another week or two, the news will be full of experts saying exactly the opposite is true."

And you know, you'd be right to say that. We're bombarded with advice, much of it contradictory, from the media. What's a poor guy or gal to believe?

Well, I'd encourage you to be even *more* cynical. I'd suggest you might like to ask some rather uncomfortable questions, like "Where did the story come from? Was it planted by a PR company (much of today's news is). If so, who are their clients? Who paid for the research? Who's paying that bow-tied, media-trained expert on TV? These are nasty, suspicious questions that demonstrate a deplorable lack of faith in human nature . . . So ask them.

Most people hate lawyers, but I have a soft spot for them. They often have witty and clever minds, can do little harm outside of a courtroom, and are mostly just frustrated authors, bless 'em. The real enemy today is the PR person.

A top PR person can handle almost any impending media disaster—for a fee, of course. They will do precisely what you want them to do, say what you want them to say. If you want them to find a doctor who will stand up at a press conference and say, "People who don't eat meat will die from moonbeam poisoning," then they will assuredly find just such a doctor. They may have to send halfway round the world to get him, of course, but if your budget's big enough, it will be done—money can buy these things. And they will do it all with a grin on their bright little faces, and not one twinge of conscience in the place where their hearts used to be. That, incidentally, is pretty close to a definition of a psychopath.

Now, the scientists who undertake epidemiological studies don't employ PR people, of course, so when their research is published in the professional journals, it rarely makes headline news. The headlines go to the PR merchants and their clients. I happened to be in the offices of one of the world's biggest PR practices a year or two ago, speaking to the account director for a big meat client (by day, I'm a literary agent, and I was there on unrelated business concerning one of my own authors). The "Mad Cow" crisis had just grabbed the headlines again. Meat sales were plummeting, and I wondered aloud how she was going to handle it all. She turned to me, and sighed deeply. "We can handle most disasters and emergencies," she said. Then she paused dramatically. "But even we can't polish shit."

POLISHING IT

This is how they do it. As the "meat crisis" in Britain lurched from one disaster to the next, the *Meat Trades Journal* gave the game away. "*SHOWDOWN!*" it screamed in huge letters across its front page. "Top Nutritionist Joins Forces with the Meat Promotions Executive to Quash the Health Lobby." The story continued: "One of the world's top nutritionists has joined forces with the Meat promotions Executive in a bid to kick the health lobby's arguments into touch."[24]

The scientist's name was Derek Miller, and he was no ordinary hype merchant. One of the world's top nutritionists, he occupied many senior positions as an advisor to governments, the United Nations, and other highly influential bodies. So when the meat industry succeeded in "taking him on as an advisor," they couldn't contain their glee. And there it was, in black and white. Miller's job was to "quash the health lobby" and to "kick their arguments into touch." It couldn't be much plainer—this man, a world-respected scientist, was now going to be used to suppress the truth about meat eating and health.

Further into the story, an even more outrageous statement was made: "He believes that meat is not only good for you, but that it is impossible to live without it."

Impossible?

There's no risk of confusion here. No chance of differing interpretations, differences of opinion, differences of emphasis. A nutritionist

of Miller's reputation and expertise would certainly be aware of studies similar to those you've just seen. He must have known that millions of vegetarians worldwide were living healthier lives than meat
eaters. So we're left with just one conclusion.

It was a lie, and he was a liar. Worse than that, in fact: a man *paid*
to lie. A man who should certainly have known better. A man whose
reputation as a nutritionist would guarantee him access to television,
radio, the press—and whose expert status would rarely be questioned
by ever-respectful journalists. What a great find for the meat industry,
indeed.

"I personally am all in favour of having a go at the vegetarian
lobby," said Mr. Miller. "Their moral arguments are not on [target]
and their nutritional arguments are rubbish."

Moral arguments? Mr. Miller was singularly ill-qualified to talk
about morals.

PRIME TIME

The subtle art of molding the public's perception (that's yours and
mine) of your product can take many forms. Sometimes, it's as simple
as changing the name you call your product. For example, when the
word "fat" acquired a negative image among consumers, the meat
trade simply decided to ban the word.

"Fat lambs are now being called prime lambs. Fatstock is known as
primestock, and fattening cattle are known as finishing cattle,"
reports the *Meat Trades Journal*. Commented a livestock auctioneer,
"There's no doubt that fat had become a nasty word in many people's
minds."[25]

And it's not just the "F word" that arouses nasty associations, as
the following news report makes clear:

The editor in chief of the *Meat Trades Journal* urged that the
words "butcher" and "slaughterhouse" be eradicated and
replaced by the American euphemisms "meat plant" or "meat
factory." Alternatively, butchers could adopt the Irish word
"victualler." This would distance consumers from awareness of
the "bloodier side" of the meat trade. . . . [The editor argued

that] the meat trade's cause was not helped by the "blood-spattered whites" of Smithfield porters as they strolled "in front of the secretary birds." They and butchers should be put into velvet overalls. "It will reduce cleaning bills and any adverse reaction from the fainthearted." These days the word "butcher" was spread over newspaper headlines about the Ripper or the aftermath of bomb attacks. A change of nomenclature might only seem a verbal difference but it would "conjure up an image of meat divorced from the act of slaughter."[26]

But the "newspeak" (should that be "meatspeak"?) doesn't stop there. The Meat and Livestock Commission now wants terms such as "hormone-free," "chemical-free," and "additive-free" prohibited when used to describe organically produced meat, because they "can be confusing and sometimes misleading and inaccurate," and lead to legal problems, bad publicity, and lack of public confidence.[27]

It goes on and on. Pig farmers are now being encouraged to stop using the words "growth promoters" to describe the drugs they give to their animals to (guess what?) promote growth. And the names given to the cells that these poor animals spend much of their lives in, "flat-deck cages" and "farrowing crates," are now considered to be "too emotive." They're going to be replaced by "nurseries" and "maternity units."[28]

Maternity units?

George Orwell would be proud.

MEAT NAZIS MUST DIE

Since the meat industry has untold millions to spend on advertising and promotion, it is perhaps surprising that their track record isn't better. Sometimes, their advertising slogans seem to be downright counterproductive. In Britain, they adopted a slogan that shouted "Where's the Meat?," which reminded millions of people that meat eating was a declining habit, and another, "Meat's Got the Lot," which emerged at the time that food poisoning, antibiotic, and hormone contamination were also hitting the headlines. At other times, they have seemed unconsciously humorous, such as the "Slam in the

Lamb" slogan, which to me seems like an Australian euphemism for sexual intercourse. But of course, that's just me and my funny mind.

The American meat industry is equally cursed. When they spent a fortune on a series of very high-profile advertisements featuring star names, they burned their fingers not once, but twice. "Sometimes," Cybill Shepherd was depicted as saying, "I wonder if people have a primal, instinctive craving for hamburgers. Something hot and juicy and so utterly simple you can eat it with your hands. I mean, I know some people who don't eat burgers. But I'm not sure I trust them."

Frankly, I'm not at all sure I trust Cybill Shepherd, especially when she's being paid to peddle me a burger, and it is indeed gratifying when such fatuous copywriting gets its comeuppance, as it duly did when Cybill subsequently confided to *Family Circle* magazine that one of her own beauty tips was trying not to eat red meat.[29,30] Shepherd later maintained that she had not, in fact, made the statement, attributing the error to a misinformed publicist. Nevertheless, the beef barons who had paid for the $23 million ad campaign must have found the whole thing rather heartbreaking.

When James Garner agreed to appear promoting "Real Food for Real People," his reward was even worse—prompt admission to a hospital for heart surgery. Members of the Farm Animal Reform Movement thoughtfully sent him a vegetarian cookbook, a rather brilliant publicity coup that seemed to get more high-profile media coverage than Garner's original advertisements.[31] And to add insult to injury, the Beef Industry Council had a "Hubbard Award" (named after a nineteenth-century advertising shyster) bestowed on it by the Center for Science in the Public Interest, for "misleading, unfair, and irresponsible" advertising. "Popular beef products, such as hamburgers, are, by definition, not lean and contain large amounts of fat," said Bonnie Liebman, director of nutrition for the CSPI. "Real beef isn't so healthful when it's eaten by real people."[32]

One of the biggest Freudian slips of recent times was spotted when college student Erik Pyontek from Trenton, New Jersey, saw a poster promoting meat products in his supermarket.[33] Entitled "America's Meat Roundup," it depicted a tall blond cowboy proudly holding the American flag, hand on hip, his firm-jawed gaze courageously meeting the horizon. Pyontek went away and dug up a picture in a high school history textbook he'd been reminded of and yes, there it was, a tall blond Aryan proudly holding the Nazi flag, hand on hip, his firm-jawed gaze courageously meeting the horizon—the same all but for the Swastika. "We're not trying to send out any subliminal Nazi messages," screeched a spokesperson for the ad agency that created it. Nevertheless, the common symbolism of the two images is very telling.

The art of advertising copywriting is a fine one. On the one hand, you have a responsibility to be accurate in what you say. On the other hand, you have to sell the product. Sometimes, the distinction between accuracy and salesmanship is blurred, as in the recent British "Meat to Live" advertising campaign. The advertisements typically feature a selection of male models doing typical he-man stunts, hand stands, and so on, thus trying to create a masculine, athletic image for their product—all very predictable and bland. However, the accompanying text is more interesting. "Without a regular supply [of iron]," one of the advertisements claims, "you could well suffer from listlessness or, in extreme cases, anemia. . . . This, on its own, is a powerful reason for eating meat." Is it? The British Advertising Standards Authority considered that this turn of phrase might give the impression that meat was essential to a healthy diet, and warned the Meat and Livestock Commission not to create this impression in future advertisements.[34]

"Healthwise," said another meat ad, "it'll steel you against the elements too." Again, the Advertising Standards Authority considered the wording to be ambiguous, and asked the Meat and Livestock Commission not to imply that eating meat could provide health benefits that couldn't be obtained by eating a balanced, meat-free diet.

But if their public aspect has been less than irreproachable, at least the Meat and Livestock Commission appreciate the benefits of a vegetarian diet where it counts—at the very heart of their organization. For when a journalist from *Marketing* magazine had lunch there, he was relieved to discover that "the staff canteen offers a vegetarian option every day for those who prefer not to ingest what they sell."[35]

Nothing like a little hypocrisy, is there?

MEET THE MAD COWBOY

Howard Lyman will probably break your arm if you ever meet him, not because he's a dangerous person (although the American beef industry thinks he is) but because his handshake is like putting your hand into a vice and tightening it very hard indeed.

Howard is an amiable giant, a real all-American cattle rancher and fourth-generation cowboy from Montana and, oh yes, he just happens to be vegan.

One day, he found himself on *Oprah*. This is what happened in Howard's words:

A funny thing can happen when you tell the truth in this country. You can get sued. In April of 1996, I was sitting on the stage of the The *Oprah Winfrey Show*, looking into the shocked faces of a studio audience that was learning for the first time that we were turning cows into cannibals. "Right now," I explained, "we're following exactly the same path that they followed in England— ten years of dealing with [Mad Cow Disease] as public relations rather than doing something substantial about it. A hundred thousand cows in the United States are fine one night, then dead the following morning. The majority of those cows are ground up and fed back to other cows. If only one of them has Mad Cow Disease, it has the potential to affect thousands." Oprah herself was taken aback, and said quite simply, "Cows are herbivores. They shouldn't be eating other cows. . . . It has just stopped me cold from eating another burger." Sitting next to me on the stage was a representative of the National Cattlemen's Beef Association, Dr. Gary Weber, whose job it was to reassure the viewing public of the absolute safety of meat. I felt sorry for the guy; he had an extremely difficult hand to play. He couldn't deny my assertion that we'd been feeding cows to cows, but belittling the fact didn't sit well with a gasping audience. During commercial breaks he privately agreed with me that we shouldn't be adding chopped-up cow to animal feed.[36]

I think you know what happened. Howard and Oprah were sued for "food disparagement"—surely one of the most ludicrously biased, unconstitutional, and nakedly self-interested pieces of legislation ever to be concocted. Between 1996 and 1997 some thirteen states enacted food disparagement laws, and similar laws are pending in other states as well. In legal jargon, food disparagement suits are called SLAPPs, for Strategic Lawsuit Against Public Participation. Actual court victories are not necessarily the goal of a SLAPP suit. They primarily aim to chill speech by forcing defendants to spend huge amounts of time and money defending themselves in court. "The longer the litigation can be stretched out . . . the closer the SLAPP filer moves to success," observes New York Supreme Court Judge Nicholas Colabella.

On the February 9, 2000, the U.S. Court of Appeals for the Fifth Circuit unanimously affirmed the trial court's decision, rejecting the claims of the cattlemen that their beef had been "disparaged." In doing so the court ruled that the plaintiffs had failed to show that Oprah Winfrey, Howard Lyman, and King World Productions had "knowingly" disseminated false information tending to show that American beef is not fit for public consumption.[37]

Said the court: "Lyman's opinions, though strongly stated, were based on truthful, established fact, are not actionable under the First Amendment." Notably, the court added: "Stripped to its essentials, the cattlemen's complaint is that [Oprah's] 'Dangerous Food' show did not present the Mad Cow issue in the light most favorable to United States beef. This argument cannot prevail."

Food disparagement laws and the SLAPP lawsuit are two additional weapons available to those who would prefer you not to know what's really going on.

SO WHAT'S REALLY GOING ON?

I'll tell you. We've looked at some of the scientific evidence, considered why the medical profession is still so reluctant to universally endorse the vegetarian lifestyle, examined some of the naughty tricks the bad boys of the meat trade get up to, and seen how repressive legislation may be used to silence critics. But there's more. And it's nothing to do with PR executives, lawyers, or doctors. It's to do with us—*you*—and how you think about yourself.

Alarmed by the growth of vegetarianism among young people—the consumers of tomorrow—the meat industry is busy spending its vast resources launching its propaganda into schools and other places where young minds can be influenced. In its thinly disguised advertising material, you will find many astonishing statements, such as: "Modern man does not need to hunt but he still needs a balanced diet—of which meat is an essential element."[38]

This is, as you may have begun to suspect by now, utterly untrue. Meat is not "an essential element" of a balanced diet, as millions of healthy vegetarians will testify. And as a parent, I find it outrageous that the meat industry (which claims to have "established a good reputation among teachers for providing credible and well-balanced classroom resources"[39]) should be allowed to go into schools with such misleading propaganda masquerading as fact. Yet many of us still mistakenly believe that humans are somehow "genetically programed" to eat flesh foods, and cannot thrive without them; that we are, in essence, carnivores.

All right, then, let's look at the evidence.

Scientific evidence suggests that our ancestors probably originated in the east African Rift Valley, which is a dry and desolate place today, but would have been very different two to four million years ago. The habitat was very lush then. There were large, shallow freshwater lakes, with rich open grassland on the flood plains and dense woodland beside the rivers. Fossil evidence shows that foodstuffs such as *Leguminosae* (peas and beans) and *Anacardiaceae* (cashew nuts) were readily available, as were *Palmae* (sago, dates, and coconuts). Evidence gained from the analysis of tooth markings indicates that our ancestors' diet was much the same as the Guinea Baboon's is today—hard seeds, stems, some roots, plant fiber—a typically tough diet requiring stripping, chopping, and chewing actions.

Our ancestors also had very large molars and small incisors, unsuited to meat consumption but ideal for consuming large quantities of vegetable matter. By 2.5 million years B.C., however, evidence shows that the land began to dry out, forcing Australopithecus (the name of one of our early ancestors) to desert this idyllic "Garden of Eden" and to try and survive on the savannahs, where he was poorly prepared for the evolutionary struggle that was to come.

Before this crucial point, there is little doubt that our ancestors had largely followed a vegetarian diet, typical of primates. Studies of minute scratches on the dental enamel of an Australopithecus fossil suggest that his diet consisted largely of hard, chewy seeds and berries, although a few eggs and small animals may have been consumed, too. Most scientists consider it unlikely that Australopithecus was a systematic hunter, or "killer ape," as this species has sometimes been depicted.[40]

So we were forced by our rapidly changing environment to eat anything and everything we could get our hands on, which of course included some flesh. As our old habitat receded, we had to make some quick decisions. We had been used to eating a mainly fruit and nut diet. As this became increasingly scarce, we had to adapt to eating whatever we could find. There wasn't much. We found roots and grasses, and made do with them. We would have stumbled across some partly rotten carrion flesh, and gratefully ate what we could salvage. We would have chased easy-to-catch small game. We ate it all, no questions asked. Interestingly, we still preserve some ability to digest and utilize leaves and grasses, which recent scientific work has discovered, and probably dates from this period of our existence. We became not carnivores, but omnivores—actually, I would argue in favor of the word "adaptivores," because it conveys a more accurate impression of what was going on at that point in our history. In his book *The Naked Ape*, the zoologist Desmond Morris made an interesting observation about this period when he wrote: "It could be argued that, since our primate ancestors had to make do without a major meat component in their diets, we should be able to do the same. We were driven to become flesh eaters only by environmental circumstances, and now that we have the environment under control, with elaborately cultivated crops at our disposal, we might be expected to return to our ancient primate feeding patterns."[41]

If we as a species can be characterized by just one word, it would be "adaptability": we have learned how to survive in almost any environment, no matter how seemingly hostile. It is our passport for success in any situation, no matter how desperate, and unquestionably the key to our survival. We were forced out of our original habitat, and miraculously we survived. We were forced to learn how to live on the plains in competition with other animals that were natural carnivores, and again we met the challenge.

So here we have a picture of a species that was originally vegetarian, and then, due to force of circumstances, adapted to become omnivorous. This reality is a long, long way from the "meat is an essential element of the diet" myth propagated by the meat trade. It is clear from recent analyses of human remains that even during this period of our development, plant food was still by far the most important source of food. The level of strontium present in bones is an accurate guide to the amount of plant food consumed, and scientists at the University of Pisa, Italy, who have analysed the bones of early Europeans have found that they were eating an "almost exclusively vegetarian diet" right up to the time agriculture was developed.[42]

So, to what extent should our omnivorous adaptation influence our modern food habits? The first point to understand here is that the word "omnivore" does not mean "carnivore," as some seem to think it does: "We humans are biologically omnivores," says the Meat and Livestock Commission in the propaganda it gives out to our schoolchildren, "and an omnivorous diet is one which includes a whole range of foods—meat, in various forms, prominent among them."[43]

This is utterly misleading, for it implies that meat is an essential part of our diet. The fact is that meat is optional—we can choose to consume it, or not. Either way, we should know what the implications are.

The second point to understand is that our genetic constitution has changed very little for several tens of thousands of years. But, of course, our diet has changed—unfortunately, for the worse. Basically, our bodies are still in the Stone Age, and expect the sort of nutrition they were getting then. They're just not used to getting the kind of junk food we give them today. No wonder so many diseases are related to our modern pattern of food consumption.

As you might imagine, modern Westernized humans consume vastly more animal flesh than we have ever done in the whole history of our species. And we don't even have to exercise to get it—the exertion of the chase has been replaced by the flick of the credit card as it slides from our wallet.

In 1912, the first ever medical observation was made of a heart attack. In less than a hundred years, heart disease has soared away to become one of the leading killers of the Western world. But why? What has changed in such a comparatively short space of time? I put this question to Professor Michael Crawford, a recognized authority in the field.

"What has happened," he told me, "is that we all started from a common baseline of wild foods. This is the sort of primitive diet which humans have eaten throughout most of their evolution, over the past five million years. However, in the last few centuries, things have gone haywire. In Europe, our diets have gone in one direction, in Africa and India they've gone in a different direction. In Western Europe we've focused on consuming foods which are very rich in nonessential types of fat, but pretty miserable sources of essential fats. Our diets have also become rich in processed and refined carbohydrates. In fact, the problems are quite easy to identify—it's taking corrective action that seems to be difficult for some of us."

All in all, it seems as if the human race has unwittingly been playing a huge experiment on itself over the past century. In the year 1860, about one-quarter of our energy came from fat sources. By 1910, this had risen to one-third, and by 1975 about 45 percent of our total energy intake was coming from fat, much of it saturated animal fat. Thus, in no time at all, the amount of fat in our diet doubled. So it's hardly surprising if this new diet that we're eating today has some rather dreadful side effects, in the form of diet-related diseases.

Modern food animals are bred to be fat: the carcass of a slaughtered animal can easily be 30 percent fat or more. But the sort of animal that primitive people hunted was a wild animal—it had, on average, only 3.9 percent fat on its carcass.[44] So today, even if we cut our meat consumption back to the greatly reduced amount that our ancestors consumed, we will still be taking in seven times more fat than they did!

But even this isn't the end of the story. The type of fat on the carcass of the animal that our ancestors ate was different, as well. Primitive meat had five times more polyunsaturated fat in it than today's meat—which is high in saturated fat, but much lower in polyunsaturated. Also, our ancestral diet only had one-sixth the amount of sodium (salt) that the modern diet contains. And because fresh food comprised such an important part of the diet, the primitive diet was much, much richer in natural vitamins. For example, there would have been nearly nine times as much vitamin C in the primitive diet, twice as much fiber, three times as much total polyunsaturated fat.

So if you were worried that a meat-free diet might not be healthy, don't be. In point of fact, it's much closer to the kind of natural food that we've always eaten, and that our bodies have always been used to. In evolutionary terms, the meat we eat today is a *new* food for us, which means that we're actually conducting a huge experiment on our own bodies. And as you've started to see, the results don't look at all good.

Now, spend a moment looking at the table below. Here you can see typical characteristics of vegetarian animals (herbivores) compared to carnivorous animals. This straightforward evidence very clearly demonstrates the overwhelmingly vegetarian nature of our species.

CHARACTERISTICS OF HERBIVORES AND CARNIVORES

Herbivore	Carnivore	Human
Hands/hoofs as appendages	Claws as appendages	Hands as appendages
Teeth flat	Teeth sharp	Teeth flat
Long intestines to fully digest nutrients in plant foods	Short intestines, rapidly excrete putrefying flesh	Long intestines to fully digest nutrients in plant foods; flesh foods cause constipation.
Sweats to cool body	Pants to cool body	Sweats to cool body
Sips water	Laps water	Sips water
Vitamin C obtained solely from diet	Vitamin C manufactured internally	Vitamin C obtained solely from diet
Exists largely on a fruit & nut diet	Consumes flesh exclusively	Diet depends on environment, highly adaptable

Herbivore	Carnivore	Human
Grasping hands capable of using tools or weapons	No manual dexterity	Grasping hands capable of using tools or weapons
Inoffensive excrement	Putrid excrement	Offensiveness of excrement depends on diet
Snack feeder	Large meals infrequently taken	Combines worst of both worlds
Predominantly sweet-toothed	Preference for salty fatty food	Likes both sweet and salty/fatty food
Likes to savor food, experiment with variety, combine flavors	Bolts food down	Likes to savor food, experiment with variety, combine flavors
Large brains, able to rationalize	Small brains, less capable of adaptive behavior	Large brains, able to rationalize (at least in laboratory studies)

WHO DO YOU THINK YOU ARE?

Did you notice in the meat trade's propaganda quoted earlier that they spoke of "modern man," when they really meant to say "modern people"? Most people tend to dismiss unconscious sexism such as this as trivial, because it is so common. However, I now want to present you with yet more forbidden knowledge that goes straight to the heart of the modern myth of the red-blooded male meat eater.

Many of us are conditioned by our upbringings to believe that "man is a natural hunter and meat eater." Note that I—like the meat industry's propaganda quoted above—said "man," not humans. In the account of human evolution that most of us learn, women are mere appendages—accessories and mating objects for the all-powerful hunting male. According to the conventional wisdom of anthropology, it is hunting that has made us what we are today: intelligent, because hunters must be wily; tool makers, because hunters must have weapons; upright walkers, because hunters must walk and run long distances; cooperative, because hunters must work with each other to ensure a kill; and masters of language, because hunters must communicate with each other.

This is simplistic rubbish. But it is only in recent years that this ubiquitous stereotype has been challenged, by a few women anthropologists, who have become rather tired of the persistent omission and denigration of women from the accepted account of human history. Less than sexually secure males may wish to stop reading now.

"The most popular reconstruction of early human social behaviour is summarized in the phrase 'man the hunter,' " explains Adrienne Zihlman, professor of anthropology at UCLA. "In this hypothesis, meat eating initiated man's separation from the apes, males provided the meat, presumed to be the main item in early hominid diet, by inventing stone tools and weapons for hunting. Thus males played the major economic role, were protectors of females and young, and controlled the mating process. In this view of things, females fade into a strictly reproductive and passive role—a pattern of behavior inconsistent with that of other primates or of modern gathering and hunting peoples. In fact, the obsession with hunting has long prevented anthropologists from taking a good look at the role of women in shaping human adaptation."[45]

The plain fact is that the sort of hunting that our ancestors practiced was never a good enough way of providing food for everyone. Careful studies of societies who lead similar lifestyles to those of our ancestors—such as the Bush People of the Kalahari—reveal that the probability of obtaining meat on any one hunting day is about one in four.[46] Now, just how long do you think a society can exist, based on a 25 percent success record? By contrast, the women always return from their gathering expeditions with food—a 100 percent success rate. And the entire tribe could comfortably feed itself if each member put in a fifteen-hour week—rather better than our own society's achievement.

It is quiet clear that in original societies such as these, hunting is only possible when backed up by an effective, dependable, and reliable source of plant food. Once the tribe is certain of food, then those men who want to (about a third of the Kalahari males never hunted) can go off and gamble on a kill—nothing jeopardized if they come home empty-handed.

And yet, many modern people, living entirely synthetic lives in wholly unnatural Western environments, still believe and behave as if meat eating is the magic thread that keeps us in touch with the primitive, authentic humans we think we ought to be ("Real Food For Real People," as the advertising slogan tries to exploit this myth). Modern people who have never been told of the absolutely crucial role of "woman the gatherer" in human development are—to be blunt—profoundly ignorant. They are ignorant about the history of their own species, which makes them ignorant about their very own, personal identities. And ignorance leaves them wide open to exploitation.

A WOMAN'S WORK

Women, being the principal gatherers, also became the first growers. There is a significant difference between horticulture (which came first, and involved the cultivation of wild plants) and agriculture (which came later, and involved ploughing the ground, using domesticated animals). While horticulture seemed to spring up almost simultaneously in many parts of the world, agriculture was never adopted in New World original societies (the Americas). And there are still some horticultural tribes in far-flung places, whose development never seems to have progressed to complete agriculture. In these tribes, such as the Australian aborigines, it is often the women who take responsibility for plant usage and cultivation, cutting the tops off wild yams, for example, and replanting them to produce a continually cropping plant in a perfectly balanced relationship with nature.

Why did horticulture first develop? Obviously, it represents a quantum leap in the amount of food that can be amassed for a given amount of effort. Instead of wandering and gathering, it was now possible to stay in a single spot and work continuously at harvesting grain. The transformation from gathering to cultivation seems to have taken place in locations where plants yielding a lot of starch were available. Grain being particularly easy to store when dry, it was now possible to work intensively at harvesting, and to accumulate an impressive store of food that would not spoil as it was kept. Modern experiments have shown that it is possible to manually harvest about five pounds of grain an hour. If four people worked continuously for the three weeks that wild wheat was ripe, they could produce about one ton of grain—enough to feed themselves for an entire year. Interestingly, this wild wheat was of a much higher protein content (about 24 percent) than our modern, highly developed strains (about 14 percent).

Now, consider the crushing impact that ever-more-prolific female horticulture must have had on the male ego. "Man the Provider" has always been a male-inspired, self-justifying myth (think of our phrase "bringing home the bacon"). The reality of the traditional hunter/gatherer society was that it was held together primarily by the food-producing and child-rearing abilities of the females—not by the males, who contributed in total far less. With the advent of horticulture, women were further challenging the usefulness, indeed, the whole *raison d'être* of the male role. They were steadily increasing the already large contribution they made to the group's food supplies. The male contribution, if anything, would have been diminishing at this point, for a fixed home base would have restricted the amount of wild animals within easy reach.

It is a strange thing, but the cultivation of plants is a rather difficult thing to control on old-fashioned, paternalistic principles. It just isn't naturally suited to it. For one thing, there are no "best bits," no parts of the plant that are so much better than the rest. In the good old hunting days, certain parts of the dead animal were more highly prized than others, and tradition dictated that the best should go to the number-one hunter. The tail of a kangaroo, the trunk of an elephant, the tongue of a bison, the eyeball fat of a guanaco (a kind of llama)—all these things were considered to be prize delicacies in certain societies and, accordingly, should only be given to the very bravest hunter. But where were these perks in a plant? Search as you might, you just couldn't find them. It would seem that vegetable foods are innately egalitarian.

On the other hand, meat strongly reinforces the established pecking order. The smallest social divisions can be exaggerated and exploited, and great ego satisfaction can be obtained by comparing one's own position to someone further down the pecking order. Here is one fairly typical social hierarchy that anthropologists have identified in contemporary hunting societies; those closer to the top receive the most highly prized cuts of meat.[47]

Active male hunters
Net owners
Helpers of net owners
Spear owners
Dog owners
Fathers of dog owners
Beaters
Those who carried the meat
Old people
Sisters or sisters-in-law of the killer
Children
Women
Dogs

All these people would receive meat in the quality and quantity that befitted their station. In addition, tribal chiefs, "house" chiefs, and chiefs of confederacies would expect their dues as well. It is on this masculine set of values that our present society has largely modeled itself, rewarding as it does any successful display of aggression, competition, or social rivalry. It is very recently that some women have started to realize that they have been tricked into supporting this pernicious ideology, and some of them, such as the writer Norma Benney, are starting to question it. She considers that hierarchical structures such as these "involve concepts of 'higher' and 'lower' in which the former inevitably exploits the latter. Feminist thinking challenges these hierarchies, and women are starting to realise that in the process of struggling for our own rights, we should not participate in the victimisation of those even worse off than ourselves in the patriarchal pecking order. We need to develop fresh ways of seeing the world if we are to get out of the habit of ignoring the realities of how other, non-human animals are living."[48]

It can be seen, then, that flesh consumption reinforces and indeed, creates, social divisions, and further celebrates the values upon which those divisions are based. Plant cultivation, on the other hand, is stubbornly egalitarian. It is clear that if the system were changed, those with the most to lose would be those who occupied positions close to the top of the pile—those who received the tastiest treats, and those with the greatest social standing. With the advent of horticulture, there was less economic dependence on the hunter and his meat than ever before. So the hunter became a horticulturist, then an agriculturist, and brought with him the values and ideology of the hunt.

Horticulture is essentially a cooperative act with the earth. Seeds are given to the ground in an area that is likely to be well irrigated, and in return the earth will manifest her fertility. It is based on the great cycle of nature—what anthropologist Mircea Eliade calls "the eternal return."

Agriculture, however, has at its core an act of coercion; it is stamped with the symbolism of the hunter, even today. Female animals are made pregnant whenever the farmer so desires, sometimes with the use of an apparatus known as the "rape rack," whose function is precisely as it sounds. Even the crops in the fields are controlled by use of chemicals that "wage war" on other plant species with no commercial value to the farmer. And of course, in modern societies, agriculture is an operation almost exclusively controlled by males. Women have been relegated, once again, to the less important role of menials, laborers, child rearers, and food processors.

Pretty soon, animals were "agriculturalized," too. It is likely that men had already formed something of a symbiotic relationship with a few types of wild species. Dogs may have been used sometimes to track and chase the hunters' quarry. Animals, both dead and alive, would have figured prominently in religious ceremonies designed to give men control over the species he intended to hunt. Young animals, orphaned when their parents were butchered by the hunt, would have been kept as pets. And it is likely that some animals served as substitute sex objects for the male. Even in modern America, the Kinsey report estimated that one in twelve of all males had sexual relations with animals.

Some animals, too, would have been kept as tame decoys, to allow the hunters to closely approach their quarry without alarming it. This practice still exits in some modern slaughterhouses, where so-called

"Judas sheep" are specially trained by the slaughter men to lead the victims from the pens to the killing floor.

Man had, therefore, been involved in a symbiotic relationship with semiwild animals for a considerable length of time prior to the development of agriculture. The status of animals and females may have been, in the collective male mind, remarkably similar. Superfluous female babies, like young animals, would be culled, sometimes by being buried alive. Women, like female animals, produced milk that men could drink. Women were (and still are, in some societies) used as wet nurses for young animals, particularly piglets.

Some anthropologists suggest that the presumed cult of the fertility goddess shows that men venerated and worshipped the female principle, but this is only one interpretation. The whole point of evolving a religion was to better yourself, to gain control over some aspect of your existence. Early man did not worship the wild boar, the reindeer, or the bear in the same way as modern people worship their God. He carved their likenesses, painted their outlines, performed magical ceremonies, and made sacrifices for one main purpose: to gain control. In the same way, he sought (and achieved) control over the female.

So both women and animals became domesticated—enslaved to agriculture. And the new agriculture regularly and reliably produced food in more ready abundance than ever before. Nutritionally, there was less need now for flesh food than at any time previously. But culturally and symbolically, the ritual of meat production and consumption was now more essential than ever, serving as an embodiment and confirmation of the values of a society created around male dominion achieved through slaughter.

Ponder on this: each time you consume animal flesh, you make a blood sacrifice to this outmoded and evil ethic.

TOOTH AND CLAW

We have briefly touched upon the development of Western society from primate to hunter-gatherer, then to horticulturalist and finally to agriculturalist. Now we need to consider why, in a modern, post-industrialized society such as ours, the myth of the red-blooded masculine hunter-killer is still a potent image for us.

There are two fundamental reasons: First, the historical record itself colors our judgment. The garbage that is generated as a result of eating meat is pretty permanent—bones last longer in the ground than husks or seeds. Scientists, usually males, have traditionally focused their attention on the tools and artifacts of hunting, rather than the easily overlooked remnants of horticulture. And this can produce some very misleading results, indeed. For example, with only their rubbish tips to go on, archaeologists studying the Bush people of the Kalahari would conclude that they were an almost exclusively meat-eating tribe—the very opposite of the truth.

But a further, and far more significant, reason is this. The science of anthropology began as a kind of natural history, a study of the peoples encountered along the frontiers of European expansion. Such peoples—invariably called primitives or savages—were often studied, not so much for what they themselves were, but rather as a means of justifying Victorian culture's position at the apex of the evolutionary pyramid. The ideas of Darwin and Huxley, frequently misquoted and misunderstood, were similarly advanced as "proof" of our culture's superiority over the savages, of Man's rightful dominion as lord and master of Nature, and of man's proper subjugation of woman. This was not what Darwin intended; but it was what happened.

"In late Victorian society," writes Darwin's biographer Jonathan Howard, "a peculiarly beastly form of social climbing, 'Social Darwinism,' was established under Herbert Spencer's slogan 'The survival of the fittest.' The evolutionary law was interpreted to mean victory to the strongest as the necessary condition for progress. As a prescription for social behaviour it justified the worst excesses of capitalism exploitation of labour, 'reasoned savagery' as T. H. Huxley labelled it."[49]

For many Victorians, evolution started to replace religion as the justification, the rationalization, for the prevailing status quo. It was no longer necessary to believe that God had put Man at the top of the natural hierarchy; Man could now claim to have gotten there by his very own efforts. If Man was really only an animal, then he was the most successful animal—more aggressive, more dominant, and more ruthless than any other. In a fast-expanding industrial society, these values were prized beyond all others; "female" values were never less visible. And it is precisely from this period in our recent history that many serious misconceptions about our origin date.

Our notion of women's and men's role in prehistory, says Adrienne Zihlman: "derives in part from currently perceived differences in status of the sexes. Popular pictures drawn of the past are too often little more than backward projections of cultural sex stereotypes onto humans who lived more than a million years ago. Themes of male aggression, dominance, and hunting have long pervaded reconstructions of early human social life; and this had led to a belief that present-day inequality of the sexes has its roots in an ancient lifestyle and in inherent biological differences between the sexes. . . . Beginning with Darwin's discussion of human evolution, the theme of male dominance and female passivity and the use of tools as weapons has run through thinking about evolution. The emphasis on hunting, as with male dominance, is an outcome of male bias, however unconscious it may be, and this bias pervades even studies of primate behavior. In Darwin's case, given the values of Western society, especially Victorian England, and the nature of available evidence, his emphasis on males is not surprising."[50]

It really is extraordinary that so many of our conceptions about the history of our own species, and our place relative to other animals and life forms, should still be so deeply biased by the values of Victorian Britain. Let us investigate some of them.

Tennyson's clichéd phrase "Nature red in tooth and claw" perfectly captures the prevailing ethos of the period, combining as it does Tennyson's own deep-rooted fear of the chaos and disorder he believed to exist in the natural world, together with the inference that it is the proper duty of Man to subdue and dominate this wild force. Today, it is still a powerful image in the minds of many people who, in other respects, would not wish to share the values and prejudices of their Victorian ancestors. Most of us do, indeed, take it for granted that nature in the raw is cruel and merciless, showing no compassion to those who are too weak to defend themselves. And it is certainly a convenient way for us to see the world, for it proves our claim to supremacy over all other creatures; and it excuses our actions toward them, no matter how barbaric.

Tennyson himself was a typical product of his era. Born in 1809, he had a secluded childhood in Lincolnshire, where his father was a minister of the church, a manic-depressive, an alcoholic, and frequently violent. Unable to form a close relationship with his father, the young boy became very shy, very insecure, and would often seek solace in the lonely churchyard, where he would fling himself down weeping among the graves, longing to die. He grew up with a sense of embitterment, and believed that life should have given him a better position than merely being a parson's son. He was a hypochondriac, and, according to those who knew him, constantly worried about his bowels.

His attitude toward women was equally characteristic of the period. "Woman is the lesser man," he believed, "God made the woman for the man." As far back as 1860, the feminist Emily Davies was poking fun at what she described as his "bisexual theory of the human ideal." Like many others, he was deeply worried by what he saw as the dangers of too much democracy. In 1865, there was a public outcry concerning the governor of Jamaica, E. J. Eyre. A small rebellion on the island lead to Eyre taking savage retribution, hanging nearly 600 people, and flogging many more. There was an attempt to have Eyre prosecuted for murder, but Tennyson thought that Eyre's action was entirely justified, being "the only method of saving English lives." He even contributed to a fund set up to defend Eyre. "Niggers are tigers," growled Tennyson. Nice chap, yes?

He wrote recruiting poems for the army and held conventional views on the subject of Ireland, which has always been a problem for the English. "Couldn't they blow up that horrible island with dynamite," he asked, "and carry it off in pieces—a long way off?"

All this begins to tell you something about the values of the man who invented that unpleasant phrase. It should come as no surprise to learn that Tennyson found "Nature" quite horrifying. "The lavish profusion in the natural world," he wrote, "appalls me, from the growths of the tropical forest, to the capacity of man to multiply, the torrent of babies." The Victorians decided that they liked Tennyson, his poetry, and his values, enough to make him the poet laureate of his day.

Even so, some people may still feel that, bigot and racist though he was, Tennyson was essentially correct about nature, or at least, about other animals. They do kill and eat each other and that justifies our own flesh-eating habit and the values it embraces. Certainly, the meat trade wishes to perpetuate this idea for its own commercial ends. In publicity material given to British schoolchildren, it approvingly quoted the television naturalist David Attenborough: "People have become divorced from the realities of nature in their urban environment. I hope to bring back in my programmes a clear understanding that we are part of that wider system, and that animals die and are eaten."[51]

There are several points to make in response to this decidedly weird "death is good" argument. First, natural carnivores—such as hyenas—certainly need to kill to stay alive; but as you have already seen, there is overwhelming evidence that humans are not carnivores.

Second, I should point out that, equally, many animals do *not* need to rip into other animals' flesh in order to survive. To argue that hyenas hunt their prey, therefore humans should symbolically do the same, is selective logic bordering on insanity. Why should humans behave like hyenas? Why not like the vegetarian elephant? Or the dik-dik? Or the lesser-spotted Patagonian nut cracker? If you're going to pretend to be another species, you may as well make it as exotic as possible, while you're waiting for the men in white coats to arrive.

If we are going to imitate other animals in our conduct, why not imitate good-natured ones? Television wildlife documentaries are often obsessed with the eating habits of carnivores, much to the satisfaction, no doubt, of the meat industry. But why don't they show us the highly developed, altruistic behavior that some species clearly demonstrate? Consider these remarkable examples:

- When dolphinaria were first becoming big business in the United States, the normal method of "collecting" wild dolphins from the sea and bringing them into captivity was to throw a charge of dynamite into the sea among a school of dolphins, and pick up those that had been stunned. Of course, this would kill many others, but that didn't matter to the people who owned the dolphinaria; there were plenty more of them in the sea. The men who were responsible for collecting the stunned dolphins in nets would frequently report other dolphins coming to the rescue of those that were unconscious. The normal practice would be for two dolphins to arrange themselves on either side of the unconscious one, and stay there until it recovered. This would enable it to continue to breathe, for dolphins are mammals and need air; otherwise they drown. "That the action was deliberate," said one report, "is shown by the way the supporting dolphins, when they had to leave it to come up to breathe, swam in a wide arc to come back and continue to support it." Unquestionably, this is altruistic behavior of a very high order—the "good Samaritan" dolphins could not have been reacting "instinctively" to a distress call, of course, because the unconscious dolphin wouldn't be able to make one. The very latest research on dolphins again challenges the human conceit that only people are capable of showing love, enjoying sex, and thinking creatively about abstractions such as the future and the past. "I'm trying to tell people that these are cultural animals," says naturalist Ken Norris, who researches spinner dolphins off Hawaii. "We're dealing with an animal for whom cooperation with its fellows is life itself . . . they can carry on a discourse about things that don't exist, like the past and future and concepts. They also teach each other, which to me is the concourse of culture."[52]

- In Tanzania, Africa, an elephant control officer is summoned with his gun to a village where elephants have been reported to be raiding the crops. He sees the bull elephant and fires, aiming at the brain. The bull falls wounded, but is not dead—the bullet has missed the brain, hitting the shoulder. Three other elephants move in on the prostrate bull, arranging themselves on each flank, one behind. Astonished, the officer does not fire again. "They boosted him onto his feet," he says. "I was amazed by it." He returns to the spot the next day, but there is no trace of the wounded male.

- In similar circumstances, another elephant control officer decides to shoot a bull elephant, raises his rifle, and fires. He misses the brain, but breaks the bull's shoulder. The bull bellows in great pain, and two cow elephants hear his calls and come running. They start to half carry, half drag the bull into the jungle, away from danger. The officer runs closer in to the bull, trying to get a final shot in to kill it. One of the cows angrily turns on him, and he shoots her point blank. She crumples up and dies. "The remaining cow," reports the officer, "went sadly on her way, every few yards stopping to listen and look back."

- Yet another officer is tracking three cow elephants and one bull. He finds them, and fires quickly at all four. The three cows drop dead, almost instantly. The bull does not, but is badly wounded and confused. To his horror, the officer now realizes that the cows have baby elephant calves with them, which the long grass prevented his seeing. The calves rush to the bull, not for protection, but arrange themselves on either side of him and try to help him along.

There are countless other examples of animals behaving selflessly with altruism. All this is a very long way from the "Nature red in tooth and claw" myth, demonstrating as it does compassion, altruism, and courage on the part of nonhuman animals, and perhaps raising a gleam of hope for the future—a future based on shared values, shared experience, and shared environment.

A PLATE FULL OF HATE

One of the saddest, most pernicious deceptions perpetrated on men today is the notion that "If you are not able to kill"—and what more potent symbol of killing is there than a slab of animal flesh on a plate?—"then you are not really a man." This is how one modern man perfectly expresses this evil concept: "The instinct of the hunter is one of the most deeply ingrained of our inheritances from the past. Could it be said that he who had no trace of such a feeling was somewhat lacking in virility?"[53]

And that man should know what he's talking about, having participated in the deaths of thousands of Earth's most magnificent mammals, not however without some stirring of conscience: "A whale struggling in its death flurry is a really moving spectacle, even to the hardened eyes of a whaler. But no sound is heard from the whales. If they had vocal cords proportionate to their bulk, with which to express their suffering, there would undoubtedly be very few men who would have strong enough nerves to bear the last moments of a whale dying by the harpoon. A blue whale, mortally wounded by several harpoons, has been known to tow a modern 'catcher' behind it for two hours before dying. Gunners themselves, who might be thought to be quite indifferent to the sufferings of their quarry, are generally affected by an obscure and uneasy feeling that we have all experienced when the 'flurry' occurred."

So are men forever destined by biology to be murderers of their fellow creatures? Of course not. As a man, I am outraged and enraged by those who tell me that the man who gazes back from the mirror is, at heart, an unrepentant and eternal killer. As the great writer and Nobel prize–winner Isaac Bashevis Singer observed, "People often say that humans have always eaten animals, as if this is a justification for continuing the practice. According to this logic, we should not try to prevent people from murdering other people, since this has also been done since the earliest of times." I also know that contact between our species and others does not have to be brutal and deadly.

In the 1970s, humans started to explore the alien world of these gentle sea creatures, and we first started to realize that we shared common bonds with them. Divers who have swam with them frequently report feeling as if the whales were protecting and taking care of them. In one amazing incident off Hawaii, a female whale asked for human help. In March 1976, the *White Bird* was carrying divers when a giant humpback whale knocked her head on the boat three or four times, diver Roy Nickerson reported. After each knock, she would withdraw, and raise herself to look up at those on deck. He donned his wetsuit and went down to investigate. He found she had aborted, and her baby calf was stillborn, but not free of her body. Other divers then went down, lassoed the dead calf, and pulled it clear. It was a sad incident, but illustrative of the cooperation that could exist between our species, if we wanted it.

But before that happens, we have to first understand, and then overcome, the doctrine of "Meatismo," which corrupts the minds of many men. Here it is, perfectly expressed, with words so evil that they chill me each time I read them. Nazi philosopher Oswald Spengler spawned them: "The beast of prey is the highest form of active life. It represents a mode of living which requires the extreme degree of the necessity of fighting, conquering, annihilating, self-assertion. The human race ranks highly because it belongs to the class of beasts of prey. Therefore we find in man the tactics of life proper to a bold, cunning beast of prey. He lives engaged in aggression, killing, annihilation. He wants to be master in as much as he exists."[54]

Now you know the enemy. These are appalling words. They speak of life without love, without compassion, without joy. Actually, they are not describing life at all, they are portraying a kind of living death (which is precisely how most modern food animals are reared). Words such as these will serve to excuse any atrocity, any barbarism. And of course, they have done so.

But they are not true. Man is demonstrably not a "beast of prey." The greatest achievements of human history—horticulture, for example—came about through cooperation, not lethal domination.

Something to think about, isn't it?

2

APOCALYPSE COW!

I love those old black-and-white movies, don't you? There's nothing better on a cold winter's evening than curling up with a glass of something comforting, the lights turned down low, and a vintage film on the television.

The Day the Earth Caught Fire is a good one to pick, if you like British sci-fi flicks from the early 1960s. It's escapism, of course, but none the worse for that. The plot is just a little bit cheesy. Russian and American teams of scientists have, unbeknown to each other, triggered a series of simultaneous nuclear explosions, which together throw the Earth off its path, spinning into the Sun. As the temperature rises, the truth can no longer be concealed from the public, and pandemonium breaks out. At the eleventh hour a desperate rescue plan is attempted: yet more nuclear explosions are detonated, this time intended to correct the Earth's wayward orbit. The bombs go off, and the world waits in trepidation to hear its fate. The last shot of the movie slowly pans over a sweltering newspaper office, where two versions of tomorrow's paper are ready to run with opposite headlines. "Earth Saved!" reads one version. "Earth Doomed!" reads the other. Which one will be used? We never discover. Fade-out and credits.[1]

Today, that is just about the situation that applies to the "Mad Cow Disease" catastrophe. Millions of people have been exposed to a potentially lethal agent, whose sinister characteristics seem to have come straight out of a science-fiction movie, and we still don't know how it's going to end: world saved, or world doomed. This is how expert microbiologist Professor Richard Lacey puts it: "If an evil force could devise an agent capable of damaging the human race, he would make it indestructible, distribute it as widely as possible in animal feed so that it would pass to man, and programme it to cause disease slowly so that everyone would have been exposed to it before there was any awareness of its presence."[2]

Of course this is *not* science-fiction, because just such a "lethal agent" started to emerge in Britain in the early 1980s. A few years later, it had become a grim plague. "You Don't Need Meat" was the first book in the world to write about this baffling and frightening new disease. In this chapter, you're going to discover some very unsettling facts, indeed. So here is the extraordinary history of Mad Cow Disease—almost certainly more truthful, and more complete, than anything you have yet seen. There are clear lessons to be learned here, which we fail to learn only at our extreme peril.

WELCOME TO THE ZOO

The Mad Cow Disease story is important for two reasons. First, even though it's over sixteen years since the first case was detected in Britain, we still don't have any good idea of just how serious the global human epidemic will be. We *do* know that it's a global problem, not just a British one anymore, because large quantities of potentially infected material have already been sent all over the planet. "There actually has been exposure worldwide already," Dr. Maura Ricketts, of the World Health Organization's animal and food-related public health risks division, told a news conference recently.[3] And the European Union's most senior scientists recently warned that *millions* of European consumers may be at risk of catching the human version of Mad Cow Disease—despite their governments' assertions that their countries are free of the cattle disease.[4] So it's still wait-and-see time.

The second reason we need to understand the Mad Cow saga is that it can—*and it will*—happen again. How can I be so confident in this assertion? Well, it's easy. Mad Cow Disease is an epidemic that, like many others before it and like diseases yet to come, has jumped from one species (cows) to another (humans). This process actually happens all the time, although most of us would prefer not to think about it.

When people eat the flesh of an animal, they're consuming a substance that has been literally and metaphorically deconstructed. The pink, shrink-wrapped cuts of meat on the supermarket shelves don't look as if they've been hacked from anything that was once alive; city children often find it difficult to believe that "meat" and "animals" are at all connected. Metaphorically, we're sold the idea that this substance consists of protein, vitamins, and other good things—rather like taking a vitamin pill.

When you awaken from this fantasy, you're in for a nasty shock. Meat comes from living animals, and animals—like us—are creatures that are subject to sickness, and sometimes pestilence. It's all part of our common bond.

Every year millions of people become ill (and sometimes die) because they catch a disease from another animal species. One of the most common is food poisoning, caused by bacteria from the salmonella group of organisms, which live in the intestinal tract of animals. This is just one example of a "zoonosis"—the scientific term for any disease that originates in animals and can be passed on to humans (sometimes in a much more virulent form). Other zoonoses include anthrax, rabies, leptospirosis, listeriosis, toxoplasmosis, brucellosis, tuberculosis, and trichinosis—all serious, often fatal, diseases that are transmitted from animals to humans across the species barrier. But outside of the research laboratory, very few people realize just what a grave health threat zoonoses may pose to all of us.

Zoonoses behave in strange, often unpredictable ways. The process of human-animal disease transmission is going on all the time; new diseases are continually being created, transformed, mutated, and activated. Some diseases may lie dormant for hundreds of years, just waiting for suitable conditions to appear before they reemerge and decimate a population that has little or no immunity to them. The stark reality is that today three-quarters of the world's rural population suffer from one or more diseases that have been passed on to them from a reservoir of infections in the animal population. But don't make the mistake of believing that it's only people who live in

Third World countries who are at risk. Apart from a few widely publicized diseases (such as rabies and salmonella), most people—and a surprising number of doctors and scientists—are hugely ignorant of the legacy of disease that humans and animals jointly share. For example, very few people know that

- The common cold came from our ancestors' contact with horses. As a species, humans first succumbed to rhinoviruses (the group of viruses that produce the common cold) from their association with horses. The cold is a recent disease in humans—we have only suffered from it since we became urbanized, about 10,000 years ago. At that time, the rhinoviruses present in horses mutated and crossed over into the human population, where they now number more than eighty.[5]
- Measles originated in the wolf population. It emerged as a new disease in humans about 6,000 years ago. The evidence shows that wolves first passed on the distemper virus to dogs, where it then mutated and became the rinderpest virus, which infected cattle, and then once again mutated and established itself in the human population as the disease we now know as measles.[6]
- Syphilis first arose from contact with monkeys. It originated in Stone Age populations between 25,000 and 18,000 B.C. from a reservoir of infections existing in monkey populations. Originally a disease disseminated by bodily contact, it evolved to become a sexually transmitted disease as the wearing of clothes increasingly restricted skin-to-skin intimacy solely to the act of copulation.[7]
- Cholera originated from sheep and cows. It is one of the newest of all human pandemics, first making its appearance in Calcutta in 1817, from which it quickly spread all around the world. The cholera organism almost certainly mutated from similar infections present in sheep and cows, and its rapid (and opportunistic) transmission is frightening evidence that, whether we realize it or not, zoonoses are our constant companions.[8]

Where will the next zoonosis come from? As we keep our food animals in ever more intensive conditions, and feed them ever more unnatural diets, we are increasingly tempting fate. One day, a new disease may spring up that will prove incurable and lethal to its human host.

Maybe it already has.

COUNTDOWN TO PLAGUE

Perhaps there was "an evil force" controlling Mad Cow Disease, after all. Because it could hardly have chosen a better country than Britain for a beachhead. Where America has its Freedom of Information Act, Britain has its Official Secrets Act, spawned from a society that has no written constitution to safeguard the rights of the individual, and that values the commercial confidences of food manufacturers as if they were state secrets.[9]

As a result, the British people were never told the full story about Mad Cow Disease. In the heat of the crisis, some officials behaved as if their prime duty was to suppress public concern, and thereby minimize economic loss to the meat industry. Both government and the meat industry were, in effect, saying to the public "keep on eating the beef until we've figured out what's wrong with it."

At all costs, "panic" had to be avoided. But panic—or alarm—is a natural human survival mechanism. It protects us from exposing ourselves to foolish risks. And with Mad Cow Disease, so many of the risks still remain extremely unclear. What connection, for example, might it have with Alzheimer's Disease? By the age of eighty-five, one in four people will suffer from this dreadful condition.[10] In the laboratory, there seem to be some ominous similarities.[11]

The story of Mad Cow Disease has three parallel threads, which eventually converged to tie a knot of Gordian complexity in April 1985, when it was first observed on a British farm.[12] Thread One begins on January 15, 1755, precisely. It was on that day that the British Parliament was petitioned by sheep farmers to impose severe restrictions on those who dealt in sheep purchased from breeders. The reason was the emergence, in epidemic proportions, of a disease they termed "rickets" (also rather quaintly known as "goggles"), an invariably fatal affliction that was wiping out entire herds. From contemporary accounts of the symptoms, it is clear that this disease was what we now know as "scrapie." It is a horrible disease—one of its distinctive characteristics is an uncontrollable urge for the animal to rub or scrape itself until the wool is entirely worn away and the bleeding skin is exposed—hence the name. Scrapie has been present in many countries for hundreds of years. In Britain, it was responsible for the virtual extermination of at least two entire breeds of sheep, the Wiltshire Horn and the Norfolk Horn.[13]

The British Parliament responded to this early animal health request with characteristic and precedent-setting decisiveness. It did nothing.

Thereafter, scrapie waxed and waned, as epidemics do. Between 1750 and 1820, there were severe outbreaks in East Anglia, Wessex, France (around Rambouillet), and Germany (around Frankenfelde and Stolpen). In the Bath area of Britain, a contemporary agricultural writer recorded that the disease "within these few years has destroyed some in every flock around the County and made great havock in many."[14]

Then, between the years 1820 and 1910, outbreaks of scrapie declined, until, by the turn of the twentieth century, it had virtually ceased to exist in Europe. This is the way of epidemics—they run their course. Slowly, more resistant sheep are bred. But only a fool would have claimed that the disease had been conquered.

From 1910 onward, scrapie began to reemerge. In East Anglia, Southern Scotland, many areas of France, Eastern Germany, Hungary, and Bulgaria, sheep once considered to be resistant started to succumb. A very slow fuse had started to burn.

PULLING THE WOOL

Let's take a moment to consider the symptoms of scrapie. It has an incubation period that ranges from one and a half to five years, during which time there are no recognizable symptoms. All this time, the "infectious agent" is replicating in the animal, finally reaching its brain. The first outward sign that something is wrong is a general restlessness, and a fixed, fearful expression in the animal's eyes. Its pupils dilate; it hangs its head; its movements become aimless and its legs, stiff and unbending. Then it starts to grind its teeth; its lips start to twitch, which soon spreads to the muscles around the shoulders and thighs. If suddenly startled, the animal may fall into an epileptic fit. Then the intense itching begins. Finally, the animal becomes completely uncoordinated, paralysis sets it, and it dies.[15] A postmortem will reveal characteristic spongy, hole-riddled areas of brain where the infectious agent has destroyed cells. This spongelike quality gives rise to the name "spongiform," which scientists use to describe this kind of distinctive pathological feature.

So here we have an incurable disease, caused by a mystery "infectious agent," capable of great devastation of sheep flocks, strongly implicated in the development of Mad Cow Disease, and very similar to certain dementia-producing diseases in humans. And we don't know how many sheep are carrying it.

As the British Veterinary Association mildly put it to the House of Commons in a memorandum: "We can only guess at the incidence of the disease. That has been an omission."[16]

Actually, successive governments cannot share all the blame for this state of affairs. As one expert, Dr. K. L. Morgan of Bristol University, explains: "The potentially disastrous economic effect of its identification in flocks producing pedigree and breeding stock has resulted in a reticence to acknowledge the presence of Scrapie. The concealment of clinical cases is such that once the first case is diagnosed and the signs recognised, other cases may be disposed of without the knowledge of the attending veterinarian."[17]

Scrapie is bad news for everyone. And like all bad news, no one wants to know about it. Until it's too late.

A BIG, BAD BUG

What actually causes scrapie? If you look it up in a medical or veterinary dictionary, you may find it described as a "slow virus" disease. That definition is inaccurate. Scrapie is not caused by anything remotely similar to other recognized viruses. Yet for decades, scientists were happy to classify it as a viral disease for the simple reason that it was inconceivable that it could be anything else. As recently as

1989, the Academic American Encyclopedia wrote: "Slow viruses are disease agents *not yet identified but assumed to exist*, because the diseases resemble virus diseases in their epidemiology" (my emphasis).

But the scrapie "virus" has never behaved like a virus should behave. No viral particles could be identified from infected tissues. No viral antibodies could be recovered in the laboratory.[18] The scrapie "virus" also violated one of the three golden rules of biology known as "Koch's Postulates," which were established a century ago by the German physician Robert Koch. Koch's third postulate states that, in order to prove that a given infection is caused by particular agent, the agent must not only be isolated from the patient but must also then be capable of being grown in a culture.

But that's not all. Sinisterly, the scrapie resisted the most prodigious efforts to kill it, such as being bombarded with radiation, being cooked at high temperatures, and being doused with strong disinfectant chemicals. None of these lethal assaults could kill the thing that causes scrapie. As one expert commented with justified exasperation: "The fourth decade of my association with Scrapie ended in 1978, with the causal agent still obscure, and virologists as adamant as ever that theirs was the only worthwhile point of view. To explain findings that did not fit in with a virus hypothesis, they re-christened the causal agent an 'unconventional virus.' Use of this ingenious cover-up for uncertainty made 'virus' meaningless—for is not a cottage an unconventional castle?"[19]

THREAD TWO: THE LAUGHING DEATH

The place is Papua New Guinea, mostly unexplored by Westerners until the second half of the twentieth century. Before then, nothing but the occasional gold prospector, the odd missionary, motivated by greed or creed, had risked death by malaria to penetrate its secret interior. And there were rumors of cannibalism among the indigenous population.

It is in the distant interior of this island where the Fore tribe make their home. The Lutherans were the first to reach them, in 1949, and the Australians followed two years later with a patrol outpost at a place they called Okapa. The temperature here in the hills is a comfortable 68 degrees F. all the year round, although the humidity can sometimes be disagreeable for a Westerner. The hills and the valleys, once extensively wooded, are now a mixture of trees and grasslands, the result of 11,000 years of continuous human habitation. It may not be paradise, but on first inspection it seems pretty close.

And how deceptive appearances can be. If you had journeyed here some thirty years ago, you would have noticed men, but mostly women, standing and sitting in a distinctive way, their feet spread wide to give them a broad base, a stout wooden pole or spade tightly grasped between both hands, planted firmly in front of them, never relaxing their grip. They sit and stand like this because they must. Without a physical support, they will simply keel over, like an uprooted tree. You see, their spongy brains can no longer be trusted to keep them upright.

These people are dying, and what is killing them is remarkably similar to the "infectious agent" that causes scrapie in sheep.

THE TRUE MEAT OF WOMEN

The Fore tribe cannot be described as living in a state of natural bliss. Sadly, this is no Garden of Eden. if we discount, for a moment, the scrapielike disease that killed up to 80 percent of all women in some villages,[20] we find a society that has several strikingly miserable parallels with our own.

Overpopulation has rarely been a significant problem here, because of frequent tribal wars. In addition, a taboo against copulation while the tribe was engaged in warfare ensured that the birth rate was often low or declining. But the really evident similarity between us and the Fore is the universal malevolence among males toward their womenfolk.

Fore males live together in houses that are strictly segregated from the women and children. Male children are taught from an early age to be disdainful toward females. Adolescent boys periodically go into seclusion to cleanse themselves from the polluting effects that their mothers and sisters radiate. Because the act of copulation is perceived as being fraught with danger, only a married man risks indulgence, for he alone has the power to ward off the evil consequences of such intimate female contact. Worst of all is male contact with menstrual blood, which may sicken a man, cause vomiting, turn his blood black, corrupt his vital juices, cause his flesh to waste away, dull his wits, and so precipitate his death.[21]

If you've ever been tempted to believe in the myth of the "noble savage," the Fore people will bring you down to earth with a bump. It is this deep-rooted hatred of Fore women that, anthropologists believe, led to the outbreak of "kuru"—as this form of scrapie was called. Cannibalism—in particular, the eating of human brains—appears to have surfaced in the Fore tribe for two main reasons: First, the threat of population decline may have resulted in an association being made between cannibalism and increased fertility. Therefore, the more human flesh a woman consumed, the more likely she would be to give birth again, and so replenish the population stock that the belligerent males had thoughtlessly decimated.

And second, as the forests and their animal populations disappeared and hunting became less and less successful, there was a corresponding increase in the domestication of pigs, and the consumption of pig flesh—but only by males. The women, on the other hand, were strongly discouraged from eating highly prized pig flesh, and they therefore resorted to flesh of an altogether different type, which the men would never seek to expropriate. This is why, among Fore males, the human corpse is disparagingly referred to as "the true meat of women."[22]

THE UNNATURAL HISTORY OF KURU

"I break the bones of your legs, I break the bones of your feet, I break the bones of your arms, I break the bones of your hands, and finally I make you die."[23]

This is the curse which, the Fore believe, when recited by a sorcerer with appropriate gestures and artifacts, will inflict kuru upon his enemy. As a clinical analysis of the course of the disease, it demonstrates an intimate knowledge of its progressively degenerative nature, starting first with increasing difficulty in maintaining balance ("I break the bones of your legs—") and resulting in complete incapacitation ("I break the bones of your hand") before death intervenes.

The first Westerners to encounter kuru were mystified, and made copious clinical records and case studies. Very often, the earliest dreaded sign of the impending tragedy would not even be noticed by the sufferer herself; a friend or family member would remark upon her shaky balance while crossing a narrow log bridge or climbing over a palisade fence that separates agricultural plots. This stage may last for six to twelve months, during which time the woman's general physical and mental health gradually deteriorates. Eventually, it becomes obvious that walking is difficult and clumsy; the rhythmic and confident swing of her plaited bark skirt is replaced by an unsteady swaying. As the disease progresses, something called the "kuru tremor" takes hold, a rapidly repeating contraction of opposing muscles resembling shivering, sometimes of the whole body, sometimes just the muscles of the face—hence the label "the laughing death." Twitching and shaking make it all but impossible to speak, and she becomes effectively mute. At this stage even sitting upright becomes impossible, and friends may drive a stake into the ground in front of her to grasp, or suspend a rope from the ceiling of her hut so that she may pull herself upright with it. Soon, paralysis and incontinence set in, food cannot be swallowed, and death comes as a sweet release.

Because of its occurrence within families, and its predilection for women, it was first thought that kuru was an inherited genetic disease. However, clever scientific detective work proved beyond doubt that kuru was clearly infectious. How kuru first arose among the Fore tribe is an unanswerable question. What is certain, however, is that the disease was transmitted by eating meat—in this case, human meat.

Yet even at the height of the devastating kuru epidemic, the proportion of people infected with the disease in the population was *five times less* than the calculated incidence of Mad Cow Disease in the British adult cow population.[24] That tells you something about the breathtaking dimension of the plague among our animals.

Of course, it would be easy to dismiss kuru as an isolated, freak disease, of no possible consequence to anyone in the modern world, if it were not for one fact: We in the West also have our own form of kuru.

THREAD THREE: BRAIN DEATH

There is a disease that is so feared by some members of the medical profession, that pathologists have refused to perform autopsies on patients who are suspected of dying from it. Operating room technicians have refused to be present when these patients are operated on; recently, the director of a pathology laboratory was so worried about the possible risk of contagion that he ordered the destruction of histology slides taken from infected patients. Astonishingly, some hospitals have even refused to admit patients suffering from it.[25]

What possible disease could cause so much terror among doctors? It is, of course, a disease caused by that familiar "infectious agent"— an "agent" that cannot be destroyed by boiling, is immune to ultraviolet and ionizing radiation, resists most common forms of disinfectants, and can survive for long periods in apparently hostile conditions. Tissue samples taken from humans, fixed in formalin (a powerful disinfectant and preservative), and then embedded in paraffin have still been found to be capable of causing fatal infection.[26]

The name of this dreadful affliction is Creutzfeldt-Jakob disease. "Creutzfeldt" (pronounced "kroytz-felled") after the scientist who diagnosed the first case in a twenty-two-year-old woman in 1920; "Jakob" (pronounced "yack-ob") after the physician who diagnosed the next three cases in the following year. It is often abbreviated to just its initials, CJD.

The disease shares many familiar symptoms with those already described. The time between infection and commencement of the first symptom can be very long indeed—up to thirty-five years has been recorded.[27] On the other hand, in cases where infected material has been placed in direct contact with a patient's exposed brain (for example, during brain surgery with contaminated instruments), the disease can manifest itself within two years.

Forgetful periods are common at first. Poor concentration, difficulty in finding the right words, depression, inexplicable feelings of fear, and aggressiveness are all frequent initial symptoms. Patients complain that objects look "strange," attacks of vertigo and dizziness occur, and so does ringing in the ears. There is widespread tingling or numbness. It becomes more difficult to walk, an effort to climb stairs, fine movements such as writing or sewing become difficult or impossible. The patient may fall down while turning around. And all this is simply the first stage of the disease.

The second stage is characterized by a lack of control over bodily movements. Trembling, writhing, and uncontrollable jerking spasms occur. At the same time, the body, or parts of it, may become very rigid. Visual disturbances and hallucinations occur.

The final stage of CJD consists of an appalling decline into a vegetative state. Patients become mute and unresponsive, incontinent, and unable to feed. In medical language, they appear "decerebrate"—as if the brain stem has been cut to eliminate brain function.

You can see why some health workers are so fearful of this terrifying and incurable disease.

TYING THE THREADS TOGETHER

So there we have it: an unholy trinity of three very closely related diseases, two of them present in humans, one in sheep; all fatal and all caused by an unknown agent that challenges the most basic concepts of modern biology. After all, just how can a disease be transmitted from one person to another without the help of DNA or RNA (chemical substances involved in the manufacture of proteins and essential to the genetic transmission of characteristics from parent to offspring)? "It's the stuff that Nobel prizes are made of," says Charles Weissmann, a leading researcher in infectious brain diseases.[28]

For decades, however, there was comparatively little mainstream scientific interest in this baffling group of diseases. That which cannot be smoothly explained is all too often ignored, even by scientists who should know better. And there was no overriding urgency to the problem: The incidence of Creutzfeldt-Jakob disease in the population was considered to be very low, kuru had been slowly dying out ever since cannibalism had been outlawed among the Fore tribe, and scrapie, well, scrapie had always been with us. Why should increasingly hard-pressed scientific resources be allocated to this peripheral area of interest? A strict cost-benefit analysis, much beloved by those officials who control today's science, would not justify the investment.

In November 1986, all that changed forever. In that month, brain tissues sent to Britain's Central Veterinary Laboratory, by puzzled veterinary surgeons, were scrutinized by experienced neuropathologists. Under the microscope, the distinctive hole-riddled areas of brain could be clearly distinguished and photographed. They had seen it before, of course, in specimens taken from diseased sheep. But this was something very new indeed—the samples under the microscope weren't from sheep, they were from cows.

Something rather strange seemed to have happened. Scrapie, present in the sheep population for hundreds of years, appeared to have crossed the species barrier and had mysteriously infected cows. Suddenly, decades of work by a few dedicated scientists on kuru, Creutzfeldt-Jakob disease, and scrapie acquired a new and urgent relevance. Because, as Dr. Tony Andrews, a senior lecturer at the Royal Veterinary College, put it: "Now we know that Scrapie has jumped from sheep to cattle there is nothing to suggest it may not, in future, wind up in people."[29]

JUMPING THE SPECIES BARRIER

It has been known for decades that scrapie, kuru and Creutzfeldt-Jakob disease are all extremely similar—so similar, in fact, that scientists term them all "spongiform encephalopathies." *Encephalopathy* is a word used to describe any degenerative illness of the brain: in this case, one that causes parts of the brain to resemble a sponge riddled with holes.

It has also been established beyond any doubt that many spongiform encephalopathies possess the ability to cross the species barrier. For example, if you take tissue from a human suffering from Creutzfeldt-Jakob disease and infect goats with it, they will die from scrapie.[30] Now consider this evidence:

- The agent that causes Creutzfeldt-Jakob disease in humans has been experimentally inoculated into chimpanzees, capuchin monkeys, marmosets, spider monkeys, squirrel monkeys, woolly monkeys, managabey monkeys, pig-tailed monkeys, African green monkeys, baboons, bush babies, patas monkeys, talapoin monkeys, goats, cats, mice, hamsters,

gerbils, and guinea pigs. Subsequently, all these animals succumbed to spongiform encephalopathy.

- The agent that causes scrapie in sheep has been experimentally
  inoculated into mink, spider monkeys, squirrel monkeys,
  cynomolgus monkeys, goats, mice, rats, hamsters, and voles.
  Subsequently, all these animals succumbed to spongiform
  encephalopathy.

- The agent that causes kuru in humans has been experimentally
  inoculated into chimpanzees, gibbons, capuchin monkeys,
  marmosets, spider monkeys, squirrel monkeys, woolly monkeys, rhesus monkeys, pig-tailed monkeys, and bonnet monkeys. Subsequently, all these animals succumbed to spongiform
  encephalopathy.[31]

I want to make it clear that I don't approve of experiments such as
these. They are often needlessly repetitive and horribly cruel for the
poor animals concerned. The traditional justification for vivisection is
that it advances human knowledge, but in the case of these experiments, that excuse is less valid than ever. Because in the public debate
that arose after Mad Cow Disease—later known as bovine spongiform encephalopathy (BSE)—was diagnosed, officials went to great
pains to stress the extreme implausibility of BSE being passed from
cows to human beings, even though they must have known that scientific findings such as those above proved nothing of the sort.

Concealing the truth about spongiform encephalopathy was nothing new for British officials, however. They'd done it before.

A BREACH OF TRUST

In the United Kingdom during the period 1959 to 1985, several thousand children were injected with human growth hormone, a treatment
for dwarfism. At that time, human growth hormone was extracted
from pituitary glands removed from the brains of corpses. A considerable number was needed, about 100 glands to treat one child per year,
and in order to achieve this quantity, mortuary technicians were
offered a cash incentive.

"We were given 10 pence (about 14 cents) per pituitary," said one technician, "and you never sent away less than twenty or in some cases forty depending on how quickly you could gather them." While some technicians were careful not to take glands from patients who had died from infectious or dementing diseases, others were not so painstaking. "All they were interested in was the cheque when it came in," said the same technician. "The more you sent off, the more money came in. You could pick up twenty-five to thirty pituitaries and not argue about it, just take the whole lot and send them off, and that was £3 (about $4.25)."[32]

During the course of research for this book, I interviewed Dr. Helen Grant, one of Britain's most experienced neuropathologists. She explained to me in graphic terms what would happen: "I was one of the pathologists who did postmortems in those days," she told me. "And I remember when I was about to drop the pituitary I had just removed into formalin, the mortuary technician would say, 'Just a minute doctor, do you want that pituitary?' And I would say, 'No, I don't think I do, why?' 'Oh well, can I have it?' he would ask. 'You can have it,' I'd say, 'but what are you going to do with it?' 'Well,' he'd reply, 'we've got to collect them for research.' Well of course I'd let him have it. It was for 'research,' you see. Never for one instant did I suppose that it was going to finish up being used in a therapeutic way—being used as a treatment on children. As far as I knew, these pituitaries were going for research, and research only."

Because the supervising authorities failed to implement sufficiently stringent procedures for the collection of pituitary glands, an unknown number of children became infected with Creutzfeldt-Jakob disease. To date, seven patients who were given growth hormone have died from CJD.[33] Not all recipients of human growth hormone treatment were (or will be) affected and no recipients of the treatment after autumn 1985 are at risk (the time when the manufacturing process of human growth hormone changed; an entirely pure form is now genetically engineered from the bacterium *Escherichia coli*).

But now comes the most outrageous part of this sad history. When evidence of the disaster began to emerge, the British Department of Health decided not to tell the patients that their lives might have been put at risk. They decided that to inform the patients who might have been injected with Creutzfeldt-Jakob disease would only cause panic.

So there was no public enquiry into this unfolding tragedy. . . . Just silence.

In the United States, the patients and families affected were notified as soon as the full significance of the situation was recognized. But not in Britain. Dr. Grant explains: "There was pressure to inform the families at the time the problem was first recognised. But it was decided not to. Why did they sit on it for seven years? Why did they sit on it at all? I suppose because it looks bad. And the effect of it was, you see, that some of those children may later have become blood donors. How about that?"

In justification of its policy of secrecy, the Department of Health stated, "The right to know was balanced against the anxiety that would be caused to these patients about a condition which is invariably fatal."[34] A blood-curdling statement indeed, and one that makes you wonder what other unpleasant facts have been concealed from us in an attempt to protect us from "anxiety."

After mounting pressure, it was eventually conceded in late 1991 that recipients of the injections should, after all, be contacted and informed of the risks. And what of compensation? There simply are not words to describe the profound personal suffering involved in this dreadful business. Surely, there is no possible excuse, and no honorable pretext, for not generously compensating both patients and their families?

"Any legal action would be defended on the grounds that as regards clinical factors at the time it was administered the treatment conformed with knowledge then available about good clinical practice," said the department in a statement to journalists working on a television program.[35]

"WE THOUGHT WE WERE SAFE, BUT WE WERE WRONG"

In the 1970s, the British Medical Research Council wanted to ensure the safety of the procedure for extracting human growth hormone from the pituitary glands of corpses. Professor Ivor Mills, professor emeritus of medicine at Cambridge University, was a member of the Endocrine Committee, whose task it was to advise on safety.

"I was on the Endocrine Committee of the Medical Research Council in the 1970s," said Professor Mills, "when we had to consider whether it was safe to extract human growth hormone from human pituitaries, because you know the pituitary is attached to the brain and it seemed to us that there might be some possibility that Creutzfeldt-Jakob disease would be in a form that was in the pituitary and we might transfer that to the children who had to be injected with growth hormone. We took advice from many experts, including Scrapie experts, because we thought there might be some relationship between the two diseases and we were advised at that time the technique was safe. We have since been proved to have been wrong and I feel rather guilty myself that this happened and two children in this country, and rather more in the rest of the world, have been inflicted with dementing fatal illness. I am anxious since there is a relationship between Creutzfeldt-Jakob disease, I think, and Scrapie that the same sort of mistake should not be made a second time because, as Professor Southwood pointed out, the results could be very serious indeed."[36]

As a result of the human growth hormone tragedy, Professor Mills became so concerned that the mistakes of the past should not be repeated that he personally testified in front of the British parliamentary committee inquiring into BSE. His evidence makes arresting reading, due in part to his distinguished scientific credentials, and in part to his obvious depth of concern. In a memorandum to the parliamentary committee, Professor Mills described how the experts at the time of the human growth hormone disaster had judged the procedure to be safe.

"We took advice from several experts including Scrapie experts and thought the technique was safe. Yet two children in this country got Creutzfeldt-Jakob disease. It is now known that this disease is very similar to Scrapie.

"We thought we were safe but we were wrong. We have made a mistake once and as a result two children got a fatal disease. We cannot afford to make the same sort of mistake again because the result would be much more disastrous. We now know much more about the agent which causes Scrapie and CJD and similar neurological diseases in man. The agent is unique and, in my opinion, highly dangerous to spread widely."[37]

In his evidence, Professor Mills made four important recommendations. First, and most important, he wanted to prevent potentially infected material (lymphoid tissue, brains, and spinal cords from cows, sheep, and goats) from being fed back to food animals. Second, he wanted to see controls extended to include calves of six months and younger. Third, he wanted to make sure that potentially infected material was not allowed to contaminate other meat in the slaughterhouse or anywhere else, and last, he proposed that calves born to cows known to be infected with BSE should not be used for breeding.

All eminently sensible precautions, in view of the devastating and enigmatic nature of the infectious agent. The human growth hormone tragedy had already proved that even the country's top experts could be terribly wrong about this disease. As Professor Mills had written previously in a letter to *The Times*: "What I think we should learn from this is that it is not good enough to say the chances of harm, we think, are very small."[38]

That is a sensible, cautious attitude, based on hard-learned experience. But it was not the position of the British government, which constantly sought to reassure the public that there was no risk. As John Gummer, the minister for agriculture bluntly put it when testifying before the parliamentary committee: "The plain fact is that there is no evidence that BSE poses any risk."[39]

That, of course, was a politician's statement.

A JOURNAL OF THE PLAGUE YEARS

No evidence? Here is the chronology of BSE. Read it, and make up your own mind.

On December 13, 1985, a portentous report appeared in the British press that, with hindsight, could be considered a curtain-raiser to the whole BSE saga. "It's Dog Eat Dog on Swedish Farms," exclaimed the headline.[40] "Many of the Christmas hams now on sale here have come from pigs fed on the minced carcasses of sick animals," wrote a journalist from Stockholm. The story had particularly revolting aspects. For several years, the rotten carcasses of diseased cows and pigs, as well as formerly loved pets, had been covertly processed to make food for cows, pigs, poultry, and domestic pets. Dairy farmers began to suspect the wholesomeness of their animals' feedstuff when their cows started to fall ill and decrease milk production. Despite attempts to conceal the size of the scandal, news eventually reached Swedish consumers, who were predictably outraged that their pets were being recycled with quite so much ruthless efficiency. With great prescience, the report also queried the wisdom of turning "the traditionally vegetarian cow" into a carnivore, not to say a cannibal.

For the average British reader, it was a relatively trivial story. What the Swedes were up to on their own farms was their own business. And in any case, it couldn't happen here, could it? There were probably laws to prevent that sort of thing. Yes, indeed. Ignorance could be so blissfully comforting.

By the time this report appeared, the first cows were already dying from BSE on British farms. But as yet, very few people realized what was happening.

Nine months later, another strangely prophetic article appeared in the science pages of a British newspaper.[41] Headlined "The Disease That Bugs Biochemists and Sheep," it described how the "exotic, utterly mysterious agent" that causes scrapie mystified scientists. How could a lethally infectious agent exist that possessed neither DNA nor RNA? "Future work in this field is sure to be immensely interesting," the piece enthusiastically concluded, with massive understatement. Quite so.

THE RENDERERS SURRENDER

Meanwhile, dire things had been happening to an obscure part of Britain's meat industry. Rendering is a little-known but essential element of the strange economic equation that holds together all the diverse sections of the flesh trade. Renderers take all the bits and pieces of animals from slaughterhouses that no one else wants, boil them up, and produce fat and protein. The fat is then turned into products such as margarine and soap, and the protein makes animal feed. Thus, they serve two essential functions: they act as a garbage disposal service for one and a half million tons of mangled corpses every year, and they act as a cheap source of feedstuff for the next generation of food animals, which in due course are fed to the following generation, and so on. As the chairman of their trade association put it, "If there is no rendering industry, there is no meat industry."[42]

No one really seems to have considered whether it was such a good idea to force naturally vegetarian animals such as cows to become carnivores and cannibals. It made sound economic sense; so they did it. But as former British Minister of Health Dr. Sir Gerard Vaughan explains, when you monkey around with nature, it is wise to expect some nasty surprises: "One of the main areas of fault is the processing of animal food using parts of the same animals. It's not a natural instinct for one animal to eat its own species, in fact it's totally foreign to it. That seems to be nature's understanding of the bacteriological and biological dangers, because if one animal starts to eat its own stock, then the dangers of infection increasing are very great indeed."[43]

By the middle of the 1980s many renderers were themselves close to the brink of extinction. The low price of vegetable oil on the world markets had made the renderers' own animal fat product uncompetitive, and the drive toward healthier eating had made edible animal fats increasingly unpopular among food manufacturers. Denied income from this vital market, the economic equation just wouldn't hang together any more. In 1986 alone, 10 percent of the industry went bankrupt.[44] The industry appealed to the government for help, but in vain. Then they tried charging slaughterhouses a fee for the disposal of animal waste, to the considerable ire of the slaughterhouses, some of whom illegally took waste disposal into their own hands. "I know of abattoirs in the North West of England and the Midlands," the then-chairman of their trade association was quoted as saying, "that minced up offal and started spreading it on fields rather than pay for it to be disposed of by renderers."[45]

Survival in a harsh economic climate is largely a question of efficiency, and the rendering industry had already started to take steps to modernize its methods and reduce its costs. The old procedure for rendering animal flesh and bone was a two-stage operation: first, the foul brew would be cooked up in a huge vessel and the fat separated from the solid (known as "greaves"), then, the greaves would be further processed, often with a solvent such as benzene or petroleum spirit, to draw off more fat, and finally leave a meat and bone meal product.

The new procedure differed in several ways: it was a continuous process, not a batch system, and the use of solvents to extract fat was discontinued in favor of mechanical pressing and centrifuging. It would later be speculated that these changes in the rendering process were the root cause of the BSE epidemic.

PUTTING THE LID ON

Sources indicate that another case of BSE was seen in January 1986, and this triggered the involvement of the government's own veterinary experts. We shall never know precisely when BSE was recognized as a scrapie-like disease, although the chief veterinary officer for the Ministry of Agriculture said on television that it was diagnosed "within a few weeks."[46] The visible effects of spongiform encephalopathies are quite distinctive—no other disease leaves such a dramatic, hole-riddled brain as evidence of its infection. And the government's veterinary experts would certainly have seen this type of disease in sheep, under the name of "scrapie." Now, the key question is, why did it take so long—over two years—for the government to begin to take any effective action? After all, here we have an entirely new disease of cattle, very similar to the lethal and incurable scrapie in sheep. If a disease of this severity and lethality suddenly starts crossing the species barrier, shouldn't that be taken as an extremely disquieting development? Surely, the alarm bells should have started ringing as soon as those government experts saw the warning signs?

Well, perhaps they did. Neuropathologist and fellow of the Royal College of Physicians Dr. Helen Grant believes that there was a policy of official silence on the matter. And since she has spoken to many of the key scientists involved, she ought to know. She told me:

"A lid was put on it. As soon as they figured out what the disease was likely to be due to, they should have stopped feeding cattle with contaminated feedstuff. But the government didn't. They let it go on, until the Southwood committee finally stopped it."

Professor Richard Lacey agrees. Much reviled in official circles ("he seemed to lose touch completely with the real world," sniffed the 1990 parliamentary inquiry into BSE[47]), Professor Lacey was one of the most outspoken critics of government policy during this period.

And his views could not lightly be dismissed: as a clinical microbiologist with a worldwide reputation, and a fellow of the Royal Society of Pathologists, he was well placed to comment. Professor Lacey believes that money was at the root of official inaction:

"The available evidence suggests," he wrote, "that there has been a carefully orchestrated manipulation of public opinion by the Government in order to avoid taking action. The main reason for this is the sheer scale of the action that would be needed. The cost of compensation for replacing say six million infected cattle could run into billions of pounds. Moreover, the adverse international publicity this would generate might effectively put the UK into quarantine with loss of food exports, tourism, and even a substantial part of our industrial base."[48]

THE STORY BREAKS

In November 1986, the official record shows that the government's Central Veterinary Laboratory formally identified bovine spongiform encephalopathy, but ministers within the government were not informed until June the following year.[49] And even then, it took ten more months—until April 1988—for the government to decide to appoint a committee to look into the disease (known as the Southwood committee). Why all these delays?

Again, we can only speculate about the real reasons. The official justification is that "transmission experiments" were needed, in which infected tissue from cows would be injected into mice. You might think that it was already painfully established that the new disease had almost certainly been transmitted—from sheep to cows. More cynical observers might conclude that, in reality, a gamble was being taken that the outbreak was small and containable, and that it could be quietly dealt with before it blew up into a major "food scare." If this was the case, the bet failed miserably.

In October 1987, BSE finally went public—but in a very demure and modest way. A brief paper, barely covering two sides, appeared in the professional journal *The Veterinary Record* in the section entitled "Short Communications," just above an advertisement for magazine

binders.[50] It described the disease in clinical terms, showed some photographs of diseased brains, and proposed the official name for the
disease: bovine spongiform encephalopathy. The paper concluded
with a careful warning—despite BSE's striking similarity to other
spongiform encephalopathies (such as scrapie and Creutzfeldt-Jakob
disease) its cause was unknown, and "no connection with encephalopathies in other species has been established."

The response of other media was appropriately low-key, most
treating it as something of a scientific oddity. "There have been suggestions," wrote the agriculture correspondent of *The Times*, a couple
of months later, "that it could be linked to a sheep disease called
Scrapie," but the short article concluded by quoting another expert as
not yet seeing BSE as a serious threat to cattle health.[51]

By April 1988, it must have become excruciatingly obvious to those
in authority that BSE was not going to go away peacefully. By now,
over 400 cases had been reported in Britain, even though the disease
was still not officially notifiable. Clearly, the world was on the verge
of an epidemic of unknown magnitude, and something had to be
done. The shrewd political response to this sort of tricky situation is
to appoint a committee. Committees give politicians breathing space:
their advice is not binding, and they provide an effective shield with
which to deflect criticism. And that is what the government did—on
April 21, the Southwood committee was announced to the world. "A
working party headed by Sir Richard Southwood, professor of zool-
ogy at Oxford, has been set up by the Ministry of Agriculture and the
Department of Health," reported the *Sunday Telegraph*, "after com-
plaints from vets that the Government has been dragging its feet."[52]
Sir Richard had the advantage of also being chairman of the National
Radiological Protection Board, and was therefore accustomed to a
high-profile, controversial position. Tagged onto the official announce-
ment was some typical public relations baloney. "The Ministry of
Agriculture said there was no evidence of the disease being transmitted between animals and no evidence of it being passed on to people
through meat and milk," the newspaper reported.

THE SUBTLE ART OF DECEPTION

The propaganda battle had now begun in earnest. At stake was a market for beef and veal worth about $3 billion and, as in all battles, truth became the first casualty. It became impossible, for example, to establish just how hard the market for beef had been knocked.

At the worst of the crisis, the head of Britain's largest chain of retail butchers was quoted in their trade journal as saying there had been "no reduction" in beef sales.[53] However, the parliamentary committee said the market had dropped by 25 percent,[54] and newspaper reports indicated that it might have plummeted by as much as 45 percent.[55]

Official statements began to be peppered with the sort of evasive language normally only used in times of war. Defensive phrases such as "no evidence" and "no proof" recurred time and time again in official proclamations. In particular, the defense of "no evidence" would be used repeatedly to quell rising public concern.

When the Ministry of Agriculture claimed that there was "no evidence of the disease being transmitted between animals" they were, of course, being economical with the truth. The evidence already strongly suggested that there had indeed been "transmission between animals," inasmuch as cows had almost certainly contracted BSE from scrapie in sheep, and extensive experimental work had already established that scrapie could be transmitted to many other mammals.

And as far as transmission between cows was concerned, it was simply too early to make any kind of prediction. As the government's own vets rather embarrassingly pointed out within a few days of the ministry's nonsensical proclamation quoted above, "Until it is known whether or not the cow is an end host, it is not possible to say if the offspring of affected animals will themselves be infected."[56] The two announcements were, of course, directed toward totally different audiences—the government's vets were speaking to other professionals, and the Ministry of Agriculture was addressing the public at large.

Thus do our rulers deceive us.

By now, intelligent people were starting to ask some penetrating questions. A thoughtful paper appeared in the *Veterinary Record* under the title "Bovine Spongiform Encephalopathy: Time to Take Scrapie Seriously."[57] It was written by K. L. Morgan, a lecturer at

Bristol University, who pointed out that tissue taken from patients dying from Creutzfeldt-Jakob disease could infect goats with scrapie, and also cause a similar disease in cats. And scrapie could also be transmitted from sheep to monkeys. In addition, it had been experimentally demonstrated that passage through animals could alter the "host range" of the scrapie agent—in other words, if scrapie had jumped from sheep to cattle, it might now become more directly infectious to human beings. This, of course, would be the ultimate "nightmare scenario."

A couple of weeks later, the government's own veterinary service also published an article in the same journal, which included the following memorable passage: "BSE must be seen in perspective. The number of confirmed cases (455) is very small compared with the total cattle population of 13 million. The number of cases is expected to increase but if as is anticipated, it behaves like similar diseases in other species only small numbers of incidents relative to the total number of cattle disease incidents are likely to occur."[58]

Did you follow that? The logic is, to say the least, convoluted. What they appeared to be saying was this: "There are currently only 455 cases of BSE, so don't panic. And even if that number increases, it will probably be a small fraction of the total number of sick cows around, so there's still no need to panic." Four years later, we are well on the way to 100,000 cases of BSE, but presumably there are still lots of sick cows who *don't* have BSE. Apparently, we are supposed to find this reassuring.

BRAIN FOOD

To their credit, the Southwood committee worked quickly, although there was criticism that none of its members were familiar with spongiform diseases.[59] In June 1988, BSE was at last made a notifiable disease, and a six-month ban was imposed (effective from mid-July) on the feeding of "animal protein" to cows and sheep. For six months, at least, these animals were to be allowed to live like vegetarians again—cannibalism was no longer compulsory—although poultry and pigs still continued to be flesh feeders. By August, it was announced that cattle known to be infected with BSE (i.e., already in the terminal stages of the disease) were to be slaughtered and their carcasses destroyed. While it was clear that the Southwood committee was spurring the government into some action, it was inexcusable that the full committee's report would not be made public until February 1989.

Furthermore, the action taken was far from adequate. Following an article in a British medical journal, the *Times* pointed out in June that there was still no legislation to stop manufacturers from adding cows' brains to meat products intended for human consumption, and no requirement for appropriate labeling.[60] "It seems odd," said Dr. Tim Holt of St. James Hospital in London, "that they have banned cattle from eating these cattle brains, but they have not banned humans from eating cattle brains."[61]

Odd? Or scandalous?

So here was the position: because the disease could not be detected by any test in the living cow, only those cows who exhibited symptoms—and who were therefore in the last stages of the disease—had to be destroyed. Other cows—and in particular, meat from the most suspect organs—could still enter the food chain.

It was now more than eighteen months since the official identification of the disease by the government's Central Veterinary Laboratory.

WHISTLING IN THE DARK

In August 1988, the Ministry of Agriculture announced that it would pay farmers 50 percent of the market value for cows that had to be slaughtered following infection with BSE.[62] This penny-pinching compromise pleased no one. Farmers were outraged that they were being denied full compensation; consumers were worried that farmers would be tempted to sell infected cows into the food chain rather than destroy them for half their value. About this time, too, concerned voices began to be heard on the subject of scrapie. Dr. Tony Andrews of the Royal Veterinary College, for one, was quoted in a newspaper interview as saying: "There is evidence to suggest a link between scrapie and Creutzfeld-Jacob disease, which causes premature senility in people. There have been experiments where tissue from the brains of dead victims of this disease has been put into goats which then contracted scrapie."[63]

Dr. Andrews wanted the government to introduce an eradication policy for scrapie, starting with the establishment of a register of scrapie-free sheep. The Ministry of Agriculture was characteristically cool about the idea, saying that "in the light of known medical evidence" it could not be justified. An anonymous ministry spokesman then outlined the official line: "Scrapie has been known about for 400 years and there is no evidence that it has ever spread to people."

The Department of Health also got in on the act, echoing the belief that there was "no proof" of a link between scrapie and human diseases. This hypothesis would later be given ministerial weight when John Gummer testified before the parliamentary committee enquiring into BSE.

The ministry's propaganda machine seriously lost credibility a few days later, however, when Dr. James Hope, head of a government-funded but independent research unit studying the disease, seemed to contradict their unctuous reassurances. While agreeing with the government's position that there was "no evidence" that humans could catch the infection from eating beef (indeed, how could there be with such a slow-developing disease?) he went on to say: "Of course there is alarm because it's potentially a great threat to the livestock industry as well as to human health. Because it jumped from sheep to cow, it might better be fitted to jump from cow to human."[64]

Yes, indeed it might. And that was a possibility that no amount of official whistling in the dark could exclude.

By now, several countries had decided to ban the import of British cattle. And in October, the results of the government's "transmission experiments" to mice showed that BSE could indeed infect other species—extremely bad news for the public relations blowhards. Then in December, legislation came into force prohibiting the sale of milk from "suspected" cattle, and the ban on recycling animal protein back to cows in their feed was extended for twelve months.

Also in December, scientists from the government's Central Veterinary Laboratory published damning evidence showing that the source of BSE was contaminated cattle feed.[65] "The results of the study," the scientists wrote, "do, however, lead inevitably to the conclusion that cattle have been exposed to a transmissible agent via cattle feedstuffs." In other words, cows had been eating scrapie-infected sheep.

PICTURES FROM THE END OF THE WORLD

So began a strangely apocalyptic period in recent British history, dramatically illustrated a decade later by some extraordinary contemporary photographs. As I write, I am looking at some of the most surreal pictures I have ever seen in my life—pictures of the farming folk of Merrie England, busily burning hundreds, eventually thousands, of their own cows.

Here is a photograph that is both ludicrous and chilling: It shows a secret Ministry of Defence location, where cows are being burned. Operatives dressed in nightmarish chemical warfare suits are clambering over earth mounds, digging ditches, maneuvering heavy-duty Army cranes from which dead cows swing. It looks like a science fiction nightmare: doomsday Lilliputians swarming over a herd of upturned bovine Gullivers. The very notion that vast herds of British cows should receive secret military funerals is beyond farce, beyond satire. While some cows go to make meat pies, other cows receive state funerals. For services unrendered, perhaps.

Another widely reproduced photograph of the time starkly conveys the surreal, Götterdämmerung-like quality of it all. It is simply a picture of Armageddon. There they lie, like vanquished warriors, a herd of supine cows, legs splayed, carcasses bloated with gas, while the flames of hell lick around them and ghostly clouds enshroud them. If you were to photograph the end of the world, it would probably look something like this. This was a disturbing, archetypal image that millions of people saw all over Britain's national media; maybe it reminded them of the evil forces that modern agriculture had unleashed on the world, and how very close we all might be to biocataclysm.

But perhaps the most widely seen image of all was that of four-year-old Cordelia, daughter of Britain's then minister of agriculture, John Selwyn Gummer. No history of BSE is complete without mention of Cordelia, the little girl who, for a few awkward minutes in 1990, was conscripted into service for the ministry, and posed with daddy before the world's media, cow burger in hand—a spectacle that one seasoned journalist movingly described as a "deeply distressing sight."[66] Today, as politicians increasingly demand that the intrusive media leave their personal lives unexamined, and threaten oppressive legislation to enforce their "right to privacy," it is appropriate to remember poor Cordelia.

What possessed the minister of agriculture to involve his little girl in such a public relations exercise is hard to fathom. Perhaps it was intended to reassure us all that, if the minister was willing to expose his own family to British beef, then all must be well. But to many, it must have seemed a cheap and cynical publicity gimmick. This "televisual pantomime"—as the science editor of the *Independent* newspaper called it—"of the Minister of Agriculture attempting to force feed his daughter with a beefburger" was all too easy to see through. "This is the man," wrote the science editor, "or to be charitable, the successor to the men, who acquiesced in turning cattle into carnivores and chickens into cannibals. And he is surprised that the public does not take his word on food safety."[67]

It was also a particularly capricious hostage to fortune. If, in later life, Mr. Gummer's daughter should ever fall ill with any meat-related disease (and I sincerely hope she does not), then you can be sure that those press photographs will reappear to haunt her. In the apt words of Shakespeare: "Upon such sacrifices, my Cordelia, the gods themselves throw incense."[68]

AN OFFAL YEAR

Things were looking decidedly bleak for the meat industry, and in 1989 they got even worse. The year started with a lambasting for the government from a very surprising source—Lord Montagu of Beaulieu, one of England's most prominent landowners. One of his tenant farmers reported having a cow with BSE in 1987, which, Lord Montagu learned with astonishment, could legally be sent to market. "I am amazed at the slow reaction of the ministry and the complacent attitude it had at the beginning," stormed his lordship, who also wrote to John MacGregor, then minister of agriculture. With an inevitable turn of phrase, a ministry official once again answered the charge of complacency by repeating the official mantra: "There is no evidence to suggest that BSE can be transmitted to humans through meat."[69]

"They are guessing, and hoping," said Professor Richard Lacey. "They have a public voice which is trying to reassure everyone, but an inner fear. I think they know there's a real problem much worse than they're letting on."[70]

"THE IMPLICATIONS WOULD BE EXTREMELY SERIOUS"

Public and professional disquiet was steadily mounting. In early February, the *Guardian* newspaper ran a front-page report headlined "Meat risks report 'held back,' " which alleged that a report into the risks of BSE to human transmission was being officially expurgated; this was subsequently officially denied.[71]

A few days later in the same paper a letter from expert neuropathologist Dr. Helen Grant of London's Charing Cross Hospital was published, which pointed out: "There are no laboratory tests to identify such [BSE-infected] animals: the only way to establish the diagnosis is to examine the brain. Such animals, thought to be healthy, will be slaughtered and enter the food chain . . . there is no doubt that animals harbouring the virus but seeming healthy have finished up as beef."[72]

The next day, *The Times*'s medical correspondent, Dr. Thomas Stuttaford, echoed rising medical concern: "Neither Mrs. Thatcher nor her scientific advisers can be sure that these organisms [BSE] . . . have not been already picked up by people as they enjoyed a piece of marrow in an Irish stew, or ate a meat pie which had contained brains or meat from an infected, but not yet stricken, animal."[73]

The Southwood report was published at the end of February, and its main conclusion was: "From present evidence, it is likely that cattle will prove to be a 'dead-end host' for the disease agent and most unlikely that BSE will have any implications for human health. Nevertheless, if our assessments of these likelihoods are incorrect, the implications would be extremely serious."[74]

Officials responded warmly to the first part of the conclusion. The Southwood committee had also described the risk to humans as "remote," and this now became the official buzzword, largely replacing the "no evidence" slogan used up until then.

But quite soon, it would be demonstrated that cattle were not, in fact, the "dead-end hosts" the committee had proposed, and that the disease could be further transmitted to other species (cats for example). Nevertheless, the Southwood report would now be used to give additional substance to the assertion that "beef is safe." As Professor Lacey pointed out: "Even after the cat deaths, the only official action seems to be the parrot-like claim from ministers that our beef is completely safe."[75]

The key concern now was this: it was known that the "infectious agent" was concentrated in certain organs, notably the brain, spleen and thymus glands. Cattle could be infected with BSE, but not show obvious signs, and there was nothing to stop their organs ending up in the food chain as offal. The Southwood committee had wondered whether meat products containing brain and spleen should be labeled as such, but "did not consider that the risks justified such a measure."[76]

However, they did suggest that offal—brain, spinal cord, spleen and intestines—should not be used in the manufacture of baby food—a rather contradictory recommendation, in view of their basic postulate in favor of the safety of beef.[77] In addition, it was announced that the government's chief medical officer advised mothers not to feed infants under eighteen months on this material.[78] This contradiction was spotted by one member of parliament, who promptly asked the Prime Minister (Margaret Thatcher), "If, as appears likely, BSE is a threat to humanity, why not ban it [offal] for all human food—or, if it is not a danger, as it is not according to the Minister of Agriculture, why ban it for babies?" The Prime Minister dodged the question, saying there was no point setting up a committee and then not taking their advice.[79]

Period	Chance of Eating Infected Beef
1986–1988	1 in 10,000
1988–1990	1 in 1,000
1990–1993	1 in 200
1993–2000	1 in 1,000

Estimated Likelihood of a Meat Eater Consuming a BSE Infective Agent[80]

HOW NOW, MAD COW?

Meanwhile, some startling revelations were coming to light. On March 13, a question was asked in the House of Commons to establish whether the Ministry of Agriculture had commissioned research to find out whether BSE would infect human cells. Donald Thompson, the parliamentary secretary to the Ministry of Agriculture, answered, "No, but trials are under way using marmosets, which are primates."[81]

This was a staggering admission. The official line had always been that there was "no evidence" that BSE posed any risk to human health. Well, of course there was "no evidence." If you don't commission the research, you don't have the evidence!

This Alice in Wonderland logic had surfaced in parliament a few days earlier, when Mr. Thompson was asked how frequently the Ministry of Agriculture had tested samples of cattle feed, to check that the ban on cows and sheep in cattle food was actually working. He replied, "Ministry officials are empowered to take and test samples of ruminant feedstuffs if they have reason to believe the ban on the use of ruminant-derived protein is being broken. To date, there has been no reason to believe the law has been broken and such action has not been necessary."[82]

In other words, the Ministry had never tested cattle feed because there was no evidence of wrongdoing. And if you don't look, you don't find.

On March 16, the ministry of agriculture was asked an all-too-explicit question in parliament by MP Ron Davies. Would he now ban the sale of those organs from all cows and sheep that are known to harbor the infectious agent? The parliamentary secretary to the Ministry of Agriculture made it clear that they had no intention of taking any such action. In justification, he presented two arguments. First, carcasses of BSE-suspected cows were already being destroyed. Second, scrapie had been present for two hundred years "without any evidence of a risk to humans." Therefore, it would not be "appropriate" to ban these organs from sale.

But, he was asked, the Southwood committee recognized that there was a danger to human health from the consumption of infected organs. And as far as scrapie was concerned, now that it had demonstrated that it can leap across the species barrier (implying a dangerous new mutation), surely this should mean that all organs that act as a reservoir of infection should now be banned from sale? Mr. Thompson disagreed, reiterating that "the Southwood report concluded that it was most unlikely that BSE would have any implications for human health."[83]

This issue was yet another hostage to fortune, when the government abruptly decided, just four months later, to reverse its policy and ban cow offal from sale. In retrospect, it seems obvious that policy was being made "on the hoof." As one policy position after another became untenable, it was unceremoniously dumped.

On April 13, Mr. Thompson was asked whether he would introduce restrictions on the movement of calves born to cattle infected with BSE. Mr. Thompson said he had no such plans. This hygiene measure was important, because as long as there was a possibility of "maternal transmission" of BSE (i.e. from cow to calf) the transport of BSE-infected calves around the country might spread the disease.

Again, this reveals an extraordinary inconsistency in the government's policy. One of their key policy justifications was the similarity of BSE to scrapie. Since scrapie hadn't infected humans—they argued—BSE wouldn't, either. But scrapie was clearly transmissible from mother sheep to lamb—there was no doubt at all about this. As Dr. James Hope explained: "In a flock of sheep, the disease is transmitted principally from mother to offspring, that is, from ewe to lamb. That's not to say that it is a genetic disease. We believe infection either occurs in utero before birth, or immediately after birth via the placenta. The placenta is highly infectious, and poses a threat to the newly born lamb and other members of the flock."[84]

The following day, evidence emerged that diseased cattle were being sent to slaughterhouses; Mr. Thompson stated in reply to a question from MP Ron Davies that forty cases of BSE-infected cows were detected in abatoirs.[85] No one could say, however, how many cows had slipped through undetected.

THE FIX

In May, the Women's Farming Union added their voice to rising public demands for a complete ban on the use in any food products of brain and spinal cord material from cows and sheep.[86] The government must take steps, they said, to ensure that BSE and scrapie could not be spread through the food chain.

The government's position had now become universally discredited. An opinion poll for *Marketing* magazine revealed that only 2 percent of the population believed the government completely on matters of food.[87] The "no evidence" defense was now seen by most people for what it was: a sad and pathetic attempt to keep people buying the dubious products of the British meat industry.

The Southwood committee had spawned another committee, under the chairmanship of Dr. David Tyrell, a retired virologist. This time, its members included scientists with experience of spongiform diseases. Again, they worked with commendable speed, and presented a report to the government in June. Disgracefully, it was not made public for seven more months.[88]

However, a few days after receiving the (still secret) Tyrell report, the government abruptly reversed its position on the sale of offal, and a total ban was announced on the sale for human consumption of all cow's brain, spinal cord, thymus, spleen, and tonsils. It was a victory, of sorts. One of the problems was that the ban would not come into effect for five more months in England and Wales, and in Scotland not for seven months. Said Dr. Hugh Fraser, a neuropathologist at the Institute of Animal Health, in Edinburgh, "They could have introduced a ban six months ago. They ought to have a ban as soon as possible. It doesn't seem right to delay it."[89]

While he welcomed the ban, Member of Parliament Ron Davies, who had asked so many penetrating questions in the House of Commons, demanded more drastic and immediate action—such as random testing on cow's brains in slaughterhouses to determine the true size of the epidemic. This eminently sensible measure would be steadfastly opposed by the government.

There was no denying that it was a fix. Just three months earlier, they had told the House of Commons that a ban on the sale of offal would not be "appropriate." Now, it looked very "appropriate," indeed. But would it be sufficient to reassure an increasingly leery public?

THE COWS COME HOME

Nineteen ninety was the year that the cows came home to roost, or whatever it is that cows of ill omen do. As Professor Richard Lacey wrote, "During the last weeks of 1989 and early in 1990, findings of spongiform encephalopathy in, first, zoo animals such as antelopes, and then domestic cats, were published completely invalidating the Southwood committee's hope that BSE was a 'dead-end host,' that is, it would not spread beyond cattle."[90]

So the key question was no longer "can BSE spread to other species?" but rather, "how many other species can it infect—and is *homo sapiens* one of them?"

A few days into the New Year, a report from trading standards officers revealed that cattle infected with BSE were still being sent by farmers to market—hardly surprising, in view of the low level of compensation being offered by the Ministry of Agriculture. Flying in the face of common sense, a Ministry official commented that compensation was "not an issue" in safeguarding the public from BSE-infected animals. "We have no evidence," the official all-too-predictably commented, "to suggest that farmers are dishonestly sending animals to market knowing they are infected."[91]

Nineteen ninety was also the year of the spin doctor. From now on, the disquieting results of animal "transmission" experiments would start to emerge. Yet, with sufficient ingenuity, even the worst results could be made to seem encouraging. For example, in early February, results were published showing that BSE was capable of being transmitted from one cow to another.[92] Gloomy though this might at first seem, a positive "spin" could point out that the cattle concerned were injected with infected material, and this artificial technique would never occur naturally. When another experiment showed that mice (a different species) could contract BSE simply by *eating* infected cow brains, it was pointed out that the amount given to the mice (.32 ounce) was proportionately far higher than the amount likely to be eaten by a human being.

Well, it was supposed to *sound* like good news.

"SO WHAT?"

In February, the investigative television program *World in Action* examined BSE and included a pugnacious interview with Britain's food minister, David Maclean.[93] He gave a truculent performance, but it must have done little to reassure the public that their food was in safe hands. "Your critics say that meat inspectors simply aren't as qualified as vets to spot BSE suspect cattle at abattoirs," commented the interviewer.

"Well, maybe they aren't," declared Mr. Maclean. "I wouldn't expect them to be as qualified as vets; vets after all, do a five-year training course. I wouldn't expect them to spot them. So what?"

"Well," said the interviewer, "they're missing a good many BSE-suspect cattle, it is suggested."

"Well, so what?" snapped Maclean.

The thrust of his argument was that since the most suspect organs from all cows were now being removed at slaughterhouses, it didn't matter if some BSE-infected cattle were reaching the slaughterhouses undetected. "We're cutting the offals out of every cow, not just the BSE suspect ones, every single cow," he said. "And that's the final preventative measure."

But the program also included evidence from an experienced environmental health officer that graphically revealed that this "final preventative measure" was by no means the absolute guarantee of safety the government evidently hoped it would be. "When you split down the carcass," he said, "there will be bits of the central nervous system tissue that get scattered all over the rest of the meat. And when the carcass is sawn down, what they do is to hose that off. But again, that in itself is a compromise, because how do we know we get rid of it all? And how do we know what we produce is satisfactory? The whole animal is full of nerves; it's impossible to remove it all. It is the job of my meat inspectors to make sure that none of the banned offal gets through. But there will be some central nervous system that is left behind that is not covered by the banned offal, anyway."

"So suspect tissue is going into the human food chain?" asked the interviewer.

"Yes, certainly," was the unequivocal reply.

HEAVY PETTING

In April of 1990, as the number of detected cases of "mad cows" passed the 10,000 mark, the government announced the commissioning of a study to examine the connection between BSE and Creutzfeldt-Jakob disease in humans.[94] This action was taken at the behest of the Tyrell committee's report, which stated, "Many extensive epidemiological studies around the world have contributed to the current consensus view that Scrapie is not causally related to CJD. It is urgent that the same reassurance can be given about the lack of effect of BSE on human health. The best way of doing this is to monitor all UK cases of CJD over the next two decades."[95]

Professor Lacey was scathing: "In two sentences, the government's intent is revealed in absolute clarity. Its action is intended somehow to reassure, rather than to take any curative action."[96]

What happened next was totally unforeseen. If an evil alien intelligence had indeed been plotting the next move of the infectious agent, it could not have contrived anything better than what followed: A cat called Max died.

The British, as is widely known, are besotted with their pets. Although we are content to allow our food animals to live mean and miserable lives—out of sight—we will not tolerate any insult or injury to our beloved companion animals. So when the first pet cat died from a uniquely distinctive BSE/scrapie-type disease, the nation was appalled and outraged.

With hindsight, it was entirely logical that, if the infectious agent was present in cattle feed, the same infectious material could also be present in pet food. However, the reality of the pets actually dying, and all the negative public relations implications, doesn't seem to have been considered—there hadn't even been a routine "no evidence" statement from the government. But once the diagnosis was made, officials acted quickly to put this right, saying there was no evidence "at this stage" of a link with pet food or, indeed, with BSE.[97]

No evidence. Remember those two words. Whenever you hear an official spokesperson use them, run as fast as you can in the opposite direction.

Remarks made by the president of the British Veterinary Association raised the possibility that many more cats might be infected, when he was quoted as saying, "Vets are presented with cats showing nervous disorders like this one every day. Some can be treated, some can't and have to be destroyed. But in 90 percent of cases when they do have to be put to sleep owners don't want us to carry out a post mortem."[98] Wisely, the Pet Food Manufacturers Association had already advised its members not to include cattle offal in their products, but in view of the long incubation time of spongiform diseases, there could be no guarantee that many more cats would not subsequently be discovered to have "mad cat disease."

There was now something close to a state of panic in Britain. Within days, beef had been removed from the menus of more than 2,000 schools across the nation. The parliamentary opposition called upon the beleaguered minister of agriculture to take immediate further action or to resign. In an amazing public admonishment, a former chief veterinary officer broke the customary silence imposed on civil servants to lambaste successive governments' policies concerning the recycling of sheep and cows in cattle feed: "No one was more alive to the potential risk involved in tampering with the eco-system than I was," said Alex Brown. "I continually drummed it into everyone around me that we should never, never forget that nature has a right to do funny things to man. You should also never dismiss the unknown, because it is unknown."[99]

That, of course, is precisely what officials had been doing when they continually asserted that there was "no evidence" of any risk. Clearly, the government and the meat trade were losing the propaganda war, and they had to counter attack. The Meat and Livestock Commission decided to launch a $1.4 million advertising campaign. "It is not a response to the latest scare over BSE," said their marketing director. "It reflects our concern about the general pressure to eat less meat."[100]

Colin Cullimore, managing director of the Dewhurst chain of High Street butchers, laid into Professor Lacey. "Professor Lacey is being alarmist," declared Mr. Cullimore to *The Times*. "He is a scientist, but he is making statements without any evidence."[101]

In a broadcast to the nation, the minister of agriculture, John Gummer, condemned "scare mongers." "The public has absolute confidence that I am not going to be pushed off what is the right action merely to curry favour with one or two people," he said.[102]

In parliament, David Maclean, the food minister, lashed out at "so-called experts" who failed to submit their evidence, and another back-bencher complained of "a bogus professor."[103] While speaking in the British Houses of Parliament, members are protected by parliamentary privilege against the laws of libel.

IMPROPER SUGGESTIONS

On Wednesday, May 23, 1990, the Agriculture Committee of the House of Commons opened its proceedings on BSE. For the minister of agriculture, it was to be a fateful day. As an astute politician, John Gummer must have realized the crucial importance of a favorable verdict—if the committee vindicated his handling of the crisis, it would provide him with some sorely needed political backing. But if, on the other hand, it censured him, then who knows what might happen?

There was always the possibility that events could take a disastrous turn, but as John Gummer prepared to testify that afternoon, he must have felt a certain degree of quiet confidence. He was not, after all, alone. On his left sat Keith Meldrum, chief veterinary officer at the Ministry of Agriculture. Next to him sat Elizabeth Attridge, head of the Animal Health Division of the ministry. And on the minister's right was Dr. Hilary Pickles from the Department of Health, joint secretary to the Tyrell committee. All in all, a high-powered team, combining political acumen with scientific erudition. It would be difficult for things to go too far wrong.

The minister kicked off with a long introductory statement, expressing his pleasure with the committee's decision to hold an inquiry, outlining the course of the disease since its detection, and summarizing the government's response. It was, as one would expect, executed with proficiency, and the formal nature of the proceedings precluded any awkward interruptions or cross-examination until the minister had finished speaking.

He started well. Although Mr. Gummer could never be accused of Churchillian oratory, his mind was sharp, and the structure of his speech was logical, stressing the government's deep concern, its swift response to the crisis, and the firm grasp his ministry had over the problem. It was a good beginning, and he must have felt increasingly confident.

Perhaps he should have left it there. He certainly could have done that, because he had already said enough to create a favorable impression. But he didn't. He was well into his stride when something altogether astounding happened:

The official line had always been that, since there was "no evidence" that scrapie could infect humans, it therefore followed that BSE couldn't infect humans. This was a central tenet of the government's policy position. But that afternoon, John Selwyn Gummer, minister of agriculture, went much, much further than that. This is what he said: "The plain fact is that there is no evidence that BSE poses any risk. Some may argue that BSE is a new disease, so how can we be so sure. Well, there is good historical evidence because BSE is very similar to sheep Scrapie which has been in the sheep population for over 250 years without any suggestion that it poses a risk to humans. Neither have extensive studies shown a link between Scrapie and the human disease CJD."[104]

To the assembled members of the parliamentary committee, it must have sounded very persuasive. As Mr. Gummer spoke, flanked by experts, he must have appeared both impressive and credible.

There was just one problem: He was absolutely wrong.

SCRAPPING OVER SCRAPIE

Whatever possessed Mr. Gummer to make such a breathtaking assertion, we may never know for certain. He could just as easily have used the formulaic weasel words so beloved of politicians—"no conclusive evidence," "no proof," and so on—which would have adequately conveyed his message without putting his neck on the line. But he didn't.

He'd now gone on record, before a committee of the House of Commons, claiming that scrapie had existed in the sheep population "for over 250 years without any suggestion that it poses a risk to humans." "*Suggestion*" is defined by the *Oxford English Dictionary* as "*the putting into the mind of an idea . . . an idea or thought suggested, a proposal.*"[105] In effect, he seemed to be implying that the very notion that scrapie might pose a risk to humans was so inconceivable that no scientist would even propose the idea.

But this was rubbish. For at least fifteen years, there had indeed been "suggestions" from scientists that scrapie might play a part in the development of CJD, Creutzfeldt-Jakob disease. It was unthinkable that the minister's experts were not aware of this. But that afternoon, the experts were on Mr. Gummer's team. They were there to support him, not to cross-examine him.

It is, of course, conceivable that Mr. Gummer had been misinformed by his expert advisers. This is highly unlikely, however, as a close examination of his words reveals. For immediately after claiming that there hadn't been "any suggestion" that scrapie posed a risk to humans, he alluded to "extensive studies" examining the link between scrapie and CJD. The obvious question that arises from this is: if there hadn't been "any suggestion" that scrapie might pose a risk, why had "extensive studies" been performed? There is a conspicuous error of logic here.

What would have happened that day if the Agriculture Committee had taken steps to widen their inquiry and examine this new area in detail? We can only speculate, of course. They might have come to the same conclusions, in any case. Then again, they might not.

From the government's point of view, the worst possible outcome of the committee's inquiry would have been a failure to exonerate their conduct of the BSE disaster, coupled with a widening of the inquiry into the related area of scrapie and sheep. Given the existing high level of anxiety among the British population, it was conceivable that such a chain of events could have precipitated a governmental crisis of uncontrollable dimensions.

Perhaps in his desire to avoid opening this particular can of worms, Mr. Gummer simply went over the top, and abandoned the careful language of politicians. If so, it was an astounding mistake, and he was indeed fortunate not to have been challenged about it.

Until this book came along.

THE FIRST "SUGGESTION"

The first major "suggestion" that sheep scrapie might be linked to Creutzfeldt-Jakob disease in humans was presented to thousands of the world's scientists on November 29, 1974.[106] That day, an issue of the widely read journal *Science* was published, carrying a letter signed by six distinguished scientists, including D. Carleton Gajdusek, the kuru expert and later, Nobel prize winner.

The letter was in response to a research paper published in the same journal earlier in the year. The authors of the earlier paper were intrigued by the preponderance of CJD among certain population groups within Israel. Jewish families who had emigrated from Libya were particularly susceptible—up to seventy-eight times more likely to suffer from CJD than the general population. In response to this strange finding, the six scientists wrote:

"This finding may be related to the dietary habit of eating sheep's eyeballs, which are a gastronomic delicacy among Bedouin and Moroccan Arabs and also Libyans. A disease of sheep, Scrapie, has clinical and histopathological features similar to those of CJD . . . If the CJD agent is found in the cornea, retina or optic nerve, the ingestion of eyeballs of sheep harbouring the Scrapie agent might possibly lead to the development of CJD in susceptible individuals and thus account for the high incidence of the disease in Libyan Jews."[107]

This "suggestion" wasn't simply idle speculation. It had recently been tragically proven that CJD could be transmitted from one person to another when the recipient of a corneal transplant, unwittingly taken from a donor suffering from CJD, subsequently contracted CJD and died from it. Therefore, if the CJD agent was present in human eyeballs, it might also be present in sheep's eyeballs.

One of the authors of the original study replied to this suggestion with some interesting evidence: "We knew that brain and spinal cord, mainly from sheep, was a delicacy among Libyan Jews," he wrote. "Inquiries even revealed that a favourite method of preparation is light grilling, which could conceivably leave an infectious agent viable."[108]

However, he went on to say that having considered the idea, they then rejected it, on the grounds that the consumption of sheep's eyeballs was not limited to just the Libyan Jewish population, "so we deleted reference to it in our final manuscript," he explained, concluding that "brain is a more likely source of the putative CJD agent than eyeballs."

And so the ongoing debate began—not in public; but among scientists, and in the rarefied pages of professional journals. Evidence would be produced in favor of the theory, and evidence would be produced against it. But no one could now claim, with any truthfulness, that there had not been "any suggestion" that scrapie posed a risk to humans.

ON THE TRAIL

Let's stay with the scrapie/CJD story for a little—not to further discomfit the poor Mr. Gummer, but so that we can understand some aspects of these enigmatic spongiform diseases.

After the publication of the initial report in *Science*, more research was conducted into the Libyan Jewish population. It produced more tantalizing evidence, but not clear proof. One piece of research, for example, showed that the vast majority of CJD patients had indeed been known to consume sheeps' brains—but so did other "controls," without apparently succumbing to CJD.[109] What did this mean?

It simply meant that a clean-cut, cause-and-effect relationship could not be easily established. While it was notable that the CJD sufferers were more often exposed to animals than the control group—and, significantly, they ate brains that were far more lightly cooked—this was not in itself strong enough evidence. Another study summarized it like this: "The results suggest either a common source of exposure or a genetic influence on susceptibility to the virus."[110]

The science of epidemiology, which is really detective work by numbers, is at its strongest when a clear cause-and-effect relationship can be proven. In order for the scrapie-CJD theory to be proven beyond doubt, it would have to be shown that people suffering from CJD differed significantly from the general population in their exposure to the scrapie agent in sheep meat. As long as there were people in the population who didn't contract CJD, but who were similarly exposed to sheep meat, it could not be conclusively demonstrated that scrapie caused CJD. So, although the evidence so far didn't *prove* the connection between scrapie and CJD, it didn't *disprove* it either.

Let's take a moment to consider these six links in the chain of disease transmission:

1. Characteristics of the agent
2. A reservoir
3. Portal of exit
4. Mode of Transmission
5. Portal of entry
6. Suspectibility of host

In a way, this chain looks rather like a game of Russian roulette—you have to be rather unlucky to lose and become infected. Before anything can happen, the infectious agent itself must be one of a strain capable of causing disease (there are several different scrapie strains). Then, there has to be something that acts as a reservoir of infection. This in itself is a powerfully suggestive argument in favor of a connection between scrapie and CJD, because CJD would have died out by now if it was purely confined to human beings—there is almost certainly a natural reservoir of it outside our own species, which periodically reinfects us when conditions are right.

Next, there must be a way of getting the disease out of the natural reservoir—in the case of scrapie, the most infectious parts of the sheep are the brain, placenta, spleen, liver, and lymph nodes. Then, there has to be a method of carrying the infection to the new host. Well, in the case of sheep, that's easy enough—we eat them. So far, so good—or bad, as the case may be. But all this still isn't enough to infect the host. Two more essential steps are necessary:

The first is the route into the host itself. Now, we know that the effectiveness of different routes of entry to the host are extremely variable. At one end of the spectrum, we know that scrapie can sometimes be transferred very easily from one sheep to another simply by allowing the healthy sheep to graze on pasture previously grazed on by infected sheep—no other contact is needed.[111] At the other end of the spectrum, it has been demonstrated that sometimes only direct inoculation into the brain with infected material will succeed in transferring infection. So between these two extremes, there is a huge variety of routes, some far more successful than others. This is a significant point, because there is evidence to suggest that eating scrapie-infected meat may not, in itself, be sufficient to produce an infection—there may also have to be some kind of accidental inoculation, such as biting the skin of the mouth at the same time, or lesions of the lips, gums, or intestines.

Finally, there has to be an existing susceptibility to the disease in the new victim. Some breeds of sheep are far more susceptible to scrapie than others. By implication, some humans may be more susceptible, too. As we will see later, this is the "joker in the pack," because Scrapie/CJD is peculiar in having both a genetic and an infectious component. Tricky stuff, indeed.

You can see that there are many, many possible factors that can affect the transmission of disease—and its subsequent detection. Because of this, it is not always possible to tease out a clear cause-and-effect relationship from the numbers. For example, in one study of thirty-eight American CJD patients, it was established that at least ten of them had eaten brains within the previous five years—apparently, a very significant finding.[112] However, nearly as many people in the "control group" had also eaten brains, and didn't get CJD.

"The chance of a person's getting the disease depends on a complex sequence of events . . . ," one scientist commented, while reviewing the results. "It is important to remember that exposure to a suspected mode of transmission may not be enough to result in disease, and some ingenuity in the method of inquiry will have to be introduced. For example, in this study, a high but equal proportion of both patients ate brains. What could be critical is that the patients may have experienced some coincidental events, such as concurrent trauma or acute respiratory infection which caused a break in the skin or mucosal lining thus allowing the CJD agent a portal of entry."[113]

The fact is, even with the best team of scientists available, it could be next to impossible to ever provide the sort of conclusive epidemiological proof that would convince everyone that scrapie can cause CJD. One major stumbling block is the sheer length of time between infection and onset of disease: how many people can accurately remember what they had to eat twenty years ago? Also, bear in mind that many CJD patients are not properly diagnosed until after death, and scientists have to question their next of kin—which makes it even more difficult to get accurate responses.

There are problems, too, simply recognizing CJD. Until 1979, the International Classification of Diseases (a system used to codify causes of death) didn't even include a specific category for Creutzfeldt-Jakob disease.[114] In Britain, approximately 75,000 people die every year from "dementing" diseases. Yet the official statistics show that only thirty to forty people die from CJD. There is good evidence to believe that the true figure is far, far higher—probably in the region of 9,000 cases.[115]

And here's yet another problem. In America, it has been found that areas with the largest number of reported outbreaks of scrapie (Illinois, Texas, Indiana, Ohio, and California) have no more cases of CJD than the national average. Is this reassuring evidence? By no means. It actually tells us very little at all. As one reporter commented, "Such a comparison is of limited value, since Scrapie-infected material may have been widely disseminated throughout the country in processed meat."[116]

Today, most of the food we eat has been transported hundreds, sometimes thousands, of miles. Therefore, a local outbreak of scrapie might result in a cluster of CJD cases far away in another continent!

Another report reveals that we can't even be certain that sheep with scrapie will be accurately diagnosed. Examining the marketing of sheep in Pennsylvania, scientists concluded that "sheep were usually marketed before central nervous system signs of Scrapie were expected to appear"; that "opportunities to detect the disease were limited"; and "sheep producers in the area knew little about Scrapie despite the fact that the disease has been reported in the area."[117]

All these difficulties present formidable obstacles to epidemiological surveys. In France, a twelve-year study of scrapie in sheep revealed that the disease had been diagnosed "in virtually every region where sheep are raised."[118] It also found that lamb consumption among some growing population groups correlated with an increasing frequency of CJD. A year later, a continuation of the same study still found that "there is a correlation between lamb consumption and CJD mortality rates in different nation-wide population categories."[119]

However, five years later, the scientists had identified a total of 329 patients dying of Creutzfeldt-Jakob disease, but were unable to conclude there was a clear connection with lamb consumption, or with any other single factor.[120] Such equivocal evidence is hard for scientists to come to grips with. Therefore, when something more substantial comes along, it is eagerly seized upon, and previous theories are forgotten. And that is precisely what happened next.

BAD GENES?

"Clusters of CJD have long been known," declared *The Economist* magazine two months after Mr. Gummer testified to the House of Commons Agriculture Committee. "The most famous was among some Libyan Jews in whom CJD was almost 40 times more common than normal. Since they ate sheep, it was thought that Scrapie might be to blame. Further research showed that the sufferers were related. . . . Although it may be worrying that such clusters of CJD exist," the writer explained, "the good news is that they seem to have been caused by bad genes, not bad mutton."[121]

Well, maybe it wasn't such good news, after all. Initially, it had been proposed that there was a simple family connection between the Libyan Jews who suffered from CJD—in other words, it was a hereditary disease. Subsequent work, however, failed to confirm this.[122]

What *was* subsequently established by genetic detective work was that the Jewish CJD patients displayed a specific genetic mutation.[123] So were "bad genes" the cause of CJD? The answer would come from the largest—and for us the most worrying—cluster of CJD cases yet discovered; right in the middle of Europe.

A PLAGUE IN SLOW MOTION

Cases of Creutzfeldt-Jakob disease among Libyan Jews were forty times more common than normal—and that was considered to be extraordinary. Today, in Slovakia, an epidemic of CJD is developing. I use the word *epidemic* deliberately, because in certain areas, the incidence of CJD is more than *three thousand times* the ordinary level.[124]

It seems strange to think of an epidemic with an incubation time measured in decades. When people drop like flies—from cholera, for example—the drama momentarily hits the headlines, and we are all horrified, until we forget about it. But with CJD, there is no instant, three-minute tragedy, conveniently prepackaged for the evening news bulletins. There is no news angle for a plague that is running in slow motion.

Whatever is developing in Slovakia is a matter of intense interest, and deep concern, to many scientists. Some experts believe that we are now seeing the beginning of a worldwide epidemic of "kuru virus"— encompassing the sudden appearance of BSE, an upsurge in scrapie in sheep, and CJD in humans. "We have a major problem in human disease," grimly warns one authority.[125]

When a conventional epidemic strikes, time is the enemy. You need time to identify the causative agent, time to study it, and time to develop countermeasures. When the period between infection and death may be just a few days, you never have enough time. But that's not the case with CJD. Which is why the Slovakian epidemic is the best-studied, most investigated outbreak of CJD ever. In the past few years, we have learned more about the cause of CJD than we've ever known before.

COMPELLING NEW EVIDENCE

This chapter began with a film plot in which Russian and American scientists battled to save the world from annihilation. A real-life parallel has been going on in Slovakia, as both Americans and scientists who were formerly under Communist jurisdiction now cooperate to comprehend the nature of the epidemic now in progress. Here is a summary of this little-known but crucial research work, to date:

- The epidemic has two centers. One is located in the rural Lucenec area of south-central Slovakia, with some cases being reported from across the Hungarian border. The other is based further toward the north, in the Orava area, to the west of the High Tatra mountains on the Polish border. The two areas differ significantly in some key respects. In the south, the disease progresses steadily, continuing to claim about the same number of people every year. In the north, however, it suddenly erupted in the late 1980s—two small villages, with a combined population of less than 2,000, have had more than twenty cases of CJD in the last three years alone.[126]

- Once again, initial research first suggested that the disease had a genetic origin.[127] Nine CJD victims from the north, and six from the southern cluster had their DNA sequenced, and it was found that they all had a similar mutation. This discovery led some scientists to claim that CJD was "caused" by a genetic mutation—back to the "bad genes" theory described above. However, subsequent evidence has shown that as a comprehensive explanation, it simply isn't tenable, for the following reasons:

- Genetic screening has established that the mutation in question was present in people living in the northern Orava region at least as far back as 1902, and probably much earlier. Yet it was only recently—in 1987—that CJD suddenly exploded in frequency there. Obviously, if "bad genes" was the root cause of CJD, there would have been cases of CJD as long as people had been carrying the genetic mutation. This clearly points to another "triggering" factor in the environment, such as the emergence of scrapie.

- When scientists studied families in which CJD had claimed more than one victim, they found that CJD occurred more or less at the same time—but not at the same age. If the disease was purely genetic, it would be more likely to occur after a certain number of years. This evidence also suggests that suddenly, an environmental source of infection appeared, with tragic consequences.

- After extensive genetic screening, it was established that many people could carry the genetic mutation, but remain perfectly healthy.[128] Further research work with CJD outbreaks in Chile has now established that among one identified group of people with the mutation, only half the expected number actually developed CJD.[129] This is very convincing evidence that an environmental factor triggers the disease in those susceptible to it.

- A case history illustrates the importance of an environmental factor with great clarity. Three children were all found to be carrying the genetic mutation. Two of the children grew up in their birthplaces, within the southern cluster of CJD. Both of these children subsequently contracted CJD and died. The third child, however, didn't contract CJD—even though she carried the mutation. The difference was that she was taken away from the area while still an infant, and lived and grew up in Bratislava, well outside the danger area.[130] But why should there be "danger areas," in any case?

- The answer to this lies in recent agricultural history. In an attempt to stimulate the Slovak sheep farming industry, sheep were imported from 1970 onward from England and France—and the breeds chosen (Ile de France and Suffolk) are both highly susceptible to scrapie.[131] Furthermore, careful research work has revealed that most of these sheep went into regions that are now suffering from CJD.

- The evidence becomes more incriminating still when you examine the jobs that the CJD patients had. Well over half of them worked in livestock farming or meat processing.[132] Further laboratory work has now confirmed that scrapie definitely exists in these flocks of sheep—and, equally troubling, scrapie infection has now been identified there in sheep not manifesting any clinical symptoms of the disease.[133]

To summarize—this evidence strongly supports the theory that the most recent epidemic of CJD is the lethal result of genetically susceptible people being exposed to the scrapie agent in sheep.

NEWS FROM WONDERLAND

Early in 1992, it seemed as if the "all clear" had sounded.

"Beef given a Clean Bill of Health," proclaimed the headline in the *Meat Trades Journal*.[134] "The results of the latest batch of tests on BSE suggest the disease cannot be passed from cattle to humans." The report continued, "British beef has been given a clean bill of health by a government scientist claiming tests on monkeys may have proved BSE cannot be transmitted from cattle to man. . . . 'I am absolutely convinced BSE can't be transmitted easily from cows to humans,' " the government scientist was quoted as saying. " 'I don't believe the meat of any cow is a risk to man and am certain that the meat arriving at any butcher always has been and still is fit to eat.' "

Reassuring words, indeed. Based on an experiment that involved transmitting BSE to marmosets, small monkeys belonging to the same biological family as humans, two marmosets were injected with tissue taken from BSE-infected cattle, and another two were injected with material taken from scrapie-infected sheep. The two marmosets infected with scrapie both died, but the other two lived on. "I feel certain that the monkeys have passed the danger period," the scientist was quoted as saying. "I would have no worries if butchers told any customers still refusing to eat beef that there is little or even no chance of them developing the disease."

Just two months later, the *Meat Trades Journal* carried the following stark, doom-laden headline:

"Primates are affected by BSE."[135]

What had happened? Why, one of the two BSE-infected marmosets had died, and the other one was only expected to live for a few more weeks. Yes, they'd both got Mad Cow Disease.

So did this change everything? Did the government scientist quoted above now consider that BSE was more of a threat to human health? Not at all. The article quoted the scientist as now saying; "We now know that BSE is even less of a risk."

And the Ministry of Agriculture commented (Do I really need to write this for you? I mean, by now, you know what's coming, don't you?) that there was no cause for concern about human health.[136]

So that was all right, then.

MILESTONES ON THE ROAD TO HELL

And the saga continued:

- In May 1994, Germany threatens to ban British beef imports but retreats under political pressure.
- In October 1994, the national Creutzfeldt-Jakob disease surveillance unit announces, "We see no evidence of an emerging CJD epidemic."
- In October 1995, the Spongiform Encephalopathy Advisory Committee orders an investigation into the cases of two British teenagers who developed CJD.
- In December 1995, Prime Minister John Major says, "I am advised that beef is a safe and wholesome product. The Chief Medical Officer's advice on the point is clear: there is no evidence that eating beef causes CJD in humans."
- In February 1996, the food minister, criticizing a "British beef could kill" campaign, says, "This campaign is outrageous."
- In March 1996, the agriculture minister tells Parliament, "British beef can be eaten with confidence."[137]

With confidence.

- On Wednesday, March 20, 1996, the British government finally admitted that Mad Cow Disease could be passed to humans by eating beef.
- The official report into the Mad Cow disaster states, "The Government did not lie to the public about BSE. It believed that the risks posed by BSE to humans were remote. The Government was preoccupied with preventing an alarmist overreaction to BSE because it believed that the risk was remote. It is now clear that this campaign of reassurance was a mistake."

So that was that.
Very gentlemanly. Very British. And no one carries the can.

EARTH SAVED? EARTH DOOMED?

I wish I could tell you what the final impact of Mad Cow Disease on the human population will be, but I can't. No one can. Projections by British experts in 2000, based on recorded deaths so far, suggest that as many as 500,000 Britons could die over the next thirty years.[138] Vegetarians and vegans can't afford to be smug or consider themselves immune: meat products are so ubiquitous in our society that it is inevitable that we will consume them in one way or another, either as gelatin, in vaccinations, as a blood transfusion, or in a host of other ways.

Is Mad Cow Disease present in America right now? Officially, no. But data from the U.S. National Veterinary Sciences Laboratories BSE Surveillance Program from 1990 to 2000 show that of approximately 900 million cattle slaughtered, only 11,954 brains (approximately 1 in 75,000) were examined for BSE. And brain examinations have generally been prompted by the presence of neurological symptoms. However, the symptoms of BSE do not commonly manifest in cattle until they are about five years of age, which is *after* the usual age of slaughter. For example, most U.S. dairy cows are slaughtered before four years of age, when even an infected cow may appear healthy. In the U.K., 70 percent of dairy cows remain alive past this point, making identification of infected animals much easier.[139]

A number of American experts believe that it is probably here, at low levels.[140] How did it arrive? Unfortunately, there are a multitude of ways. For example, British export statistics show that twenty tons of "meals of meat or offal" that were "unfit for human consumption" and probably intended for animals were sent to the United States in 1989. In an exception to the import ban, many health supplements have contained glandular material from animals whose health status could not be determined.[141] Tourists to Europe would certainly have been exposed to infected beef, just as the locals were. Military records reveal that millions of U.S. military personnel stationed in Europe before 1996 would have eaten British beef on base during the height of the epidemic.[142] As I'm writing this, today's *New York Times* reports that U.S. pharmaceutical companies have been using animal ingredients from cattle raised in countries where there is a risk of Mad

Cow Disease, even though the U.S. Food and Drug Administration asked them not to.[143] In today's global economy, no nation is an island, and the arrogant failings of the British political administration don't jeopardize just the health of Britons: they potentially affect everyone in the world.

We also know that CJD is seriously underdiagnosed at present, the most common misdiagnosis of CJD being Alzheimer's disease.[144] In fact, the brains of the young people who died from the new CJD variant in Britain look like Alzheimer's brains.[145] Four million Americans are currently affected by Alzheimer's;[146] it is the fourth leading cause of death among the elderly in the U.S.[147] Epidemiological evidence suggests that people eating meat more than four times a week for a prolonged period are three times more likely to suffer a dementia than longtime vegetarians.[148]

My own experience of watching the progress of this epidemic is that we would be very, very foolish to write it off as gone away. Time and time again the British government seems to have done exactly this, and like a monster from a horror movie, the thing you think you've killed gets right back up and keeps coming at you.

So what can we do?

WHAT AMERICANS MUST DO

"Our government has been frighteningly slow to react to the very real threat of CJD in America," said Dr. Neal Barnard in a critique of U.S. government policy in January 2001. Dr. Barnard is president of the Physicians Committee for Responsible Medicine, and he talks a lot of good sense. He continued, "The protective measures taken so far are grossly insufficient. We should learn from Europe's mistakes and implement tough precautionary measures—now, before it's too late." Here are his five recommendations for protecting the American public against Mad Cow Disease:

1. Ban the use of animal-derived livestock feeds for any species, given the likelihood that animal by-products will, in turn, be recycled to ruminants (that is, cows, sheep, and goats).

2. Prohibit animal by-products in all medications, supplements, and cosmetics.

3. Label all foods containing animal by-products (such as gelatin or "natural flavorings"), indicating both the presence of animal by-products and the species of origin.

4. Provide warning labels on all foods that carry a risk of CJD, using standards similar to those for tobacco and alcohol products.

5. Institute comprehensive monitoring programs to check for diseased animals and humans in the U.S.[149]

And what can you, as an individual, do? The Mad Cow Disease crisis is a stupid, self-inflicted epidemic caused by the greed of an agricultural system that puts profit ahead of all other considerations. If we turn a naturally vegetarian species, the cow, into an intensively reared cannibal, then something nasty is likely to happen. It did, and we're only beginning to count the cost. My advice to you is simple: go vegan. You will greatly reduce your risk of coming into contact with infected material, and you will also stop supporting a greedy, grossly unnatural, and deeply unethical food production system that is good for neither man nor beast.

3

PIG TALES

As a kid, I'd come to the conclusion that my personal obstinacy in regard to meat eating was a lone and unique eccentricity, an abnormality in a world where meat eating was the universal rule. I had grown up in close contact with many kinds of animals, and I grew to like them and understand them. This is unusual today; most children now grow up in big cities, and the only contact they have with animals is with pets, or with the processed animals on their dinner plates.

If you have a companion animal, you'll know that he or she has a personality, probably quite a strong one. Actually, *all* animals have individual personalities; it's just that most of us never have the chance to get to know them.

One snowy January, my parents bought some goslings (baby geese) with the intention of fattening them up and selling them just before Christmas. But a strange thing happened over the next few months: every goose (and gander) got a name, and as I observed them, I became increasingly involved with their rich and complex lives, which are every bit as multilayered as the average human's. There was the "alpha male" (Thomas), who was a typical male chauvinist. Bossy and domineering, he tried to control everything, but in doing so was embarrassingly subject to frequent pratfalls, causing him to lose much of his dignity and prestige. There was Janet, a small and very pretty female who was jumpy and quite literally flighty: flapping her wings in excitement would often lead to unexpected takeoffs, and even more bizarre landings, such as the time when she alighted on my mother's head—a major surprise for both of them. And there was Simon, an outcast, raised inside the farmhouse and believing himself to be a human, not a goose. Simon surprised all of us one spring when "he" laid an egg.

Come Christmas, it would have been as murderous to think about sending our geese to market as it would have been to kill a close family member. Yet, when visitors came to stay with us, they always said, "How on earth can you tell them all apart? They look exactly the same!" I could never understand this comment: for me, each goose was clearly and obviously a distinct individual.

Both the geese and the chickens, ducks, and other assorted family members we seemed to accumulate had their own very understandable languages. I quickly learned, for example, the language that chickens used to tell each other where food was found, or the "words" that mother geese use to summon their goslings. To eat creatures that were, in effect, my friends seemed to me to display all the moral superiority of the cannibal. As George Bernard Shaw once remarked, "Animals are my friends, and I don't eat my friends."

I don't know how you feel about these things. You might feel I'm just being squishy and sentimental, and in the real dog-eat-dog world (have you ever actually seen a dog eat another dog?) there isn't time for these cuddly, warm thoughts. Maybe. All I know is, my life as a kid was made richer and deeper from my "friendships" with the animal world, and it's permanently broadened my range of experience. But maybe you're right, and I should have spent my time watching Schwarzenneger videos and playing "killer" videogames, like kids these days do. It might have toughened me up a bit more.

When, many years later, I discovered that mine was not an isolated and freakish persuasion, that countless other people shared my qualms about slaughter, and that vegetarianism had a long and mightily distinguished history, I was frankly astonished. I no longer considered myself to be simply "squeamish": now, I walked in some pretty good company: Da Vinci, Empedocles, Gandhi, Lincoln, Paine, Plutarch, Pythagoras, Schweitzer, Shaw, Tolstoy, Voltaire . . . all these and many more were either vegetarian themselves, or resoundingly endorsed the meat-free ethic.

That vegetarianism was not merely a "food fad," but had a rock-solid ethical basis was indeed wondrous news to me. With this revelation, I began to wonder how any educational system that is worthy of the name can allow children to emerge without at least some basic exposure to the ideas of the great ethical thinkers of history.

PAY ATTENTION—THIS IS INTERESTING

Today, ethics is one of the hottest fields of study in higher education. It's not a remote, academic subject only of interest to professional philosophers: increasingly, the application of practical ethics will determine the future of our world. Just think about a few of the advances that science is on the brink of offering us:

- The chance to permanently alter the human germ line
- The ability of parents to specify a new baby's characteristics just as easily as they might order a Big Mac
- The possibility of life extension offering some of us near immortality
- The creation of artificial life that is to all intents and purposes identical to us
- The likelihood of coming into contact with other intelligent life forms in the universe

Increasingly, the question will not be "*can* we?" . . . It will be "*should* we?" And that is why the study of ethics is absolutely crucial. Luckily, the basics aren't too hard at all.

Ethical theory can be divided into two main schools of thought: one is called Consequentialist, the other Nonconsequentialist.

These wordy labels disguise ideas that are basically pretty simple (as is too often the case with philosophy). Consequentialist ethics are based on the idea that an action's "rightness" or "wrongness" depends on the consequences of the action. For example, if you steal your friend's watch, thus causing him to miss an important meeting, then the act of stealing would be wrong, because the consequences of your action were detrimental to your friend. However, if your friend never missed his watch, then it might be argued that what you did was not wrong, because no negative consequences ensued, indeed only positive ones to you—a "victimless" crime.

Nonconsequentialist theories take a different point of view. They hold that, regardless of the consequences, an action may be either morally right or morally wrong in itself. Stealing, for example, would generally be considered to be a bad thing according to many Nonconsequentialist schools of thought, even if there was no harm as a result. Stealing your friend's watch is wrong, whether he misses it or not.

Now, what is most interesting is this: within both major ethical theories, there are highly developed arguments in favor of vegetarianism—it is *not* the exclusive property of one or the other major (and mutually antagonistic) school. Let me explain:

Within Consequentialist ethics, we find the doctrine known as Utilitarianism, which had its origins among the British philosophers of the seventeenth and eighteenth centuries. Again, it is a straightforward enough idea, simply expressed in the words of eighteenth-century philosopher Jeremy Bentham, who believed that an individual should seek "the greatest happiness of the greatest number."

Utilitarian philosophers therefore judge an action's rightness or wrongness by its overall impact on the balance sheet of happiness: if it creates more happiness than suffering, the action is good; but if it creates more pain than pleasure, then it is wrong. Consequently, Utilitarianists advocate vegetarianism for the very good reason that the trivial amount of pleasure created by eating meat is more than offset by the huge amount of suffering inflicted on the animal population. Within the Utilitarian school, Peter Singer (who wrote *Animal Liberation*) is one of its chief modern advocates. Note that Utilitarians rarely talk in terms of absolute "animal rights" or even "human rights." Professor Singer, for example, could foresee certain restricted circumstances in which even vivisection would be right. As he says, "If one or even a dozen animals had to suffer experiments in order to save thousands, I would think it right and in accordance with equal consideration of interests that they should do so. This, at any rate, is the answer a Utilitarian must give."[1] The attraction of Utilitarianism lies in its coherent and flexible basis; it sees morality as a human creation with the aim of increasing the amount of happiness in the world.

Nonconsequentialist ethics, on the other hand, include those philosophers who argue in favor of animal (and human) rights. Rights are absolute things—they are not subject to a cost-benefit analysis. For example, according to some people, dropping the atomic bomb on Hiroshima shortened the course of the Second World War, and therefore saved lives on both sides. Some Utilitarians might argue that this was on balance a good thing, but those philosophers representing the rights viewpoint would disagree, saying that killing is always wrong, whatever the circumstances or putative benefits. Those Nonconsequentialist philosophers who advocate vegetarianism (such as Professor Tom Regan, who wrote *The Case For Animal Rights*) do so on the principle that the basic moral right possessed by all beings is the right to respectful treatment. They also hold that animals, like humans, have inherent value in themselves; they have the potential to lead fulfilling lives, and should be allowed to do so. Where the inherent value of an animal is debased—as, for example, in the case of the degrading conditions in which factory farm animals are kept—then their rights have also been violated. Similarly, if an animal can be either treated fairly or unfairly, their basic right to justice dictates that we must treat them fairly. The attraction of the philosophy of animal rights is that it provides clear and unambiguous guidelines about the way we should treat animals; and anyone who accepts the philosophy of human rights must, logically, also accept the validity of animal rights. If they do not, then they are acting as speciesists, sibling to racists and sexists.

As a little boy of eleven, I knew nothing of these vast ideas. For me, then, and for countless numbers of other little boys and girls who are upset at the thought of killing animals, not eating their carcasses seemed to be the very least one could do. Adults, of course, often resort to trickery in their attempt to make children eat meat. They may stuff it inside a banana-shaped casing and claim it's a "hot dog," or even lie barefacedly to their kids ("the little piggy-wiggy *wants* you to eat this, darling").

But it's the lies that adults tell to *themselves* that are the most interesting.

A MIND SPLIT ASUNDER

Schizophrenia is the most common form of psychosis in our society. It literally means "split mind," and it is used to describe an abnormal splitting of psychic functions so that ideas and feelings are often rigidly isolated from each other. For example, a sufferer may express frightening or sad ideas in a happy manner.

Meat eaters also demonstrate a kind of "split mind." When you think about it, the whole point of eating meat is to obtain pleasure (there is no other valid justification). Listen to the conversation of gourmets—folk who often take their pleasures with frightening seriousness—and you will hear people engaged in nothing else but the earnest pursuit of indulgence, as they debate, with great feeling, the comparative delights of such delicacies as veal, goose liver paté, frogs legs, and an endless agenda of even more recondite morsels.

Well, there's nothing wrong with taking pleasure in what you eat. Food is, after all, one of humanity's greatest delights and sources of comfort, is it not?

Indeed it is. But what puzzles me is this. When savoring a tender mouthful of veal, or deliberating over those oh-so-succulent *cuisses de grenouille*, how do you stop yourself from thinking about the misery and pain that the animal experienced? I mean, doesn't the thought of a baby calf, crying in fear to be reunited with its mother, upset you— just a little? Doesn't it take the edge off your appetite?

Meat eaters do not allow such unpleasant thoughts to interfere with the weighty processes of ingestion and digestion. But actions have consequences. When someone eats veal, the consequence is that the market for veal increases, and more baby calves will be born and live sad and wretched lives.

Yet in the divided mind of the meat eater, no connection between his action and the inevitable consequence has been made, because unpleasant thoughts like that are simply not permitted. And so he or she learns to live in a kind of dream world, where actions don't have consequences, and self-gratification takes precedence over everything.

A split mind.

THE NAZI INSIDE

"American slaughterhouses," says Dr. Alex Hershaft, a prominent campaigner for animals, "are our Dachaus, our Buchenwalds, our Birkenaus. Like the good German burghers, we have a fair idea of what goes on there, but we don't want any reality checks. We rationalize that the killing has to be done and that it's done humanely. We fear that the truth would offend our sensibilities and perhaps force us to do something."

Does this offend you? Do you think that it is wrong to compare the deaths of the victims of the Nazi holocaust to the way animals are treated in present-day America? Actually, I agree with you. It *is* offensive. But the fact that the comparison gives offense doesn't in itself make it incorrect. In fact, Dr. Hershaft wasn't the first to make this comparison. The first to do so was the great Jewish writer Isaac Bashevis Singer, winner of the 1978 Nobel Prize for Literature. Singer put these thoughts into the mind of one of his characters in his short story, "The Letter Writer":

> "In his thoughts, Herman spoke a eulogy for the mouse who had shared a portion of her life with him and who, because of him, had left this earth. 'What do they know—all these scholars, all these philosophers, all the leaders of the world—about such as you. They have convinced themselves that man, the worst transgressor of all, is the crown of creation. All other creatures were created to provide him with food, pelts, to be tormented, exterminated. In relation to them, all people are Nazis; for the animals, it is an eternal Treblinka."[2]

Singer himself narrowly escaped Treblinka, widely regarded as the second most important German wartime extermination center, where a total of 870,000 Jews were killed.[3] It hardly needs to be added that Singer was vegetarian. But why is it, I wonder, that we find the comparison of a slaughter house to an extermination camp so disturbing?

Is it because Treblinka was a place where humans were massacred like animals (in which case, why is it acceptable to massacre animals, but not humans?). Is it because it defiles the memory of the victims of the Holocaust to be compared to the innocent victims of today's slaughterhouses? Yet that is precisely what the death camps were: vast industrialized killings machines that treated people just like animals. If we minimize this, then we deny the horror and enormity of the Holocaust itself.

Or perhaps it is, as Dr. Hershaft suggests, the fact that it is all simply too close for comfort. While six million Jews were being systematically and brutally massacred by the Nazis during World War II, most of the world stood by silent. While eight billion farm animals are killed in the United States each year, most of us stand by, equally silent.[4]

Perhaps that reaction is, in truth, the most painful of all reactions . . . a twinge of conscience.

THE BEST OF THE BEST

I wanted to see the best, not the worst, that the world's meat industry could show me, so I went to a celebrated farm in southern Britain on a squally spring day. This is a very special farm, because the animals here are treated better than anywhere else in Britain, probably the world. Their meat is sold for high prices at the best shops in London. If you can't quite go vegetarian, but you care enough to avoid cruelly raised supermarket meat, this is the farm you buy it from.

So here we are, in our Wellington boots, walking and talking with Richard, one of the younger generation of farmers who try to produce their meat in a kinder and more ethical way. First, I want to raise the question of terminology.

"You describe your meat as 'high welfare,' " I say. "Is that the same as 'cruelty free'?"

"I suppose so," he answers. "It's terminology, isn't it? I think, all in all, our welfare standards are the highest in the country, if not in Europe, if not the world."

"So are you saying there's actually no cruelty involved at all in your method of meat production?"

"I think that would be tricky, wouldn't it? I don't think you possibly could say that, really. I mean, it depends what you mean by 'cruel,' doesn't it? What I'm seeking to do is to rear the animals much the same way as any one of our customers would do if they did it themselves. In other words, I don't think a customer would, if you gave them ten porkers, they wouldn't build a mini–factory farm with gridded floors, cut its tail off, medicate it, choose a growth promoter. They'd find an old coal shed or something and put some straw in it, and feed it scraps. That's what we're doing. That's a fascinating question. You remind me of a guy from BBC TV who asked much the same thing—he asked if animals have rights or not, and I think it's a difficult one, it's a long discussion, you need more than half an hour's continuous chat, and probably as long to think about it."

"But you must have thought about it."

"Not exactly in those terms. I think my farm is undoubtedly high welfare, and I agree with you that's not the same as cruelty-free. I mean, supposing you have a pig that doesn't want to get on the lorry. We will pick it up and carry it on. If you wanted to be utterly cruelty-free, I think you'd have to let it go, and hope that it wanted to go next week. So at the moment, I'll say we are definitely high welfare, but to say that we are absolutely cruelty-free, 100 percent, would be difficult."

"What about the rights argument? Do animals have rights?"

"You'd have to talk to a priest about that."

"I'm asking you. Do you think animals have rights?"

"I think they deserve respect and kindness, particularly if you're using them as a source of food. I think they do anyway, but particularly, I say particularly because in a way you're then using them, as opposed to living with them. It's not as if they're performing some other function, such as a guide dog."

"It could be said that what you're really doing is just being kinder to meat eaters, rather than being kinder to the animals. Because it avoids the unpleasant thought in their mind that the animal they're eating has suffered."

"I wish that thought was stronger in their mind in the first place," says Richard. "I mean, I actually think that thought doesn't lurk much in people's minds."

We stop talking, and tour the farm. The wind is bitterly piercing, and the driven rain is turning the chalky soil the same leaden gray as the sky. I am grateful for the shelter of the first farm building we are herded into; but I am not prepared for the sight that meets my eyes. It is dark, but in the gloom I can see three vast sows, confined by metal frames, their teats exposed and constantly available to the baby piglets that run and squeak as we enter. The sheer bulk of these sows is breathtaking, even majestic. But these are not just female pigs, they are mothers, too. In the narrow farrowing crates in which they lie imprisoned, they are all but denied access to their own babies. They cannot even turn round. I catch one of the sow's eyes, and I understand the particular distress she is experiencing. When we resume our conversation, I tackle him about this.

"I wanted to talk to you about some of the things we've seen today. Now the first thing that we saw was the farrowing crate, which has been criticized by various organizations. Can you tell us why it's been criticized?"

Suddenly, he has become very distant.

"I presume because it restricts the freedom of the sow. For the period of giving birth to the piglets."

"And what's your feeling about that?"

"I think if you don't, and the sow then treads on the piglets, or savages them, or they suffer in any other way, then it can create more problems than it solves. It remains a totally unsolved concept in this company. We allow all forms of farrowing, and both have advantages and disadvantages, and after six years we have no clear policy. And any honest welfare person wouldn't have, either."

"I must say I found it quite disturbing to see those sows like that. The first thing that hit me, when I went into the building to see those sows lying down, completely immobile, was what a common bond there is between the human animal and the pig animal. It seems to me that the meat trade is founded upon the exploitation of the female reproductive qualities of animals. Have you ever thought about that?"

"Well," he replies, "I think one of the saddest things in this country is that people are so far apart from all methods of production, and to anyone not used to keeping animals I'm sure it all seems terrible. I mean, those pigs are actually having a lot easier time than my own wife had during the birth of our children."

"Really?"

"Well, because they don't seem agitated, actually. I mean, they actually are not in the crates for very long, and they go in them very freely."

"But you are perverting natural maternal instincts, aren't you? Because you're confining that sow. You're stopping her from leading the full life of a mother, which all mothers, whether human or pigs, are entitled to. Surely that is a fundamental right?"

"I don't think so. Life is more complicated than that. That's too naive. That's dangerous stuff."

"What about veal. Isn't that inherently much more troubling? Killing a small, baby animal is surely one of the most horrible things that anyone can do. Doesn't that upset you?"

"Well, it upsets a lot of people, and I have to remind myself that it's similar to lamb. And objecting to killing a calf aged six months to a year is similar to killing lambs, which doesn't give me a problem, really."

"Why not?"

"If it's to die, and has lived a decent life, probably the length of time it's lived is irrelevant. It's a bit like one of the free-range chicken definitions, which actually gives a different echelon to an animal which has lived longer, in fact thirty days longer. I think that is absurd. I mean, you may accuse me of being an evil man for killing animals at all."

No, I don't think he's evil. After all, he has recognized some of the inherent cruelty in meat production, and is trying to do something about it. But I do think that he—in common with most farmers and butchers—hasn't thought through all the moral issues involved in the business.

"Your male cattle are castrated," I say. "Are you quite happy to do that?"

"As long as it's done with anesthetics."

"But essentially, it's still a mutilation."

"Yes, of course," he replies.

"But you think it's worth doing?"

"Well it doesn't actually harm the animal. I mean it depends what you call a mutilation. I've got a pierced ear; that's mutilation. I don't see it as a big problem. I mean it's part of keeping animals."

"How do they feel afterwards?"

"That would be an interesting research project. I've no idea."

"You've got no idea?"

"With beef animals, if you don't castrate them, you can't keep them outside. You're terribly stuck then. I would say that the choice between being able to get out in a field and the castration weighs in favor of letting it be outside, rather than keeping it in all the time. Very difficult decision."

Difficult, indeed. Now I want to raise another "difficult" issue, the question of human rights and animal rights. In common with many people of his generation, this young farmer was, at one stage, involved in antiapartheid demonstrations.

"Why do you feel that's an important issue?" I ask.

"Because there is discrimination in South Africa between two sorts of human beings, based entirely on color."

"So it's wrong to discriminate between the same species, on the grounds of color or genetic constitution, but it's OK to discriminate between species? That's OK?"

"I don't have a problem with it," he replies.

"What makes it all right?"

"I go back to the simple fundamental fact there is no moral problem, for me, with eating meat. It's every man's choice, and I'd love to spend hours arguing the philosophical point, and heaven knows, eventually one might be convinced. But my gut feeling tells me that eating meat's all right, as long as the animal's not abused."

"But surely," I reply, "there's no greater abuse than taking a life unnecessarily?"

"I mean during its life."

"So it's OK to commit the ultimate abuse—taking a life—but it's not alright to commit lesser abuses along the way?"

"I would say," he answers, "that living torture is probably worse than death. Isn't making an animal suffer during its life worse than killing?"

"I think it's better if the animal had never been born." I feel I have to push him now, to make him explain precisely how he justifies what he does. "But tell me, in your mind, is the pleasure you get from eating a lump of steak worth X amount of suffering to the animal?"

"That's what you call a loaded question."

"No, it's not a loaded question. I'd like a clear answer."

"The clear answer is this, that I do not believe that the way we rear animals involves suffering during their lives. Nor even their death. So it doesn't suffer. So I'm not balancing the pleasure against the suffering, I am balancing it against the life of an animal. And I square that simply because I do not see the eating of meat, and therefore the killing of an animal that has lived properly, as fundamentally wrong. And that's where you and I differ."

"The only difference is that I view the taking of a life as murder," I say. "But you don't, do you?"

"Not of animals. Do you?"

"Yes, of course."

There is an iciness in the air now.

"Are you prepared to do violence about it?" he asks me. His eyes have narrowed, and his lips are pursed. His question takes me aback.

"What do you mean?"

"I mean," he says, "there are those who burn lorries and blow people up because of it. What about that? You answer that, you owe me that much."

"Of course not," I say.

We stop talking.

THE SCIENTIST

I'd first met Dr. Alan Long at the Vegetarian Society. One of the most renowned organic chemists of his generation, he is not the kind of person to take an overly sentimental view of animals. I went to talk to him.

"Are you an animal lover?" I ask.

"I wouldn't call myself a great animal lover," he says. "I'm a great respecter of animals, and I think that when they die, they're entitled to be treated with respect, just as when human beings die."

And Dr. Long certainly knows about death, and how it comes to our food animals. For several decades, he has visited livestock markets and slaughterhouses, witnessed and recorded events there, and used this information to become one of the most informed and respected critics of our process of meat production.

"What made you get involved in this area?"

"My mother was involved with a campaign in the 1930s to abolish the pole-axe," he says. "Because of that, there was always an interest in animal matters in my family. I was very much influenced by the parable of the Good Shepherd, and I couldn't equate the allegory with the dead lamb on my plate. I decided that I preferred to see lambs in fields rather than mutton on the dinner plate. My parents were understanding, and said, 'All right, you don't have to eat lamb if you don't want to,' and so we thought it through, and gradually all of us became vegetarian.

"My mother was still concerned with animal welfare, and I went to see livestock markets with her. I suppose I was an inquiring little boy, and I asked more and more questions and eventually decided that something ought to be done about the things I saw.

"So I started to collect facts, and I became a campaigner for what was then generally perceived as a really nutty cause. I decided that the best way of dealing with this perception was to get the facts, and use them in an unemotional way."

"Now, your scientific background is quite significant, because many within the meat trade and the farming industry accuse people who feel concerned about the plight of food animals of being over-emotional."

"Yes, I thought that the animals should speak for themselves. And I don't believe in accumulating facts without making them work. I don't believe in collecting facts like stamps, just to look at and admire. I was, if you like, a self-appointed shop steward for the animals, constantly putting out all the facts I could uncover."

"Some farmers have said to me that the animals in their care are really quite happy for most of their lives, and that people like you and me are just being overemotional. How do you react to that?"

"I would say that they have no real grounds to make that assertion; in fact, they're being emotional by saying that. You have to ask, 'How do they know? Where is their evidence?' On the other hand, we certainly have scientific evidence that many animals suffer very considerably—you can do lots of experiments on stressor hormones, you can look at dehydration, that sort of thing. And I think that many farmers would privately agree that animals sent to market suffer very greatly."

"But when a farmer says to you, 'prove that my animals suffer pain,' what would you say to him?"

"Well, a lot of work has been done on this. The first thing you can point to is the general condition of the animal: many of them look quite poorly, their coat isn't in good order, that sort of thing. Then there's the environment—they suffer from the cold and the wet, just as we do. You can see cows in hot weather that are so thirsty that they try to lick the urine off the concrete, and that to my mind is definitely a sign that they are suffering. You can analyze the concentration of stressor hormones, the concentration of sugar levels in blood—all of these are signs of stress. There are 30 cases of mastitis for every 100 cows in a dairy herd. Mastitis is an inflammation. It doesn't take much imagination to think that an animal doesn't like mastitis any more than a human being does—inflammations hurt. Lameness is another prevalent problem. And you can survey the health of animals arriving at the slaughterhouse. One study has shown that 30 percent of all chickens have sustained broken bones being transported to slaughter. There's a dumpster at one market I visit where they throw the bodies of pigs that have actually died on their way to market. This sort of evidence is really incontestable."

"Pigs are particularly susceptible?"

"Yes. With modern breeding, you can see that they have been bred to be fleshy—they're really travesties, these animals. And that puts a strain on their hearts, because their organs haven't been adapted to meet the demands of intensification; they are ill-equipped to deal with the effects of stress."

"But farmers say that it's in their own commercial interests to keep the animals happy, otherwise they don't put on weight, or produce enough eggs."

"That's an old, discredited argument. Of course, they do put on weight—unhappy people will put on weight. Unfortunately, cows will continue to give milk, even though they're in a very bad way. This is understandable, because Nature's way of survival is that certain processes will go on, right to the end. The other point you have to remember is that these animals don't have to live very long. Nearly all the animals that are in production in this country are killed off in one way or another before they reach puberty. Sadly, what farmers do instead of looking after their animals with 'tender loving care' is to shovel in loads of drugs to keep them going—growth boosters and that sort of thing."

"Tell me about your first slaughterhouse experiences."

"Well, the first I went into was a little poky place. To some extent, I'd been prepared for it, because my mother had been into slaughter-houses, of course, and she'd told me. She didn't encourage me to go in, but when I was a big boy, and ready for the facts of life and death, I went in. And I was horrified, and I am still horrified. They were slaughtering horses. They weren't stunning them first; they were just cutting their throats."

"How on earth can you cut a horse's throat without somehow immobilizing it?"

"They hoist it up by its back legs."

"So you've got this enormous horse, just struggling on the end of a chain?"

"Yes. You will see an animal in that sort of circumstance, strug-gling about for a minute or so, rather like a huge, wriggling puppy."

"Now, people say small slaughterhouses are better?"

"Well, that varies a great deal. Today, most slaughterhouses are very large; they're essentially killing factories. You can go to a slaugh-terhouse where they're killing chickens, and the enormity of the whole scale is really quite appalling. These chickens being shackled upside down on conveyor belts, and being mechanically eviscerated, and mechanically defeathered. The sheer scale of the massacre—which is what it is—is rather horrifying. And the whole smell and stench of death pervades the place. The trouble with a killing factory is, if any-thing does go wrong, then it can go very wrong indeed."

"You've actually seen religious slaughter, which very few people have. What happens?"

"At the first one I went to, the foreman said to me, 'I can tell that you find this horrifying—I do too.' Well, he was an honest man, I suppose. The Jewish law requires that you use a very big knife to cut the throat, and in one stroke. In order to do this ritual, the animal has to be prevented from struggling about too much. The biggest problem that presents itself with large animals is to get them down. So in the early days, they used to tie the animal, hobble it, and throw it on the floor. When the animal was hobbled, it couldn't struggle very much, so several men pushed it over, and it lay on the ground, and they cut its throat. It got exhausted, and eventually bled to death. Well that process was very unpleasant, and there were hygienic as well as welfare objections to that. So they invented the casting pen—with the help of animal welfarists, which I find incredible.

"It was a pen into which the animal was driven, and the sides were moved up so that it was squashed in. Then the pen was capsized, so the animal was turned upside down. Those are very unpleasant circumstances, particularly for animals with a big rumen, like bullocks and cows, because the weight of their stomach actually prevents them from breathing.

"Then there begins an appalling time of battering about and screaming and wriggling—as I say, a half-ton bullock, wriggling like a little puppy. Sometimes, it will get a leg out, sometimes both legs. It would be battering its head up and down. I saw these dreadful, blood-covered casting pens where the animals were bleeding from where they'd bashed their heads on the floor, because they were so terrified. I used to time this, and it was always over a minute before the animal's struggles died down. Then they'd put some water onto its neck, which started it struggling again. Then you'd have another bout of this awful struggling. And by that time, it was more or less exhausted, and couldn't do much more. Then, an ordinary slaughterman held the animal's head, and the Jewish slaughterman, a *shochet*, took the big knife, called a *chalof*, and cut the animal's throat from side to side. In some slaughterhouses, after the cut has been made, an ordinary slaughterman may shove a knife into the chest, through the wound, to make it bleed more plentifully. And then it's hoisted up by a back leg, and left there to bleed for a while, before it's finally butchered—dressed as they say."

"Is halal, the Muslim procedure, significantly different?"

"With *halal*, quite a number will now accept prior stunning of the animal. And there are moves afoot for both types to accept slaughter in a upright position, so that the cut has to come from below.

"Sheep and goats are the main *halal* animals. I spoke to one Iman who was slaughtering, and he was complaining that he was really a holy man, a learned man, and he really shouldn't be doing things like this. The procedures in that place were equally appalling—they were not using any prestunning, and the sheep and goats were twitching about for minutes on a cratch while they bled to death, some of them were actually falling off onto the floor. And the animals were being slaughtered within sight of one another, which shouldn't have been happening. The whole thing was dreadful. The foreman of that particular place told me that he tried to do something about it, but he had trouble with race relations. He told me that he dare not stir things up, and the meat inspector told me the same. All they had succeeded in doing was to try to improve things by severing the spinal cord immediately after the cut had been made. Well that is a very dubious procedure, and that whole process was ghastly.

"Another problem with ritual slaughter taking place in a 'mixed' slaughterhouse is that it tends to corrupt the other system. You have to remember that slaughtermen are often paid on a per-kill basis, so the quicker they can get the animals through, the more it pleases them, the more money they get. If they can cut out a 'nicety'—and I use the word rather cynically—like stunning, then that will speed things up. So the ordinary slaughtermen will look at the ritual slaughterers avoiding it, and they are tempted to do the same."

"Have you come across any slaughtermen who have had qualms of conscience about what they do?"

"Yes. I often ask them, 'Would you want to do this again?' Every foremen I've asked that has said 'No.' They've told me that they're glad their children aren't doing it. Who would want their daughter to marry a slaughterman? One told me he'd never go back to slaughtering horses, and he would never have anything to do with ritual slaughter. Yes, I find that there are men who think about it in more detail. But of course, it attracts a number of people who are, unfortunately, brutal types. Every now and then you see a case of cruelty to animals, and it often involves a butcher or slaughterman. It's not really surprising."

"Yes, I know of several unpleasant cases like that. There was a slaughterman who was recently sentenced to a maximum-security hospital for strangling a woman and then drinking her blood—a real-life vampire. He said he used to do the same thing to the animals in the slaughterhouse."

"Yes, and I've come across a bunch of slaughtermen who were tormenting a cat. They'd shoved a knife in its mouth—this is an illegal way of slaughtering animals, but it is used for poultry, to stab through the mouth into the back of the throat. It's a horrid, slow death."

"Now, one more question about ritual slaughter. Many people would avoid ritually slaughtered meat if they knew the animal had been killed like that. But there's no way of telling, is there? The meat on your plate could easily come from an animal killed like this?"

"Yes. What happens is that the hindquarters of the animal can't be 'porged'—which means taking out the blood vessels and the sciatic nerve. So butchers find it more profitable to sell just the forequarters to the Jewish trade, and to pass the hindquarters into the ordinary trade. So today, you'll find that those people who criticize ritual slaughter may in reality be sitting down to eat a bit of meat killed by the very method they abhor."

"What keeps you awake at night?"

"What horrifies me most is the thought, 'Will I get hardened to all this?' "

MEAT CENTRAL U.S.A.

What actually happens in today's slaughterhouse? Gail Eisnitz is one of America's leading experts on slaughterhouse practices and has conducted investigations for the Humane Farming Association, an organization that monitors and tries to improve conditions in slaughterhouses. Over the years, she has visited many of the nation's meat packing plants, taking detailed notes, photographs, interviews, and testimonies. She knows as well as anyone what goes on in these unseen places, where living creatures are reduced to burgers, hot dogs, steaks and grills. Her book *Slaughterhouse* caused an uproar when it was published a few years ago, because it provided such incontrovertible evidence of widespread cruelty.[5] I asked Gail to explain how she first got involved in this area. This is what she told me:

My story began back in 1989 when I received a complaint from a U.S. Department of Agriculture (USDA) employee stationed inside a beef plant in Florida. He said that the cattle at his plant were not being properly stunned and they were still alive and fully conscious when they were having their heads skinned. Not only was he concerned for the animals, but he was also worried about the workers who were getting injured by struggling animals that were kicking and thrashing as workers were skinning them. I contacted USDA headquarters to ask about conditions at that plant and was told that the allegations were not true, so I traveled down to Florida and interviewed plant workers who corroborated the allegations. Before contacting me, the whistle-blower had attempted to get corrective action from his USDA supervisors, and when that failed, he had gone to members of Congress, the Veteran's Administration, anyone who would listen. When word leaked through one of his friends that he had contacted me for help, he was fired.

The fact that he was fired was pretty ironic since the U.S. Department of Agriculture is the very agency that is charged with enforcing the Humane Slaughter Act. The Humane Slaughter Act was passed nearly fifty years ago to ensure that animals in federally inspected packing plants are not abused during handling or slaughter. More specifically, the Humane Slaughter Act requires that animals in federally inspected slaughterhouses—those are the slaughterhouses that kill 98 percent of farm animals—be handled humanely from the moment they set foot on slaughterhouse grounds; and that they be rendered unconscious with one application of an effective stunning device prior to being shackled and hoisted up on the line. Once stunned, animals must remain unconscious during shackling, hoisting, bleeding, and butchering.

Stunning is accomplished in a variety of ways. Cattle are rendered unconscious or "knocked" with a captive bolt gun, which is activated by a guy who stands over the animal's head and shoots a metal rod into the head, and then quickly retracts it. After stunning, the cow has a shackle placed around a hind leg, is hoisted up on to a moving rail, has the throat cut—that process is called "sticking" and is performed by the "sticker"—is supposed to bleed out for several minutes, and then is skinned and dismembered. With pigs, it's a little different. They are stunned with electricity applied behind the ears (and sometimes on the back), shocked into unconsciousness, shackled, hoisted up on the rail, they have their throats cut, and then, after bleeding out for several minutes, they are dragged through a long tank of scalding water to loosen their bristles for removal.

The Humane Slaughter Act has other provisions also, like requiring that disabled animals be protected from inclement weather conditions; that pipes and sharp objects not be used to prod animals; that animals are not to be dragged; that animals have access to water at all times and feed if held more than 24 hours. Humane Slaughter Act regulations authorize USDA meat inspectors and veterinarians stationed in slaughter plants, whose primary responsibility is to inspect carcasses, body parts, and meat for wholesomeness *after* animals are slaughtered, to stop the slaughter process when violations occur and are not immediately corrected.

In the last fifteen years, more than 2,000 small to mid-sized packing plants—or one-third of the nation's packing plants—had been forced out of business by a few large, high-speed operations, each with the capacity to kill millions of animals a year. Today eleven plants slaughter nearly half of all cattle in the country, and ten plants slaughter nearly half of all hogs. With fewer slaughterhouses killing a growing number of animals, slaughter "line speeds" have skyrocketed.

Today, as individual workers struggle to kill as many as 1,100 animals per hour—that's one animal every three seconds—a production mentality has emerged in which the slaughter line does not stop for anything: not for injured workers—they're just supposed to be dragged away from the moving line—not for contaminated meat, and least of all, not for slow or uncooperative animals. In an operation, a minute of "down time" can spell a loss of hundreds, if not thousands, of dollars, so workers often find themselves resorting to brutality to keep the production line running uninterrupted to keep their jobs. That translates to deliberately strangling, scalding, skinning, and dismembering fully conscious animals, all in an effort to keep up with the pace and keep the line running smoothly.

But back to my story. After I corroborated the violations down in Florida, I got a lead on another plant, this one in the Midwest, where pigs were supposedly being immersed into the scalding tank alive. Word had it that at this plant, the stunning equipment was bursting blood vessels and marking the hogs' loins, and as a result, the plant reduced the amount of electricity in the stunning equipment. Stunning the pigs without the necessary electricity was not rendering them unconscious. As a result, thousands of hogs were being shackled alive and since they were struggling, it was difficult to cut their throats properly to get an adequate bleed; then the hogs weren't given enough time to bleed fully, and so they were being immersed in the scalding tank alive, kicking and splashing water all over and squealing. Like many other violations, this is all captured as evidence on video.

After talking to a lot of workers, I also learned that frustrated stunners, shacklers, and stickers were beating pigs with pipes, poking their eyes out, chasing them into the scalding tank alive, crushing their skulls. They stuck electric prods up animals' butts and in their eyes and held them there. They dragged disabled animals with meat hooks in their mouths and anuses until their intestines ripped out. When there was down time, workers half-stunned pigs with electricity to watch them flip up in the air. They also described the routine arrival of hogs frozen solid from transport in subzero temperatures that would have to be pried off the sides of trucks—leaving chunks of skin behind—and then were ultimately tossed onto piles of dead hogs until they died. They allowed disabled animals to freeze to concrete floors, and then stay there for days; they chain-sawed hogs alive into pieces for rendering.

I believe that the people who work in these places are victims, too, of a system that brutalizes both humans and animals. Here are some notes from my records of comments that particularly stick in my mind:

"After a while you become desensitized. And as far as animals go, they're a lower life-form. They're maybe one step above a maggot. When you got a live, conscious hog, you not only kill it, you want to make it *hurt*. You go in hard, blow the windpipe, make it drown in its own blood. Take out an eyeball, split its nose. A live hog would be running around the pit with me. It would be looking up at me and I would just take my knife and—eerk—take its eye out while it was just sitting there. And this hog would just scream."

"If you get a hog in the chute that refuses to move, you take a meat hook and clip it into his anus. You try to do this by clipping the hipbone. Then you drag him backwards. You're dragging these hogs alive, and a lot of times the meat hook rips out of the bunghole. I've seen hams—thighs—completely ripped open. I've also seen intestines come out. If the hog collapses near the front of the chute, you shove a meat hook into his cheek and drag him forward."

"The preferred method of handling a cripple is to beat him to death with a lead pipe before he gets into the chute. It's called 'piping.' All the drivers use pipes to kill hogs that can't go through the chutes. Or if a hog refuses to go into the chutes and is stopping production, you beat him to death."

"Hogs are stubborn. Beating them in the head seems to work about the best. Piece of rebar about an inch across, you force a hog down the alley, have another guy standing there with a piece of rebar in his hand. It's just like playing baseball. Just like somebody pitching something at you."

Sadly, every time I thought I'd encountered the worst violations I could imagine, I'd visit another plant with even more horrendous violations. I criss-crossed the country visiting more pig, horse, and cattle plants. I met slaughter workers through the workers' union, by hanging out in post offices, employment offices, convenience stores, bars, cafés, trailer parks. Sometimes I'd find out their addresses, stake out their homes until they arrived, and then I'd literally follow them into their houses. I got to talk to scores of workers any way I could. And I devised reasonable covers that got me inside many plants as well. The workers I talked with represented 2.5 million hours on the kill floor. They let me audiotape our conversations, and most of them signed sworn affidavits about what they'd seen and done.

They told me that they routinely had to pound away at cows' and horses' heads with ineffective captive bolt guns in order to render the animals unconscious. Workers strangled cattle with cables when they were dragging them up to the stun area, they listened to bones cracking and necks popping when they dragged horses. They used saws or blow-torches to remove the legs of live cattle that were stuck in trucks in chutes, and in the stun area. They drove over the legs and heads of disabled animals with tractors; they routinely skinned heads, bellies, sides and rumps, removed legs, ears, horns, and tails, and began eviscerating cattle that were alive.

"When a cow arrives at the first hind-legger [who removes the legs], usually the legger tries to make a cut to start skinning out the leg. But it's hard to do that when the cow is kicking violently. A lot of times the leggers'll take their clippers and cut off the cow's leg right below the knee—the skinny part. The cow'll continue to kick, but it don't have that long of a reach."

"I've seen thousands and thousands of cows go through the slaughter process alive. If I see a live animal, I cannot stop the line. Because the supervisor has told us that you have to work on a cow that's alive."

"One day when I went out to the suspect pen, two employees were using metal pipes to club some hogs to death. There had to be twenty little hogs out there that they were going to give to the rendering company. And these two guys were out there beating them to death with clubs and having a good old time. I went to the USDA vet, my supervisor, to complain. He said, 'They're of no value because they're going to be tanked [rendered] anyway.' So, according to my supervisor, it was all right to club those little hogs to death. They were beating them like they do those little seals in Alaska."

"I've seen them put twenty to twenty-five holes in a hog's head trying to knock her and she was still on her feet. Her head looked like Swiss cheese. Tough gal. Sometimes they'll use a twenty-two and shoot the hog through its eye. Or you might have to hit both eyes on the same hog."

"A steer was running up the alley way and got his leg between the boards and he couldn't get it out. They didn't want to lose any time killing cattle and he was blocking their path, so they just used a blow torch to burn his leg off while he was alive."

Shockingly, it's not just the workers and inspectors making comments such as these. In 1996, the USDA commissioned its own study of humane slaughter to be conducted by an independent consultant in a handful of USDA inspected plants. Despite the fact that the USDA's study was announced—the plants were anticipating the visit from the USDA consultant—the study indicated that 7 out of the 11 beef plants visited had unacceptable stunning.

Yet, despite its clear Congressional mandate, and the fact that it's got badge-carrying law enforcing meat inspectors present inside every plant, the USDA has decided that the solution to the problem is more *voluntary* programs to be implemented by the meat industry. I believe that the USDA has enjoyed an incestuous relationship with the meat industry for years, and it is actively trying to come up with ways to further *deregulate* the meat industry . . . with what consequences I shudder to think.

I would like consumers to also be aware of the 8.2 *billion chickens* who are exempt from the Humane Slaughter Act, yet who are subject to incredible suffering at slaughter. The U.S. poultry industry clings to the myth that a dead bird won't bleed properly—so they want to keep its heart beating—yet they need to immobilize birds to facilitate neck cutting. To do this, U.S. poultry processors, on an average, use only about one-tenth the current necessary to ensure that birds are adequately stunned. The result is that untold numbers of birds are going into the scalding tank alive.

Over the course of my investigations, I have faced many roadblocks: informants were gagged and fired; one was stabbed to death; TV producers repeatedly got my hopes up that they would expose my findings only to drop the story when a top executive worries that the subject is too disgusting and will result in viewers switching channels. And yet, I still do believe that the American public truly cares about this issue, once they are fully informed of the facts. Most people are naturally compassionate, and would not want to give their money to an industry in which such atrocities are routinely perpetrated on our fellow creatures. That's why it is important for people to know the truth."

RELIGIOUS SLAUGHTER

Religious slaughter was once described to me by an official veterinary surgeon (someone who spent most of his working life watching animals being killed) as "the most revolting sight I have ever seen inside a slaughterhouse." He told me how it would sometimes take up to four slaughtermen to hold one sheep down as it struggled on the slaughtering table. The slaughterer then cuts the animal's neck open, and allows it to bleed to death. "He didn't cut so much as saw," the vet said to me. "It took four attempts by the slaughterman before the animal's arteries were finally severed."

Now there's one huge problem associated with religious slaughter, and that is the ethnic dimension. Extreme right-wing elements have already tried to use this issue as a means of stirring up hatred against both the Jewish and Muslim communities. And both communities have reacted strongly to defend what they perceive as an ethnically motivated attack on their way of life. Because of this, most animal welfare organizations have been very reluctant to confront the problem.

In fact, religious slaughter affects all meat eaters, not just those Muslims and Jews who believe it to be necessary. Because every person who eats meat will, without knowing, have eaten ritually slaughtered food at some time. It is estimated that approximately 70 percent of the meat that comes from animals that have been killed by ritual means actually ends up on the open market, finding its way into school meals, restaurants, and meat products of all descriptions.

Basically, there are two main reasons for the Jewish (*schechita*, or kosher) and Islamic (*dhabbih* or *halal*) ways of slaughtering. First, the animal must be "whole" if it is to be consumed by humans. This is taken to mean that it must not be sick or damaged in any way. It is therefore argued that prestunning, even if it occurs only a few seconds before death, is not acceptable, since it results in a damaged animal. The second reason is to exsanguinate (bleed out) the animal, since consuming its blood is not permitted.

"Blood is unhealthy," explained Dr. A. M. Katme, a representative of the Islamic Medical Association. "It is full of toxins, urea, and organisms. The consumption of blood is forbidden for Muslims. . . . It is arrogant for someone who is not a Muslim to presume that he can teach us the practice of our faith. God protect us from those who think that they know better than He."[6]

I have no wish to teach anyone their faith, but I must respectfully point out a fundamental reality of religious slaughter, which is that it is never possible to drain all of the animal's blood from its body—as any vet can testify. So if Muslims are to correctly observe the prohibition against the consumption of blood, it therefore follows that they should not eat meat. This is an often-overlooked reality, and it should be urgently and honestly addressed.

The proponents of religious slaughter claim that the loss of blood the animal suffers is so sudden that it induces rapid unconsciousness. This is how the chairman of the Shechita Committee of the board of Deputies of British Jews explains it:

"The animal's throat is cut, and the whole operation can, if done properly, take less than half a minute. People imagine that because the animal has its throat cut while fully conscious it must be in pain. But what has been found as a result of experiments conducted in the late 1970s at the University of Hanover is that the animal becomes unconscious within two seconds of its throat being cut."[7] Rabbi Berkovits, registrar of the Court of the Chief Rabbi, has defended *shechita* on much the same grounds, claiming that it is preferable to the conventional stunning and slaughtering process.[8]

But here, the supporters of religious slaughter are on very shaky ground. The majority of vets I have spoken to strongly dislike ritual slaughter for the "pain, suffering, and distress" it causes the animals (to use the words of the British government's Farm Animal Welfare Council). Research undertaken by the Institute for Food Research and the Institute for Tierzucht und Tierverhalten in Germany clearly shows that animals killed by ritual slaughter may remain conscious for up to two minutes after their throats are cut.[9] The researchers implanted electrodes in the cerebral cortex of animals to be slaughtered, and found that the animals' brains would respond to a stimulus up to 126 seconds after the cut.

Research carried out at a New Zealand university found that calves were making attempts to get up off the floor *five or six minutes* after their throats had been cut. One Birmingham vet (Birmingham has several major slaughterhouses that are devoted to ritual killing), believes that it can take up to twelve minutes for the animal to lose consciousness. "How would you feel about the same fate for your cat or dog?" he asks. "There's no difference."[10] Another vet explained to me that all animals (including humans) have several arteries supplying the brain, and not just the carotid ones that are slashed in ritual slaughter. He explained that another major artery, the vertebral one, ran close to the spinal column, and it would be quite impossible to sever this (unless the whole head was cut off). Consequently, this artery goes on supplying blood to the brain even after the others have been cut, thus prolonging the animal's agony.

Fortunately, there are compassionate people within both Jewish and Muslim communities who understand the need for immediate reform. Over the past few years, I have been fortunate enough to make a number of friends within the Jewish vegetarian movement. They have struck me, without exception, as being caring, concerned people, whose sincere approach to Judaism may provide others in their community with some serious food for thought, so to speak. An editorial in the Jewish vegetarian magazine is well worth pondering, as it relates to our treatment of food animals today:

The Sabbath day was granted to all, and Rashi comments that even domestic creatures, at least on that day, must not be enclosed but shall be free to graze and enjoy the work of creation. If now they are incarcerated in darkened containers seven days and seven nights in each week for the entire period of their lives; if they neither see the luminaries of the heavens nor experience the sweet smell and the taste of the pastures, has not the most sacred Sabbath Law been flagrantly violated, and can the flesh of their bodies be Kosher?

Would the law that states "Thou shalt not muzzle the ox when he treads the corn" acquiesce in the computerized feeding of chemical fatteners, whilst the poor beast scents the dew and clover in the meadows beyond his darkened cell?

When it is written "Thou shalt not yoke an ox with an ass" does it imply that a calf may spend its entire life standing on slats, never to lie down, and effectively chained to the sides by its neck to prevent it doing so? Is this a perversion of the Torah? And when the unfortunate victim is slaughtered, can its remains be considered Kosher?

If the law forbids one to cause distress to a mother bird by removing eggs from the nest in her presence, would it concur that during its lifetime a hen could be shut up in a receptacle of twelve square inches, its beak removed and feathers clipped? And after its throat is cut, would its body be Kosher for food?

If a cruelly treated animal shall be considered unfit for food, and if the measure of the cruelty is determined by its ability to walk, do the authorities inspect the incarcerated animals in the factory farms, and is there any record as to whether they are able to walk to their own slaughter on their own emaciated legs? And if not is their flesh Kosher?

If the law forbids the mixing of species, even of plants, and confusion of sexes, would it condone the injection of female hormones into the male beast, even though it is acknowledged to be cancerous in practice? And when this distortion of blood is covered with earth, even as is human blood, is this respect for the Creator who saw that all he created was very good? Or is this confusion, is it defilement, is it sacrilege, and is the flesh still Kosher?

Shall a certificate of Beth Din convey that Torah min hashamayim has been sincerely observed, or shall it become a license for misinterpretation, evasion, and permission to the beholder to bow down each man to the God of his own stomach?

Let all who are observant and devout remember that the responsibility is their own; no Jew can use an intermediary, whether in this case it be a Beth Din, a Board of Shechita, or just a Kosher butcher with a label on his window. If unaware of the facts, his is a sin of omission; if he is aware and chooses to ignore his personal responsibility, his is a sin of commission; he is eating Trefah.[11]

These are good and wise questions, which raise fundamental issues of conscience that all of us, Jewish or not, must urgently consider.

PIG TALES

The problem with pigs is that they are uncomfortably similar to humans in far too many ways.

Pigs, for example, know how to have fun. They will play with each other, and with humans, for hours on end, if they can. "Those who know pigs can't help but be charmed by their intelligent, social, and sensitive nature," write Melanie Adcock, D.V.M, and Mary Finelli of the Humane Society of the United States. "Yet perhaps no other species has been so misrepresented, misunderstood, and, even, betrayed. A glutton is labeled a hog, a messy person is termed a pig. The people caring for both *Charlotte's Web*'s Wilbur and his modern counterpart Babe love them one minute, yet intend to kill them and eat them for dinner the next. How can society be so insensitive—so conflicted—toward a species when it finds the individual members of that species so adorable?"[12]

Some Pig Points:

- If they can, pigs form peaceful family groups of ten or fewer members, who sleep in a communal nest.
- Pigs are more intelligent than dogs, naturally very clean animals, and discriminating eaters. Unable to sweat, they bathe in mud to cool off and to protect their skin from sun and insects.
- They enjoy novelty and are extremely active and inquisitive. When free to roam, they spend much of their day enthusiastically smelling, nibbling, and manipulating objects with their snouts. A pig's sense of smell is so keen that the animal is trained in France to unearth truffles, an edible fungus that grows underground.
- Adults in the social group will protect a piglet, leaving food or their own litters to defend the endangered youngster.
- Touch and bodily contact are especially important. Pigs seek out and enjoy close contact and lie close together when resting. They also enjoy close contact with people familiar to them and will roll over to have their bellies rubbed.
- They have an elaborate courtship ritual, including a song between males and females. Newborn piglets learn to run to

their mother's voice, and the mother pig sings to her young while nursing. After nursing, a piglet will sometimes run to "Mom's" face to rub snouts and grunt.

- Vivisectors call pigs "horizontal man" because the arrangement of their internal organs is so similar to humans.
- According to those who have tasted both, pig flesh tastes very similar to human flesh.

Yes indeed, the problem for the unfortunate pigs is that they are really far too similar to us, far too similar for their own good. Perhaps that is why we disparage and ridicule them so much—it puts some metaphorical distance between the two species, without which, our ruthless exploitation of them would be far more distressing for us.

I'd like you to meet someone who knows about pigs. Andrew Tyler is a friend of mine, a good journalist and a talented writer. He has spent a long time working incognito on pig farms. Here is an extract from the diary he kept while working on one such farm, an establishment raising thousands of animals each year for both slaughter and breeding. Tyler's diary is almost certainly the most accurate account of the secret life of today's pigs that you will ever read.

Woke up tired, burning eyes at 5:30. Got to the farrowing house to find a litter of ten piglets had been born in the night. They were still shuffling clumsily around their mother when Ed, the farm manager, demonstrated the art of teeth and nail clipping—done with a pair of steel pliers. First the teeth—two on top, two on the bottom, both sides. The piglet is seized, his jaws forced open, and the little pointy teeth clipped off, down to the gum. Such squealing! Then an inch of tail is removed and a squirt of purple antiseptic applied to the belly over the umbilical. The operation ends with the young one being chucked back in the pen. Always they are thrown, grabbed—by a back leg or ears, no matter how small.

Next I watch ten sows moved from the house where they'd been impregnated to the pens in which they'll wait out their pregnancy—all of them assumed now to be "in pig." After which I check inside the drug cabinet, a battered tin object with its doors permanently swung open, and see the staggering array of antibiotics, de-wormers, growth boosters, antiseptics used here.

At 8:30 weaning begins—among the cruelest of the host of daily cruelties. Twelve sows with 113 piglets on them are removed from their farrowing crates—tight-fitting metal contraptions that allow the mother to stand and flop down but not turn around. She has been sharing it with her young since their birth 21 days earlier. Now the sow is removed with a shout and a slap—backward, down the steep stone step into a central aisle that is slippery with shit and piss; you'd have thought they might have cleaned it out first. They are slapped on the head, pulled by the tail, and kicked out of the joint, most of them struggling to remain with their young, who stare bewilderingly at the tailboard of the crate and the direction in which their mothers are being taken. The men will be back for them soon.

Most of the sows rebel and try to return to their young while being driven across the yard to their next stop: the service house. Here they are penned up and, incredibly, an hour later, checked to see if they are ripe for another servicing. Being a mixed batch, unused to each other, and disturbed through being torn from their young, the sows fight among themselves. Simultaneously, they are howling and screaming for their young. Ed tells me that fighting and complaining go on 'for a day or two.' Another worker, Mac, goes round them, pushing and actually riding on their backs, examining their vulvas and decides one is ready to be served. He leads her out to a boar in a facing pen. When she gets there they discover her milk sac is bleeding and raw, possibly from a fight, possibly from being stood on. Mac applies the remedy—an antiseptic spray and antibiotic injection in the neck—even while she's in the boar's pen. The boar tries to mount. She screams and runs. They try her again but realize she wasn't on heat at all but "stood" for Mac's riding because she'd been trapped by the other sows in the crowded pen and couldn't go anywhere.

As well as the boars penned in the service house, there are half a dozen in individual old-fashioned brick styes just across the yard. A sow who was "served" on successive days three weeks ago but failed to fall pregnant is taken to one of these. She's mounted and, as the penis is inserted, she howls and begins bleeding, quite a lot of blood. They believe at first it's the male's sheath but continue anyway once they realize it's coming from here— Mac assisting entry with his fingers. It seems the boar has struck her bladder, a common complaint. They persist in cornering the female so the impregnation can continue but the sow eventually breaks loose making it impossible. She gets an antibiotic jab, a splash of purple marker on her shoulders and, I'm told, she'll be served again this afternoon. "Raped" is probably a more suitable word than "served."

Disease problems they have had to cope with include viral pneumonia scours (a diarrhea that in the young is often lethal), meningitis—which the owner describes as "virtually similar to the human kind," salt poisoning (an often lethal and often agonizing condition caused by them not getting enough drinking water), plus there is the memory of Aujeszky's disease outbreak some seven years ago.

I ask the owner what happens to the dead animals. He'd already acknowledged that the smaller ones at the other farm were dumped on the muck heap to be spread on the fields. But here, being bereft of straw, they have no muck heap. He says the corpses all go into a "death pit," but he looks seedy when offering this. Maybe because, as I witnessed, his death pits seem to breach the health and safety rules by not being enfenced; or maybe it's because the small ones are actually tossed straight into the lagoons. The death pit is an incredible sight; a hole about seven feet deep, about ten feet square, and clogged with the decomposing corpses of grown and half-grown animals, some beginning to go green, the skin and flesh bubbling vilely. They are in a variety of twisted positions, rear ends and snouts up but none fully submerged. Perhaps these represent just the top layers of animals, unable to sink for the bodies of their comrades.

So this is how bacon is brought into the world. Later, Andrew witnesses the conclusion of the process:

No sign declares the name or nature of the business, and it is a condition of my entry that I withhold the firm's identity. All the animals start in the lairage—a large stone area divided by bar gates into a system of pens. Before the pigs' throats are opened, they receive what the plant manager calls "electrical stimulation" of the brain. The manager has just such a phrase for every aspect of the killing process.

The "stimulation" is accomplished by a pair of hand-operated tongs, like giant pliers, that are clamped on either side of the pig's head just in front of the ears. This takes place in a stunning box, a walled-in area about fifteen feet square into which about a dozen animals at a time are corralled. The stunner himself is a lank, bony faced man, bearded, with one wayward eye, and forearms tattooed with the Reaper and wreathed skulls.

As the first dozen is driven into the stunning pen, one urinates on the trot and makes a screeching noise I hadn't heard before. Blood and mucus fly from his snout. The eyes close, the front legs stiffen, and when the tongs are opened, he falls, like a log, on his side. He lies there, back legs kicking, as the stunner turns to the next animal. He tells me that the tongs should be held on for a minimum of seven seconds to ensure a proper stun before the throat is cut. But, urged on by his mates further along the slaughter line, he is giving them one and a half or less.

When he has stunned three or four, he shackles each of them with a chain around a back leg. They are then mechanically lifted and carried to an adjoining stone room, where a colleague cuts deep into the neck and the still pumping heart gushes out blood. They are supposed to stun and shackle one animal at a time, since the delay involved in doing them in groups means they could go wide awake to the knife.

Suddenly an electrocuted animal slips her shackle, drops five feet to the stone floor, and crash lands on her head. The stunner continues jolting more creatures while her back legs paddle furiously. Without restunning her, he hooks her up again and sends her through to the knife. This crash-landing routine is to be repeated several more times in the next few minutes.

One animal slams down twice. One man curses him as he lies paddling, blood seeping from anus and mouth. Another man, meanwhile, is ear-wrestling a would-be escapee that is leaping at a small opening in the metal gate. "You can have it another fucking way then, you idiot," he cries, as he helps slap the animal down.

There is just one more waiting for the tongs, a small quiet creature which, from her position near the gate, looks me directly in the eye, breaking my heart. The stunner chases her a few steps. The tongs first ineptly clasp her neck; the eyes close in a strange blissful agony. The tongs are adjusted, and like a rock she falls.

IN PRAISE OF PITY

The farmers and the butchers say it is wrong to feel moved, to be horrified, or even to shed a tear when you read accounts of everyday atrocities such as these. They say that we are being emotional, sentimental, even hysterical. They say that our hearts rule our heads.

But what I say is this: if you do not shudder when you learn about these dreadful things, then you are missing part of your humanity. Let's examine this.

For a man, the charge of "being emotional" is particularly stinging, because emotion is thought of as a female quality. Evidently, a man who is accused of being "emotional" is also implicitly accused of being something less than male. In a world where testosterone sets the agenda, this is a grave accusation, indeed.

Think how this parallels those appalling words of hatred we uncovered in the first chapter: "The human race ranks highly because it belongs to the class of beasts of prey. . . . We find in man the tactics of life proper to a bold, cunning beast of prey. . . . He lives engaged in aggression, killing, annihilation." This sort of human being does not shudder, does not feel empathy, does not feel joy or love. The emotions of kindness, pity, mercy, and compassion are far beyond his limited experience—mere weaknesses to be eliminated.

And this is the sort of human being the meat industry implies we ought to be.

Hmmm . . .

Their motives are obvious, of course. Writer Brigid Brophy exposes them with great precision:

"Whenever people say 'We mustn't be sentimental,' you can take it they are about to do something cruel. And if they add 'We must be realistic,' they mean they are going to make money out of it. These slogans have a long history. After being used to justify slave traders, ruthless industrialists, and contractors who had found that the most economically 'realistic' method of cleaning a chimney was to force a small child to climb it, they have now been passed on, like an heirloom, to the factory farmers. 'We mustn't be sentimental' tries to persuade us that factory farming isn't, in fact, cruel. It implies that the whole problem had been invented by our sloppy imaginations."[13]

Writer Robert Bly well understands the importance of gaining access to these prohibited feelings:

"Children are able to shudder easily, and a child will often break into tears when he or she sees a wounded animal. But later the domination system enters, and some boys begin to torture and kill insects and animals to perfume their own insignificance. . . .

"Gaining the ability to shudder means feeling how frail human beings are. . . . When one is shuddering, the shudder helps to take away the numbness we spoke of. When a man possesses empathy, it does not mean that he has developed the feminine feeling only; of course he has, and it is good to develop the feminine. But when he learns to shudder, he is developing a part of the masculine emotional body as well."[14]

I was once on a radio program with a representative of the meat industry.

"What did you feel when you first went into a slaughterhouse?" I asked.

He looked at me as if I had just made a pass at him.

"I didn't *feel* anything," he said.

"Well," I asked, "what did you *think*?"

"I thought it was not well organized, and I wanted to make it more efficient."

I don't think I want to live in a world where efficiency has replaced compassion.

YOUR MOVE

I suspect we are at something of an important turning point in our species' history. A new kind of ethic seems to be emerging—a universally appropriate morality which, in the words of Einstein, will "widen our circle of compassion to embrace all living creatures and the whole of nature." A century before Einstein, Abraham Lincoln had predicted the fundamental importance of this emerging ethic, saying "I am in favor of animal rights as well as human rights. That is the way of a whole human being."

By changing your diet to refuse to consume the products of cruelty, you are actively extending Einstein's "circle of compassion." It's not a difficult process; it conveys many health benefits as you'll see in the next chapter, and it is a very powerful way of bringing about positive change.

After all, if you like animals, one of the nicest things you can do for them is not eat them.

4

THE MANUAL OF VEGETARIAN HEALTH

"Introducing the Everyday Hero. She's your mother, your daughter, your sister, your grandmother, your wife. If you're a woman, she's you. She punches a clock, washes the clothes, pays the bills, carts the kids to soccer practice (and makes every game, too). She packs lunches, picks up her husband's dry cleaning, changes the baby, checks on her aged mother, consoles her best friend, and still manages to get dinner on the table each night. She doesn't cure cancer."

Bizarre advertising material issued by the National Cattlemen's Beef Association, presumably intended to make beef entirely irresistible to women. The date is the most surprising thing of all: February 2001[1]

"If meat really was bad for you we could be sure the Government and the majority of health and diet professionals (not to mention the leaders of most religious groups) would have joined together to tell us so."

Meat & Livestock Commission, PR materials for schoolchildren[2]

The truth is out there, but it's pretty difficult to find. Organizations such as the National Cattlemen's Beef Association spend significant time and resources denigrating the vegetarian diet.[3] They do this for obviously commercial purposes: clearly, the more vegetarians there are, the fewer consumers there will be for their products of the slaughterhouse. Their material is intended to reach far and wide, and influence consumers, health care professionals, teachers and indeed, schoolchildren.

Unfortunately, there is little in the way of an equivalent commercial lobbying organization to put forth the vegetarian point of view, so it's often a rather one-sided battle. In this chapter, you will find an enormous amount of information that redresses the balance. I think you'll find it eye-opening.

ANEMIA

Vegetarians don't eat red meat, and since red meat contains iron, vegetarians are at risk of anemia, aren't they? So runs the logic of the meat industry, for whom the risk of iron-deficiency anemia is a major marketing opportunity. This is defensive marketing at its nastiest: if you can't tempt consumers to buy your product, then frighten them into believing that they will die without it. So you may be surprised to know that, despite all the meat industry propaganda, the facts reveal that a healthy vegetarian diet is an excellent way to get all the iron you need.

What Is It?

Anemia literally means "lack of blood." More precisely, the word is used to refer to a reduction in the oxygen-carrying capacity of the blood, which can be caused in three main ways:

- Loss of blood (e.g. heavy menstrual periods)
- Excessive red blood cell destruction
- Defective red blood cell formation

Oxygen is held within the red blood cells by the pigment hemoglobin, which transports oxygen from the lungs to body cells and returns waste carbon dioxide from the cells to the lungs. About 20 percent of the total oxygen used each day is used by the human brain. Fatigue and mental dullness occur when the brain doesn't get enough oxygen. If your hemoglobin level drops, your heart rate will speed up, and you will start breathing faster to try to compensate for the lower oxygen delivery. Replacement of hemoglobin requires iron in the diet, as well as vitamin B_{12} and folic acid. If any of these are inadequately present, or are inadequately absorbed, anemia will result. There are many kinds of anemias, but the most common include

- Iron-deficiency anemia. Caused by either chronic blood loss or insufficient iron absorption or utilization.
- Pernicious anemia. More often found in middle-aged and older people. Generally, it is caused by an inability to produce an enzyme (known as the "intrinsic factor") that is essential for the proper assimilation of vitamin B_{12}.

Iron-deficiency anemia is thought to be a common nutritional problem, although precise estimates of its incidence range very widely. Some suggest that up to 65 percent of all women in Western countries may have "low" iron stores in their bodies, and up to 20 percent may suffer from iron-deficiency anemia.[4] In Britain, a survey for the Ministry of Agriculture suggests that young women (ages fifteen to twenty-five) consume, on average, only three-quarters of the recommended daily allowance of iron.[5] Whatever the exact figures, it is clear that this is a widespread health problem, and vegetarians would be wrong to trivialize it. However, the meat industry is equally wrong to imply—as their advertising often seems to—that meat eaters need not worry about iron-deficiency anemia. Clearly, such exaggeration is dangerous rubbish. With up to one in five women suffering from it, the problem of iron-deficiency anemia is a real concern for meat-eating women.

How the Vegetarian Diet Can Help
Since anemia can result from an inadequate intake of three nutrients—iron, vitamin B_{12}, and folic acid—it is often alleged that vegetarians are risking their health, and are condemned to become anemic. But is this true? In a word: No! Let's examine each nutrient:

Iron-Deficiency Anemia
Iron-deficiency anemia is uncommon in men, but more widespread in women. Obviously, iron-deficiency anemia can simply be caused by not consuming enough iron in the diet, but it can also occur if the

body does not properly absorb the iron in food—for example, chronic diarrhea or the prolonged use of antacids may impair absorption.

Iron is a trace element. The adult body contains a total of about 3 to 5 grams. About two-thirds of this is bound up in hemoglobin, and about a fifth is held in storage, much of it in the form called ferritin. This remarkable protein allows animals to survive for considerable periods without dietary iron. Most of these ferritin iron stores are found in the liver, bone marrow, and spleen. However, minute amounts of ferritin are also found in the blood. One test for iron deficiency measures the amount of ferritin present in the blood, because that gives a good idea of the quantity of ferritin present at the body's main storage sites. Plasma ferritin of 12 micrograms per liter or less suggests that iron stores are becoming depleted.[6] Plasma ferritin levels will, however, naturally vary in a normal human. For example, they tend to be higher in the morning, and lower in the evening. Stress, too, can affect the results of ferritin tests, as can recent infection. But carefully conducted tests that reveal a consistent picture of steadily declining ferritin levels indicate the beginnings of iron deficiency, which if unchecked, will eventually result in anemia. Those population groups at particular risk of iron deficiency include

- Infants
- Teenage girls
- Pregnant women
- Women of childbearing years
- The elderly

Blood loss due to menstruation is the most common cause of iron deficiency among women of childbearing years. It is of great importance that people in all these groups obtain enough dietary iron to replace natural losses.

Since some types of meat (principally liver) provide large amounts of iron, and since some of that iron is in a form (heme) that is more easily assimilated than the iron found in plants (nonheme), conventional wisdom recommends the consumption of meat as the main source of dietary iron. However, there are several logical objections to this point of view:

- As already mentioned, iron-deficiency anemia is a problem that affects a large section of the population, who are mostly meat eaters. Meat consumption, therefore, does not appear to be an effective means of preventing widespread iron deficiency.
- Other primates eat a naturally vegetarian diet (a chimpanzee does not, as a rule, breakfast on sausages!) and do not suffer from iron-deficiency anemia.
- A vegetarian or vegan diet is well capable of providing normal dietary iron requirements, generally obtained from dark green, leafy vegetables, iron-fortified cereals, and whole grains.
- New evidence (see below) suggests that the overconsumption of iron-rich foods may in fact be a health hazard.

In addition, scientific fieldwork in this area paints an extremely revealing picture, which flatly contradicts the notion that vegetarians are at particular risk of iron deficiency. For example:

- A study of British vegans concludes that their iron level is "normal in all the vegans and no subject had a hemoglobin concentration below the lower limit of normality."[7]
- In their 1988 position paper concerning the vegetarian diet, the American Dietetic Association concluded, "With both vegetarian and nonvegetarian diets, iron and folate supplements are usually necessary during pregnancy, although vegetarians frequently have greater intakes of those nutrients than do nonvegetarians."[8]
- Further field studies conducted among British vegans report dietary iron intakes of 22.4 mg[9], 31 mg,[10] and 20.5 mg[11] per day. The mean figure of these studies (24.6 mg) is more than *double* the official estimated average requirement (EAR) of 11.4 mg a day!
- In Israel, a study compared the iron intakes of meat eaters and vegetarians, summarizing: "The intake of iron was significantly higher in the vegetarians . . . it is concluded that a long-term ovo-lacto vegetarian diet does not lead to mineral deficiencies."[12]
- In Holland, another study compared meat-eating and vegetar-

ian preschool children. While the vegetarian children had a good intake of dietary iron, the meat eaters "had intakes of iron below the Dutch RDAs [recommended daily requirements]."[13]

- In Sweden, yet another study compared the diet eaten by vegans to that of meat eaters, and found that the vegans' iron consumption was "nearly double."[14]

- A Canadian study looked at the iron levels of long-term vegetarian Seven-Day Adventist women and concluded, "The iron and zinc status of these . . . women appeared adequate despite their low intake of readily absorbed iron and zinc from flesh foods and their high intake of total dietary fiber and phytate."[15] (See pages 212–13 for more information about the influence of fiber and phytate on zinc levels.)

- Further—and highly significant—evidence comes from the "China Study"—the most comprehensive, large-scale study ever undertaken of the relationship between diet and the risk of developing disease. The study was truly massive, involving the collection of 367 detailed facts about the diet and lifestyle of 6,500 participants across China, from 1983 onward. It reveals that meat eating is by no means necessary to prevent iron-deficiency anemia. The average Chinese adult—who shows no evidence of anemia—consumes twice the iron Americans do, but the vast majority of it comes from the iron in plants.

- In a very carefully controlled study of the impact of high and low meat diets on iron levels, scientists from the Grand Forks Human Nutrition Research Center found, to their surprise, that subjects (in this case, postmenopausal women) given a high-meat diet had, after seven weeks, a worse iron level than people eating a low-meat diet! "The negative effect of meat consumption on iron status was unexpected," they concluded, "the results emphasize the need . . . for identifying additional dietary components that influence iron nutriture."[16] This is a point we'll return to in a moment.

This research, and more besides, disproves the fallacy that a meat-free diet can't provide enough iron. It certainly can—you've just seen some of the evidence.

But what about the other side of the coin? Although the research you've just seen demonstrates that vegetarians *can* get enough iron, does this mean that they always *do*? Aren't they, after all, more likely to develop anemia? This is certainly the implication of many medical and nutritional textbooks. Their reasoning is usually as follows:

1. Meat provides heme iron, which is more easily absorbed than nonheme (plant sources).
2. Vegetarians don't eat meat.
3. Therefore, vegetarians are likely to be anemic.

The science of nutrition, just like any other branch of human knowledge, is full of its own folklore. Opinions such as these are often passed down from one generation of practitioners to another, because they sound plausible, and because no one bothers to check or question the original research in the field. If they did, they'd be in for quite a shock.

A computer search reveals that in the period from 1966 to the beginning of 1994, a total of 7,618,328 articles were published in the world's major medical journals.[17] Of these, just 62 mentioned the word "anemia" in connection with the words "vegetarians" or "vegans." That's just under 0.000814 percent of the medical literature in 28 years. Not very much, is it?

But when these sixty-two reports are themselves analyzed, the picture becomes even more unequivocal:

- The majority (twenty-two reports) dealt not with iron-deficiency anemia, but with individual case histories of people on very restricted diets with vitamin B_{12} deficiency (see below).
- Most of the reports of iron-deficiency anemia among vegetarians (seven) dealt with the iron status of impoverished Indians, either in India itself or as immigrants to the West. Is it their vegetarianism causing them to be anemic—or more likely, their poverty?
- One report described iron-deficiency anemia among macrobiotic subjects. Most vegetarians do not eat a macrobiotic regime (which, by the way, may include flesh).
- Another report described the "marginal" iron status of a

group of elderly Dutch vegetarians, sixty-five to ninety-seven years old. Despite the researchers' judgment about their "marginal" status, their subjects were described as "apparently healthy."

- Another report described the improvement obtained by supplementing the diets of a group of anemic preschool children, not with meat, but with vitamin C. "The children who received vitamin C supplements showed a significant improvement in hemoglobin level as well as in red cell morphology," wrote the researchers.[18] Vitamin C is normally well supplied in a vegetarian diet (there is no vitamin C in meat).

The allegation that the vegetarian diet causes iron-deficiency anemia can now be firmly rejected. Nearly thirty years of published research has failed to substantiate it.

Now we come to a particularly interesting aspect of this controversy. Studies comparing the plasma ferritin levels of vegetarians to meat eaters sometimes show that although the vegetarians' levels are within the normal range, they are rather lower than meat eaters, suggesting that meat eaters store more iron in their bodies than vegetarians. Is this good, or bad?

Consider the following warning by a noted researcher on dietary iron: "Possibly, as discussed in the previous chapters, while decreasing the risk of classical iron-deficiency symptoms, the current RDA for iron is increasing the risk of infection. In this respect, nutritionists have lowered their RDAs for iron over the past decade—40 percent lower in newborn infants and 17 percent lower in adult females in 1989 as compared to 1980. Certainly, the physiology of these groups has not changed, which leads one to wonder about the accuracy of these values. . . . I foresee a continuing downward trend of RDAs for iron and an upward trend for Vitamin C as more hard data become available."[19]

It has been known for some time that very low levels of iron in the human body increase the risk of infection. It is not so well known, however, that high levels of iron *do precisely the same*. Invading bacteria require iron to grow—and the more iron made available to them, the faster they'll multiply.

But that's not all. Over the past few years, Dr. Randall B. Lauffer has proposed a theory that has been greeted in some quarters as medical heresy. Dr. Lauffer has an impressive pedigree: he's an assistant professor at Harvard Medical School, an expert on mineral biochemistry and the use of minerals in medical diagnosis and therapy, and also the director of a research laboratory at Massachusetts General Hospital. According to Dr. Lauffer:

> "Scientific discoveries are coming out every day showing new roles that iron plays in many common diseases. We are coming to recognize that there has perhaps been an overemphasis on iron deficiency in the past. Worldwide, iron deficiency is a major problem, especially in populations that are malnourished. However, in the well-fed populations of the Western world iron deficiency is increasingly rare, and is mainly observed in certain sub-groups such as pregnant women and children."

Dr. Lauffer clearly and carefully explains the danger of having too much iron in the body:

> "Iron is a key component of the free radical theory of disease. This was discovered some time ago, and more and more evidence is being laid down in support of it. Basically, the theory is this: Oxygen—which of course is good for you—is used in burning the body's fuel, that is, the foods that we eat. But oxygen also can be converted into toxic by-products. Now, most of these toxic by-products are pretty mild. However, in the presence of iron, and also, in some cases, copper, these mildly toxic forms of oxygen are converted into much more toxic forms. And wherever they are produced, they can damage the tissue that surrounds them. This is true in heart disease. The leading theory of atherosclerosis involves free radical damage to the 'bad' form of cholesterol . . . LDL, or low density lipoprotein. Then certain cells in the artery itself and the artery wall begin sucking up this damaged LDL. And this begins what we call atherosclerotic plaque development. But the most important role for iron is that excess iron in the heart creates more damage when a heart attack actually occurs.

The same type of chemical reaction that oxidizes LDL can also damage the heart cells directly. For example, when you have a heart attack, you have diminished oxygen supply to the heart. Then, when you have either coronary bypass surgery, or a procedure, such as angioplasty, where the artery is opened up and blood flow resumes, more oxygen is quickly perfused into the heart, and this generates more damaging oxygen free radicals. And the more iron present, the more damage occurs in the process."

There is a simplicity in Dr. Lauffer's exposition that indicates a thorough knowledge and understanding of his subject.

"We are now following a Finnish study . . . which shows that men who have higher iron levels are predisposed to heart attacks. We don't have enormous evidence that excess iron will cause atherosclerosis directly. We do believe, however, that the combination of high cholesterol levels—which are common in Western cultures—and high iron and/or copper levels can contribute to this process. People have wondered for years why men are predisposed to certain diseases from which women seem to be protected. For heart disease, it is not that women are totally protected; they seem to be protected only prior to menopause. The conventional medical view is that it is all hormonal, that in some mysterious way, women's hormones protect them during the childbearing years. And there's been no clear mechanism proposed as to how that would actually work. For example, the effects of estrogen on cholesterol levels are really quite ridiculously small to ever be a mechanism for this. The changes in iron metabolism, however, are dramatic, and appear to be a much more sensible explanation for the difference in incidence of heart disease in men and women. The iron levels match exactly the mortality rates of heart disease in men and women. Men get very high iron levels early in life, say twenty years old, whereas women's iron levels are held down by the natural loss of iron through menstruation. As soon as that ceases, however, their iron levels bound up quickly to that of men, and, at the same time, the incidence of heart disease increases."[20]

Luckily, the same kind of meat-free, dairy-free diet (i.e. vegan) that lowers cholesterol levels also lowers iron. Says Dr. Lauffer:

"It makes sense to look to many of the Asian cultures, where heart attacks are of much lower prevalence, and at the type of diet they eat, and try to mimic that. It's very simple. In fact, the biggest contributor to both high iron and high cholesterol levels is meat consumption. Meat is a one-two punch: it contains a certain form of iron [known as heme] that is very rapidly and easily absorbed. And it contains saturated fat and cholesterol. So every bite of meat is contributing to two problems in the body—both of which lead to heart disease and possibly other chronic diseases that are common in Western meat-eating cultures."

Dr. Lauffer also suggests that iron may play an important role in the causation of cancer:

"We have had evidence for a long time that high iron levels do increase the risk of cancer," he says, "and there are two reasons: first of all, iron's role in free radical damage is important in cancer. Cancer arises when the blueprint for the cell, the DNA, is damaged. Second, iron is known to be a key catalyst for this process. . . . The body tries to safely sequester iron away in the cell and keep it away from the DNA. However, free radical damage still occurs. The body repairs the damage as best it can, but it can't sometimes repair every little nick that occurs. And so, the more of these nicks you get, the greater chance you have of getting cancer. Iron has another role in cancer: iron is a key ingredient for cell division. If the cell doesn't have iron around, it simply does not divide. So if you can restrict the amount of iron to a cancer cell, it actually slows down cancer growth."

The possible connection between iron levels and heart disease was first proposed in 1981, when Dr. Jerome Sullivan, a pathologist at the Veterans Administration Medical Center in Charleston, South Carolina, suggested that menstrual bleeding might protect women from heart disease by reducing the amount of iron in their bodies. Although experts have traditionally blamed hormonal changes for the sudden surge in cardiovascular illness in women after the age of menopause, Sullivan pointed out that women's cholesterol levels change little after menopause, although their iron levels *do* rise sharply. Further evidence to support Sullivan's theory comes from studies that show that surgical removal of the uterus (the site of menstrual bleeding) causes an increase in heart-attack risk—even if the ovaries are left to produce estrogen.

Then, in 1992, the first major piece of practical research in support of the iron–heart disease connection was published.[21] Researchers at the University of Kuopio in Finland tracked the health of 1,931 men from 1984 until 1989, and found that men with higher iron levels in their bodies had twice the risk of heart attack compared to men with lower levels of stored iron. Men with both high iron and high cholesterol were four times as likely to be stricken.

Since then, the debate in medical and scientific circles has been raging. Iron—just like protein before it—has been a sacred cow of conventional nutrition for decades; the idea that it might be a doubled-edged sword is still anathema to many. Nevertheless, the evidence against excessive iron consumption—primarily from flesh foods—is increasing, and cannot be lightly dismissed.

In Conclusion

- Eating a meat-free diet does not increase the risk of iron-deficiency anemia.
- The body naturally regulates its absorption of dietary iron according to its needs.
- A healthy meat-free diet will include several good sources of iron (see below).
- Eating foods—or supplements—rich in vitamin C will considerably enhance iron bioavailability. Iron must be delivered in a soluble form to the small intestine if it is to be absorbed, and vitamin C can make sure that nonheme iron remains soluble in the acidic environment normally found there. Other organic acids found in fruit and vegetables, such as malic acid and citric acid, are also thought to possess this iron-enhancing attribute. This effect is substantial: adding 60 mg of vitamin C to a meal of rice has been shown to more than triple the absorption

of iron; adding the same amount to a meal of corn enhances absorption fivefold.[22] Vegetarians and vegans are fortunate inasmuch as many excellent sources of iron are also naturally good sources of vitamin C.

- Several factors can significantly reduce the absorption of iron, among them tea (the tannin forms insoluble iron compounds) and the food preservative EDTA. Both of these can reduce assimilation by as much as 50 percent.
- Use iron supplements only on medical advice. And keep them away from children—in America, iron pills are the most common cause of childhood poisoning deaths.[23]
- Too much iron may be as dangerous as too little. A vegetarian diet that allows our bodies to absorb the right amount of iron from several natural sources is the healthiest option. After all, it works pretty well for our primate relatives!
- Milk and milk products are practically devoid of iron. Worse, milk may reduce the absorption of iron from other foods[24], thereby compounding iron-deficiency problems.[25] One study has shown that 44 out of 100 infants receiving whole cow's milk had blood in their feces. This would also contribute to an iron-deficiency problem.[26] Egg yolks do contain iron, but this is poorly absorbed due to the presence of an inhibitor, phosvitin.

GOOD SOURCES OF IRON

An extensive analysis of several thousand vegetarian foodstuffs reveals that the following are good sources of this nutrient:

Food	Measure	Mg of iron
Molasses: cane, third extraction; or blackstrap	1 cup	52.8
Pumpkin & squash seed kernels, roasted	1 cup	33.91
Potato flour	1 cup	30.78
Spirulina, dried	100g	28.5

Food	Measure	Mg of iron
Breakfast cereals, e.g. corn flakes (fortified)	1 cup	20.95
Sesame seeds, whole, dried	1 cup	20.95
Molasses: cane, second extraction; or medium	1 cup	19.68
Quinoa	1 cup	15.73
Natto	1 cup	15.05
Molasses: cane, first extraction; or light	1 cup	14.1
Tofu: raw, firm, prepared with calcium sulfate	1/2 cup	13.19
Pizza with cheese topping	1 12-in. pizza	11.56
Broad beans (fava beans), raw	1 cup	10.05
Sunflower seed kernels, dried	1 cup loosely packed	9.75
Soy flour	1 cup	9.24
Cocoa powder	1 cup	9.2
Soybeans, cooked	1 cup	8.84
Endive, raw	1 head	8.72
Pistachio nuts, dried	1 cup	8.68
Hummus	1 cup	8.41
Dried mixed fruit	1 pkg. (11 oz.)	7.94
Tomato paste	1 can (7 oz.)	7.7
Miso	1 cup	7.53

Food	Measure	Mg of iron
Apricots, dehydrated dried	1 cup	7.5
Oats	1 cup	7.36
Lima beans, canned	1 can (1 cup)	7.21
Wheat, durum	1 cup	6.75
Peanuts, raw	1 cup	6.68
Barley	1 cup	6.62
Lentils, cooked	1 cup	6.59
Peaches, dried halves	1 cup	6.49
Spinach, cooked	1 cup	6.43
Wheat germ, crude	1 cup	6.26
Potato, cooked in skin	1 potato	5.94
Peas, green, canned	1 lb.	5.90
Gingerroot, crystallized, candied	1 oz.	5.88
Sesame butter	1 oz.	5.45
Beets, canned, drained solids	1 can (10 oz)	5.35
Cashew nuts, oil-roasted	1 cup	5.33
Thyme, ground	1 tbsp.	5.31
Kidney beans, cooked	1 cup	5.28
Almonds, dried, blanched	1 cup whole kernels	5.27
Cabbage, raw	1 head	5.08
Baked beans	1 cup	5
Peanut butter	1 cup	4.9

Other Dietary Anemias

Apart from iron deficiency, anemia will also result if the diet does not contain sufficient vitamin B_{12} or folic acid (which is sometimes referred to as vitamin B_9). Both of these vitamins play an essential part in the regular replacement of hemoglobin in the body.

Folic acid deficiency is a widespread problem globally. Unlike vitamin B_{12}, the body does not store appreciable amounts of it, so it is essential that the diet regularly contains goods sources. Apart from the risk of anemia, it has been shown that pregnant women whose diets are low in this vitamin are more likely to bear children with serious neural tube defects, such as hydrocephalus and spina bifida (birth defects characterized by a spinal column that does not form properly). Research shows that the simple precaution of taking folic acid supplements, especially during early pregnancy, can dramatically reduce the incidence of these afflictions. The U.S. Food and Drug Administration is so convinced of the importance of this vitamin for preventing birth defects that it wants it to be added to bread, flour, and other enriched grain products.[27]

The good news for vegetarians is that folic acid (the word comes from the Latin for "leaf") is present in many common green leafy vegetable foods (note, however, that it can be destroyed by excessive cooking). It is *not* present in most meat, milk, eggs, and root vegetables.

Of far more concern, particularly to vegans, is the question of vitamin B_{12} deficiency anemia. Those who are commercially opposed to the vegan diet cite the relative lack of vitamin B_{12} as conclusive proof that veganism is a perverse practice. On the other side, ardent vegans have been known to declare that vitamin B_{12} "simply isn't an issue." As with iron deficiency, the truth is far more complex than either of these extremes, and a little basic knowledge about the role of this vitamin in the diet, and its best sources, would calm a debate in which there has frequently been more heat than light.

There is no question that lack of vitamin B_{12} will eventually cause serious health problems, described here by two medical experts in the field (both, incidentally, practicing vegetarians):

The pernicious anemia patient was first described in the medical literature in 1849 as one who appeared pale and sallow with a shiny tongue and complained of weakness and fatigue that progressed gradually to the point of paralysis. Blood tests done on such patients today would reveal low hemoglobin levels and large, pale red blood cells. In the early stages of the illness there are numbness and tingling in the hands and feet with a loss of sensation. Gradually a lack of motor coordination develops. These symptoms are now known to be due to an inability to synthesize myelin, the fatty sheath that insulates nerve fibers. As a result, the nerves to the limbs degenerate. If allowed to proceed unchecked, the deterioration progresses into the spinal cord and ultimately to the brain. Moodiness, poor memory, and confusion give way gradually to delusions, hallucinations, and overt psychosis.[28]

Clearly, we're dealing with a very serious set of symptoms, which it would be dishonest—and dangerous—to ignore or to trivialize. However, this is only the beginning of the story. The fact is that the vast majority of cases of vitamin B_{12} deficiency occur not in vegans, but in the general meat-eating population. Comments Dr. John Lindenbaum, a vitamin B_{12} researcher and director of the department of medicine at Columbia University, "We see less than one case a year due to insufficient intake of vitamin B_{12} alone."[29] Compare that number to the fifty cases of pernicious anemia that Dr. Lindenbaum sees in nonvegetarians in the same period of time.

So if meat eaters can experience vitamin B_{12} deficiency—and meat itself contains large amounts of vitamin B_{12}—*what is going wrong?*

The answer is that although these people consume large amounts of B_{12} in their diets, they cannot absorb it due to low acidity in the stomach, disease, or the absence of an enzyme called the "intrinsic factor." In any of these cases, vitamin B_{12} is blocked from entering the body's normal biochemical pathways, and will therefore never do its work in the body. The fact is that cases of vitamin B_{12} deficiency are most often due to a defect in absorption, and not to a dietary lack of the vitamin.

Many vegans feel, quite justifiably, persecuted over the matter of vitamin B_{12}. The number of cases on record of vegans exhibiting health problems due to B_{12} deficiency is very small—certainly when compared to the millions of people who die every year of diseases linked to meat consumption. But there are, indeed, a few clinical cases on record of vegans, and their babies, developing anemia because of low B_{12} dietary intake. Such cases are rare, but because the implications are serious—particularly for babies, whose intellectual development may be impaired—they must not be ignored.

Vitamin B_{12} is itself the subject of much continuing research. The amount needed in the diet is absolutely tiny; the smallest of all the suggested daily intakes of vitamins.[30] Measuring the B_{12} content of food is difficult, partly because the quantities are so small, and partly because foods sometimes contain substances that are chemically very similar to B_{12}, but do not possess the same biological activity (non-cobalamin analogues). Vitamin B_{12} is almost always manufactured by bacteria (although, even here, the possibility exists that that some peas and beans actually produce their own vitamin B_{12}). The vitamin B_{12} in meat itself is produced by bacterial action within the gut of the animal in question; it is also likely that bacteria on the surface and around the roots of plants eaten by that animal will also contribute toward the total B_{12} content of the animal's flesh.

The obvious question has been posed that if farm animals can produce vitamin B_{12} from their internal bacteria, why can't humans, too? In all probability, we can. Bacteria in our gut, in our mouth, around the teeth and gums, in the nasopharynx, around the tonsils, in the folds at the base of the tongue, and even in the upper bronchial tree may all produce vitamin B_{12}. And if we eat foods grown in soils where the bacterial flora is rich, such as organic produce, then we will probably take in a useful dose of B_{12} from this source, too.

All these aspects of vitamin B_{12} are intriguing, and all are grounds for much additional research work and speculation. But none of these points should be used to obscure the fact that healthy vegans need to make sure they periodically eat foods that they know to contain good sources of B_{12}. Indeed, there are many, because B_{12} is often added to many of the most common foodstuffs, such as soy milk, yeast extract, textured vegetable protein foods, and most breakfast cereals. Because of this, B_{12} is one of the easiest of all nutrients for vegans to obtain: all you have to do is to check the product's label for information on its B$_{12}$ content.

In Conclusion

- Inadequate folic acid intake is a substantial hazard for many meat eaters—it is not found in most meats, milk, or eggs. Because of their high intake of green leafy vegetables, wheat, beans, lentils, and other good dietary sources, vegetarians are well-placed to avoid the health problems associated with folic acid deficiency.
- Pernicious anemia is usually caused by an inability to absorb vitamin B$_{12}$—whether or not you eat meat has nothing to do with it.
- Dietary vitamin B$_{12}$ deficiency is never a problem for vegans who periodically eat foods that contain this vitamin.

ANGINA

What is it?

In medical language, angina properly means a spasmodic, choking, or suffocating pain. For example, the complaint *angina acuta*, which sounds very alarming, merely signifies a simple sore throat. However, "angina" is now used almost exclusively to describe angina pectoris, a chronic condition of pain in the chest. The word "angina" comes from the Greek for "strangling," which sums up both the cause and effect of this serious and threatening condition. It is almost always caused by an insufficient supply of oxygen to the heart muscle, which is itself usually the result of progressive blockage of the coronary arteries. It is closely linked to both coronary heart disease and high blood pressure. Angina is most likely to strike during physical exertion or emotion, and will disappear when the excess work load or emotion is relieved.

How the Vegetarian Diet Can Help

As explained in the section related to heart disease (pages 226–42), Dr. Dean Ornish's work treating patients with a low-fat vegan diet clearly demonstrates that the plaques that build up and eventually block coronary arteries can be diminished by appropriate diet therapy. This results in increased flow of blood and a corresponding decline in the severity or frequency of angina, which has now been verified by several detailed scientific papers.[31] Rather than repeat the evidence here, I will refer you to the sections relating to heart disease and hypertension (pages 226–50), where the science is covered in some detail. It is, however, worth emphasizing that it is the vegan, not the semivegetarian, diet that can reverse atherosclerosis. "Many doctors still recommend 'lean meat' diets," comments Dr. Neal Barnard, president of the Physicians Committee for Responsible Medicine, "even though such diets do not reverse heart disease for most patients and, in fact, are too weak even to stop the progression of the disease."[32] Confirms Dr. Ornish, "Our study and now four other studies have shown that, on average, people with heart disease who only make moderate changes—less red meat, more fish and chicken, fewer eggs, and so on—overall they tend to get worse over time. The arteries become more blocked."

ARTHRITIS AND RHEUMATISM

What Is It?

"Arthritis" is a specific term describing inflammation of the joints; "rheumatism" is used more broadly and describes all aches and pains in the muscles, bones, and joints. In this sense, we have all suffered from rheumatism at some time. Rheumatoid arthritis is therefore inflammation and pain of the joints *and* the surrounding tissues. There are, in fact, some 100 different types of arthritis, including

- Reiter's syndrome, an acute form often accompanied by eye inflammation and more frequently found in young men
- Ankylosing spondylitis, a chronic complaint, affecting the spine, pelvic joints, and sometimes the heart and eyes. It causes pain, fatigue, and depression, which can last for years.
- Systemic lupus erythematosus, more common in women and characterized by skin rashes and joint inflammation
- Gout, which involves swelling and severe pain, normally in the big toe. It has long been known to be aggravated by diet, especially foods rich in purine, which produces uric acid.

Why Do People Get Arthritis?

Many different causes have been suggested including stress, aller-gies, food and environmental pollution, malnutrition, hormonal imbalance, and digestive inadequacy. In addition, our body can mis-takenly attack itself in trying to fight off foreign bacteria that closely resemble our own tissue. This is called an "autoimmune response." Relevant to all of these causes is the ever-increasing evidence that diet has a very important role to play in the onset and control of these degenerative disorders.

How the Vegetarian Diet Can Help

Medicine has conventionally treated the notion that arthritis might be responsive to the meat-free diet as unsubstantiated folklore. As recently as 1990, for example, the University of California's own health publication advised its readers that "though scores of clinical studies have been conducted, no dietary regimen or nutritional sup-plement has been shown to alleviate or prevent arthritis."[33] Neverthe-less, the evidence has steadily accumulated over the years, and at last it seems as if the testimony of countless sufferers is being given a sym-pathetic hearing by many doctors. There is, indeed, a good scientific explanation. Meat and dairy foods contain arachidonic acid, and it has been demonstrated that levels of arachidonic acid in the blood fluctuate according to the consumption of these products, and can indeed promote joint inflammation.[34] Adopting a vegan diet can sig-nificantly reduce arachidonic acid, and the subsequent pain of arthri-tis, as several studies prove:

In one early study of rheumatoid arthritis, published in 1986, patients were asked to fast for a week, and then for three weeks eat a vegan diet. At the end of this time, 60 percent said they felt better, with "less pain and increased functional ability."[35] Studies such as this, however, do not always make the medical headlines, and it was several more years before most specialists began to appreciate just how important the role of diet might be in diminishing the pain of arthritis.

Some people may be particularly sensitive to dairy products. In this well-constructed experiment, a fifty-two-year-old white woman with eleven years of arthritic suffering was tested to see which foods—if any—provoked her arthritis the most.[36] Eating her "normal" diet, she would average about 30 minutes of morning stiffness, with 9 tender joints and 3 swollen joints. After a 3-day fast, there was no morning stiffness, just 1 tender joint, and no swollen joints. However, when she was given milk (the study was "blinded"—the foodstuff she was swallowing was disguised), the arthritis returned with a vengeance, with 30 minutes of morning stiffness, 14 tender joints, and 4 swollen joints.

Perhaps the most widely publicized study appeared in the medical journal The Lancet in 1991.[37] Twenty-seven patients were asked to follow a modified fast for 7 to 10 days (herbal teas, garlic, vegetable broths, and juices), and were then put on a gluten-free vegan diet for 3½ months. The authors of the study had already accepted that "fasting is an effective treatment for rheumatoid arthritis, but most patients relapse on reintroduction of food." Their aim, therefore, was to see whether the achievements attained during fasting could be maintained. Gradually, the subjects' diet was altered by adding a new food item every other day, eventually arriving at a lacto-vegetarian diet for the remainder of the study. If the introduction of one food produced symptoms, then it would be eliminated again. A control group ate an ordinary diet throughout the whole study period. After four weeks the vegetarian group showed a significant improvement in number of tender joints, number of swollen joints, pain, duration of morning stiffness, grip strength, white blood cell count, and many other measurements of health. Best of all, wrote the scientists, "the benefits in the diet group were still present after one year."

Today, it seems that the dietary treatment of the excruciating pain of arthritis is at last finding widespread acceptance by medical specialists. Speaking at the launch of the Arthritis and Rheumatism Council's booklet "Diet and Arthritis," consultant rheumatologist Dr. John Kirwan commented, "As far as we can tell at present, low-fat diets, cutting out red meat, full-fat milk, butter and confectionery made with butter—together with an increased intake of coldwater fish or vegetable oil—may enable people to take fewer pain killers and antiinflammatory drugs."[38] And that's no bad thing. In an earlier report from 1986, British doctors estimated that nonsteroidal antiinflammatory drugs (NSAIDs) used in the treatment of arthritic pain may be causing 200 deaths and 2,000 cases of intestinal bleeding each year.[39] Almost all the victims are elderly, and most are women.

What Else Can You Do?

There are a number of other dietary measures you can consider when making appropriate lifestyle changes to reduce the pain of arthritis.

A New England horticulturist has developed a theory that solanum alkaloids, found in members of the nightshade family of plants, could cause arthritis in some people. The nightshade family includes deadly nightshade, eggplant, red and green pepper, potatoes, tomatoes and tobacco. A group of 3,000 sufferers cut this family of foods from their diet and experienced reduced aches, pains, and disfigurement.[40]

Dava Sorbel, a former *New York Times* science writer, and market researcher Arthur Klein surveyed over 1,000 arthritis sufferers aged 10 to 90 in an attempt to find out what the sufferers themselves found to be effective.[41] Forty-seven percent changed the way they ate because of their arthritis. Of these, 20 percent said the dietary changes helped their condition—in some cases, dramatically. The researchers found that the most-avoided foods were red meats (155 patients), sugar (148), fats (135), salt (98), caffeine (56), plants in the nightshade family, such as tomatoes and eggplant, (48). Most-favored foods were vegetables (204 patients), fruit (174), fish (89).

People who alter the bacterial content of their gut often experience relief from rheumatic symptoms.[42] A change of diet combined with a course of colonic irrigation and the use of acidophilus supplements is certainly worth trying.

A calorie-controlled diet is of benefit to those who suffer rheumatism or arthritis and are overweight. Excess weight only adds to the strain placed on already overstressed joints. A healthy way to lose weight is to eat a vegan diet and, at the same time, cut out all refined sugar. This diet lets you drop the pounds quickly while significantly reducing joint discomfort.

Fish oils have been shown to have some benefit for arthritis sufferers, probably because of the omega-3 fatty acids they contain. For ethical reasons (and indeed, for reasons of health—the many fishing areas are known to be extremely polluted), you should consider instead flaxseed oil supplements. Also, the linolenic acid in soy bean oil (soy lecithin) is believed to get rapidly converted in the body to the same omega-3 fatty acids found in fish oils.

Vitamin A is necessary for the body to fight infection, a key in many rheumatoid arthritis cases. To make sure you get enough of this vitamin, eat plenty of yellow, orange, and green fruits and vegetables such as spinach, carrot, papaya, pumpkin, sweet potato, watercress, and parsley.

If you are taking drugs for a rheumatic disease, it is possible that you are lacking in vitamin B complex. This is found in whole grains and brewer's yeast.

Vitamin C helps to thin the synovial fluid in your joints which leads to improved mobility. Arthritics particularly benefit from taking vitamin C because the aspirin they take to reduce pain and inflammation depletes the body of vitamin C. Fresh citrus fruit, blackcurrants, green peppers and cauliflower are all excellent sources.

Vitamins C and E and the mineral selenium are all antioxidants; oxidation is a process in which nutrients in the body are broken down before the body can use them. Selenium also reduces the production of prostaglandins and leukotrienes, both of which cause inflammation. Whole grains, vegetable oils and nuts are rich in vitamin E. Selenium is a trace mineral available from most plant foods or from supplementation.

People with arthritis sometimes have an enzyme deficiency in their small intestine, which means they are unable to absorb gluten, a protein found in wheat flour. In fact, maps of areas in the world where gluten-high cereals are eaten correspond to those areas with the highest incidence of rheumatoid arthritis.[43] And countries where rice or corn is the staple grain show a much lower rate of the rheumatic diseases than those whose staple grain is wheat. Reduce your consumption of gluten by substituting rice cakes and oatmeal or corn bread for wheat bread and cake.

Yucca is a folk medicine that has been used for more than 1,000 years in America. A study into its effects found that 60 percent of rheumatoid arthritis and osteoarthritis patients experienced an improvement in their symptoms of swelling, pain, and stiffness.[44] Yucca is available in supplement form.

An alfalfa supplement may be of particular help to you. It is rich in protein, minerals and vitamins and contains chlorophyll, an excellent detoxifier of your system that helps reduce pain and swelling. Consider taking it in tablet or powder form, or as a tea. Also, you may like to add alfalfa sprouts to your salad or sandwich.

As a last resort (and this is not meant altogether seriously), you might consider getting pregnant. Scientists have long noted that women suffering from rheumatoid arthritis often get better during pregnancy. Why this should be so is open to question, but it is possible that the body's natural defenses jump into action against what seems to be a foreign invader—the baby—which somehow relieves the arthritis at the same time.[45]

ASTHMA

What Is It?

"Asthma" literally means "panting," which rather understates the possible severity of an asthmatic attack. "Gasping" would perhaps be a better description of this acute condition, which is caused by a temporary narrowing of the bronchi (the airways branching from the trachea to the lungs). Asthma attacks can be precipitated by a sensitivity reaction to food, pollens, mold, and fungi, but may also be caused by airborne pollution or by infections of the respiratory tract. Most asthma attacks can be controlled by the administration of drug therapy, although this is in no sense a cure. Childhood asthma very often is associated with eczema or similar hypersensitivity reactions, and in many cases it disappears with age.

In the last decade, the death rate from asthma climbed by 46 percent, according to the Centers for Disease Control.[46] The greatest increases were seen among women and African-Americans. "It's generally thought that asthma is a treatable disease with no fatal outcomes," commented Dr. Jessie Wing of the CDC. "Unfortunately, we're seeing severe disease with fatal outcomes." A shocking British television documentary recently found that nearly half of the boys under the age of five in one London borough suffered from asthma.[47]

How the Vegetarian Diet Can Help

In this case, we're definitely talking about the "vegan" diet—as opposed to the vegetarian one, which may, of course, include dairy products. Food sensitivity was a subject that excited an enormous amount of publicity in the last decade, and stormy passions were aroused on both sides of the fence. Today, there seems little doubt that food sensitivity can be involved in the development of a range of problems—urticaria, angioedema, anaphylaxis, eczema, asthma, rhinitis, infantile colitis, inflammatory bowel disease, migraine, and hyperactivity, to name but a few, although it is by no means certain to what extent diet is a major causative factor. People are, of course, very different creatures, and what provokes a reaction in one person may well not do so in another. It does seem, however, that among those who experience diet-induced asthma, the most likely foods to produce this effect are cow's milk and eggs.[48] Therefore, the vegan diet seems to be a good starting point to test the diet-asthma theory.

This is precisely what some researchers did in 1985.[49] Taking 35 patients who had suffered from bronchial asthma for an average of 12 years (all of them on long-term medication, some on cortisone), the scientists prescribed a vegan diet—which also excluded chlorinated tap water, coffee, tea, chocolate, and sugar—for 12 months. Most fruit, vegetables, beans, lentils, and peas were freely allowed, although apples and citrus fruits were not, and grains were restricted or eliminated. The results were quite amazing—in nearly all cases, medication for asthma was either *totally withdrawn or drastically reduced*. Naturally, there was a significant decrease in asthma symptoms. Twenty-four patients fulfilled the treatment. Of these, 71 percent reported improvement at 4 months and 92 percent after the full year. The scientists concluded, "Selected patients, with a fear of side-effects of medication, who are interested in alternative health care, might get well and replace conventional medication with this regimen."

It is important to emphasize the long-term nature of this experiment—some patients needed the full 12 months before achieving maximum effect and freedom from medication. Speculation as to why the vegan diet should have this very profound effect probably centers around the removal of the more likely food allergens (such as eggs and milk), and also the absence of dietary arachidonic acid, found exclusively in animal products. Arachidonic acid is metabolized in the body to produce prostaglandins (which perform a wide range of hormone-like actions in the body) and leukotrienes (which are potent stimulators of bronchial constriction). It has been observed that people with asthma may have an excess of leukotriene activity,[50] and for this reason various experiments have been designed to see whether the consumption of fish oil, which is rich in omega-3 fatty acids, might somehow equalize the production of leukotrienes from arachidonic acid. However, there are conflicting studies about the effect of fish oil on asthma sufferers. Some studies suggest that it may have a useful effect,[51] others do not.[52] One investigation required 10 patients with asthma to consume a fish-oil enriched diet.[53] After 5 weeks, it was clear that the patients were doing rather badly—bronchodilator usage was up (13 puffs a day using fish oil, compared to 7 puffs a day without it). Also, their breathing was less efficient, with the maximum rate of air flow during expiration down by 15 percent—a significant amount. This hardly amounts to convincing evidence in favor of fish oil consumption and, as already mentioned, whatever beneficial effects are present in fish oil can also be obtained from plants oils such as flaxseed. On the other hand, the vegan study described above does suggest that a diet that eliminates meat products will reduce arachidonic acid and its asthma-provoking metabolites.

What Else Can You Do?

Asthma has many possible causes, and it is therefore worth trying a number of different approaches in its treatment. Some that have proven successful are described below:

Vitamin B_6 (pyridoxine) levels have been found to be lower in adult patients with asthma than in nonsufferers.[54] The same study has reported finding a significant decrease in frequency and severity of wheezing and asthmatic attacks in patients taking B_6 supplements.

"Reports of the value of Vitamin C for the control of asthma began around 1940," said Linus Pauling, twice Nobel prize winner and distinguished champion of vitamin C therapy for many modern diseases.[55] "There is now good evidence," he continued, "that vitamin C has such value as an adjunct to conventional therapy. Some of the older studies gave negative results, perhaps because of the use of too small an amount of the vitamin for too short a time. Most of the recent studies have shown that the vitamin has had an effect."

Pauling pointed to several such studies. When 6 healthy young men were given a drug (methacholine) that simulates the effect of asthma, it restricted their airflow by 40 percent.[56] Yet when they were given 100 mg of vitamin C (about the amount in two oranges) 1 hour before exposure to the chemical, it only restricted their airways by 9 percent. A double-blind test (one in which both subject and experimenter don't know who's taking the vitamin C and who's taking the dummy pill) was performed on 41 asthma patients in Nigeria.[57] In the rainy season, respiratory infections are common, and they exacerbate the condition of asthmatics. For 14 weeks, half the group (22 people) were given 1,000 mg of vitamin C a day; the other half was given a placebo (dummy pill). When the experiment was over, it was found that those who had been taking the vitamin C had suffered less than a quarter as many asthma attacks during the rainy season as those who hadn't taken the vitamin. Some of those taking vitamin C had no attacks at all for this period. However, the attacks returned after the experiment finished.

Another study looked at the effects of taking vitamin C before exercise. The bane of many asthmatics' lives are the paroxysms they suffer after exertion. "Characteristically, what happens is that an asthmatic will engage in a sport," says Dr. E. Neil Schachter, one of the researchers involved, "or some kind of exercise, and feel fine throughout the activity. But then 3 to 5 minutes after the exercise, he'll feel a tightness in his chest and will start wheezing. The attack tends to get progressively worse over the next 30 minutes." Patients in this study took just 500 mg of vitamin C before exercising and found that the severity of any subsequent attack was significantly reduced.[58]

These and other studies indicate that taking vitamin C, usually in quantities far higher than a normal diet can provide, may be beneficial for some people.

Other nutritional factors that, research suggests, help reduce the severity of asthma are carotenes (vitamin A), vitamin E, and selenium. All these substances have been experimentally shown to decrease leukotriene formation.

Certain chemicals and food additives may sometimes induce sensitivity reactions in susceptible indiduals. The most common include aspirin and other nonsteroidal antiinflammatory drugs (NSAIDs), sodium benzoate, sulfur dioxide, potassium sorbate, and tartrazine.

The food additive monosodium glutamate (MSG) can provoke asthma in certain people, although the attack itself may not take place for up to 12 hours after food containing MSG is eaten, which can present a real problem in identifying the cause of the attack for both the sufferer and doctor.[59]

Babies who are not fed allergy-triggering foods such as milk and eggs are less likely to suffer from asthma and allergies during the first year of life, according to a British study conducted on 120 families with histories of allergies.[60] Scientists restricted the diet of both babies and mothers, and found that "what the mother eats while breastfeeding can be sufficient to sensitize the baby," according to Dr. David Hide, of St. Mary's Hospital in Newport, Isle of Wight. It seems that proteins from the mother's food transfer into her breast milk and may cause babies to get allergies, even if the mother does not suffer from them. The mothers and their babies were divided into two groups: one ate "normally," but the other did not consume dairy products, eggs, fish, nuts, wheat, or soy. After 1 year, 14 percent of infants in the diet group showed signs of one or more allergies, whereas 40 percent of babies in the "normal" group became allergic. Over twice as many babies in the "normal" group showed asthma symptoms compared to those on the special diet. The diet is recommended only for those with a family history of allergies.

People who develop asthma as a sensitivity reaction to birds' feathers may also become hypersensitive to chickens' eggs, and possibly chicken flesh. One study found that 32 percent of people who developed bronchial asthma and rhinoconjunctivitis when exposed to bird feathers also developed a sensitivity reaction to egg proteins.[61]

Relaxation and stress reduction can be important parts of treating the underlying cause of asthma in some people. There is evidence to show that learning yoga, a Hindu discipline that is learned in eight steps, may have a beneficial effect—especially that part of yoga that deals with the art of breathing, *pranayama*.[62] Usually, the best scientific studies are performed on a "double blind" basis, in which both subject and experimenter are not told whether the treatment is actually being performed. To assess the effect of yogic breathing with a double blind method seems, at first glance, impossible. Yet that is just what some ingenious scientists have done. They achieved this using a device called the Pink City lung exerciser, which is a device used to teach students of *pranayama* the 1:2 ratio between breathing in and breathing out (short breath in, long breath out). The scientists used this machine, and also a look-alike device, which appeared to, but in fact did not, enforce this method of breathing on the students. Both devices were used by 18 patients with mild asthma, who spent a couple of weeks on each machine. Each patient recorded his symptoms, how much medication he had to use, and his best "deep breaths," both morning and evening. The results were encouraging, suggesting that *pranayama* exercises may indeed help to control mild asthma.

Finally, in the interest of reducing the incidence of asthma, we can all press for tighter controls on pollution and acid rain. There is a clear relationship between bronchial disease and air pollution, and children are more vulnerable than any other group to this insidious side-effect of industrialization.

CANCER

It cannot be concluded that a clear and consistent relationship exists between red meat and cancer. While some cancer prevention guidelines suggest limiting red meat intake, this implied association is not based on firm scientific evidence.

—National Cattlemen's Beef Association, *Food & Nutrition News*, Winter 1998

A Preventable Scourge
Did you know . . .

- Half of all the cases of cancer are suffered by just one-fifth of the world's population—those who live in industrialized countries.[63]
- As a leading cause of death in the United States, cancer is second only to heart disease. Colorectal, breast, lung, and prostate

cancer accounted for over half (60 percent) of all cancer deaths in 1996.

- One in eight American women will get breast cancer, and one in three people will be diagnosed with some form of cancer at some point in their lives.[64]

This is shocking. It means that, far from "winning the war" against cancer, we're actually losing it. Writers and journalists don't usually make that kind of statement. When you read about cancer, it's always the "good news" you see. We're supposed to concentrate on the fact that many cancer patients survive longer than they used to a few decades ago, and that the the new genetic technologies promise cures undreamed of just a few years ago. Let's hope they do.

But for anyone who's lost a friend or loved one to this ravaging disease, no amount of cheery optimism will convince us that the "battle" is being won. We've seen the casualties. We know the pain.

Cancer can be prevented. That's not a message that is often heard. But it's true. We already know—and have known for decades—a great deal about the factors responsible for causing cancer. Most of the cancer charities and organizations remain more interested in treating cancer than in preventing it, and so relatively few of us truly understand that many of the factors giving rise to cancer are actually within our control.

For example, it is estimated that 60 percent or more of all cancers in the Western world today are related to environmental causes.[65] This is by no means a radically new proposition. As long ago as 1775, the eminent surgeon Sir Percival Pott, one of the great names in the history of medicine, suggested that there might be a link. He was the first to notice that chimney sweeps often developed a particular form of cancer, and put forward the theory that their atrocious working conditions were responsible.

So if we have reason to suspect that our environment might be a factor in the causation of cancer, shouldn't we try to do something to control it, or at least to reduce the risk? After all, we spend huge amounts of money trying to find cures or more effective treatments for cancer. Surely we should be trying to prevent the disease from appearing in the first place?

Of course we should. But that's not what usually happens. In 1991, one of the major British cancer charities spent over $60 million on research, and barely $850,000 advising the public of how they might reduce their risks. The same charity commented in its annual report, "Although circumstantial evidence suggest that diet is linked to the cause of many human cancers, the evidence is extremely controversial."[66] Commented the director of another major cancer charity, "The basis for dietary effects on cancer is not understood."[67] What dismal, discouraging words.

Well, at least one form of preventive medicine is on the agenda. "Women worried about breast cancer should consider having healthy breasts removed before the disease has a chance to develop," one newspaper recently reported a professor of obstetrics and gynecology as stating.[68] It's rather like removing "a redundant gland and pad of fat," he said. Another proposal is to give healthy women Tamoxifen—a powerful anticancer drug—*before* they develop the disease.[69]

But let's get back to reality. In 1981, an epoch-making report was produced by the eminent epidemiologists Richard Doll and Richard Peto.[70] It assembled all the evidence they could find linking the occurrence of human cancers to specific identifiable factors. Although the authors of the 1,308-page report warn that not all causes of cancer can be identified or avoided, it does seem from the evidence collected that some of the causes of cancer they identify are well within our own control. This is what they estimate the main risk factors to be, with their best estimates of the percentage of total cancer-caused deaths that are attributable to them:

FACTORS THAT CAUSE CANCER

Factors Responsible for Cancer	Percentage of Cancer-Caused Deaths
Diet	35%
Tobacco	30%
Infection	10%

Factors Responsible for Cancer	Percentage of Cancer-Caused Deaths
Reproductive and sexual behavior	7%
Occupation	4%
Alcohol	3%
Geophysical factors	3%
Pollution	2%
Food additives	1%
Industrial products	1%
Medicines and medical products	1%

You can see that "diet" comes right at the top of the list. "Diet" means what we *choose* to eat, doesn't it? So, by informing ourselves of the evidence, and by taking steps to change our diets accordingly, we ought to be able to significantly reduce our chances of suffering from a diet-related cancer.

Now let's be quite clear. As long as there's been cancer, there have been quacks, charlatans, and swindlers who have preyed upon victims and their loved ones, selling them fraudulent "cures," or exploiting their distress to obtain some kind of advantage. So let's state here that vegetarians aren't immune to cancer. If you were the healthiest-living vegetarian in the world, who just happened to live downwind from Chernobyl, then the odds would be stacked heavily against you, regardless of your diet. There are a host of factors that can predispose us toward this ghastly affliction, and only some of them are controllable. Avoiding cancer is fundamentally about reducing your risk. The evidence you're about to see shows the vegetarian diet can do this for you.

What Is It?

Cancer is the term used to describe malignant forms of a larger class of diseases known as *neoplasms* (literally, "new formations"). It is initiated by exposure to a carcinogen (cancer-causing substance), which can be a chemical, a virus, or something physical such as radiation. Certain cancers can also arise as a result of hereditary factors.

A general characteristic of the development of cancer is the time lag between the first exposure to a carcinogen, and the subsequent development of cancer (scientists call this period the "tumor induction time"). Whether cancer eventually develops, and how quickly, is partly the result of the degree of exposure to a second class of substances called "promoting agents." Although tumor promoters do not themselves *initiate* cancer, they can have a great bearing on its outcome. This two-stage process of initiation followed by promotion is a central characteristic of the cancerous process. It introduces a wildly uncertain element into the equation, and explains why not everyone who is exposed to a carcinogen will contract cancer. It also offers us a great deal of hope, because the activity of tumor promoters can be greatly affected by a wide variety of factors—including, of course, what we eat.

Cancer begins as a single abnormal cell, which starts to multiply uncontrollably. This is the essential feature of cancer—an uncontrolled growth of cells. Malignant groups of such cells form tumors and invade healthy tissue, often spreading to other parts of the body in a process called "metastasis." Because of this fundamental ability to invade and destroy other parts of the body, the Greek doctor Hippocrates called this disorder *karkinos*, which literally means "crab," the origin of the modern word "cancer."

Neoplasms are divided into two fundamental types—benign and malignant. A benign neoplasm does not metastasize—in other words, it only grows at its point of origin—and it is usually named by tagging the suffix "oma" onto the word for the tissue concerned. For example, the Greek for "fat" is *lipos*, so a benign tumor of fat cells would be called a *lipoma* (there are, however, several exceptions to this general rule).

Malignant neoplasms (cancers) grow more rapidly than benign forms and invade adjacent, normal tissue. They are described by adding either "carcinoma" or "sarcoma" to the word for the site of the cancer (a malignancy of the fat cells would, therefore, be termed a *liposarcoma*). These two general classes of malignant neoplasms are defined thus:

- *Carcinomas* affect the skin and tissues that covers both the external and internal body, for example, breast cancer, prostate cancer, or cancer of the uterus.
- *Sarcomas* affect the body's supportive and connective tissue, such as muscles, blood vessels, bone, and fat.

It may take years for a noticeable tumor to develop, and it is undoubtedly true that speed of diagnosis can be a lifesaving factor. The American Cancer Society suggests there are seven warning signs which, even if only one is present, should provoke a prompt investigation. They are

- A change in bowel or bladder function
- A sore that does not heal
- Unusual bleeding or discharge
- A thickening or lump in the breast or elsewhere
- Indigestion or difficulty in swallowing
- An obvious change in a wart or a mole
- A nagging cough or hoarseness.

The prospects for survival depend, among other things, on the site in the body affected, the speed of diagnosis, the treatment given, and, to a considerable extent, on the attitude of the patient toward the disease.

Now, it's been suspected for a very long time—certainly over a century—that a meat-based diet is more likely to produce more cancers in a population than a plant-based one. Consider this extract from *Scientific American* magazine: "Inhabitants of cities indulge far too freely in meat, often badly cooked and kept too long; the poor and country population do not often get their meat fresh. Professor Verneuil considers something should be done to remedy this state of things. He points out that Réclus, the French geographer, has proved that cancer is most frequent among those branches of the human race where carnivorous habits prevail."[71]

Even earlier than this, we find evidence of the vegan diet being used by dietetic reformer Dr. William Lambe (1765–1846) to treat patients with cancer. In 1804 John Abernethy, a renowned surgeon of St. Bartholomew's Hospital in London (who, incidentally, gave his name to a biscuit flavored with caraway seeds), wrote the following account of Lambe's diet and its effects. Abernethy's clear-sighted description and interpretation of results would surely put many of our modern-day scientists to shame:

> Very recently Dr. Lambe has proposed a method of treating cancerous diseases, which is wholly dietetic. He recommends the adoption of a strict vegetable regimen, to avoid the use of fermented liquors, and to substitute water purified by distillation in the place of common water. . . . I think it right to observe that, in one case of cancerous ulceration in which it was used, the symptoms of the disease were, in my opinion, rendered more mild, the erysipelatous inflammation surrounding the ulcer was removed, and the life of the patient was, in my judgment, considerably prolonged. . . . It seems to me very proper and desirable that the powers of the regimen recommended by Dr. Lambe should be fairly tried, for the following reasons:
>
> • Because I know some persons who, while confined to such diet, have enjoyed very good health; and further, I have known several persons who did try the effects of such regimen, and declare that it was productive of considerable benefit. . . . They were not, indeed, afflicted with cancer, but they were induced to adopt a change of diet to allay a state of nervous irritation and correct disorder of the digestive organs, upon which medicine had but little influence.
> • Because it appears certain, in general, that the body can be perfectly nourished by vegetables.
> • Because all great changes of the constitution are more likely to be affected by alterations of diet and modes of life than by medicine.

- Because it holds out a source of hope and consolation to the patient in a disease in which medicine is known to be unavailing and in surgery affords no more than a temporary relief.[72]

Reading those perceptive and open-minded words in our profoundly arrogant twentieth-first century, one cannot help but be depressed by our lack of progress. Most of Abernethy's comments concerning the impotence of medicine when confronted with cancer are still true. To Abernethy, it made sense to experiment with diet, just to see what might be achieved. Yet the majority of Abernethy's medical successors refused to even contemplate this route, retreating instead to the paraphernalia of the exclusive medical freemasonry—the scalpel, the nostrum, and their ensuing high-tech offspring.

What damns us even more is the hard-won knowledge we now have about diet and health. In Abernethy's day, two hundred years ago, there were no epidemiological studies, no vast pools of accumulated data upon which to base decisions. Today we have that information, but for the most part choose to ignore it. I wonder what Dr. John Abernethy would have thought of us.

The Evidence

As researchers studied facts and figures about mortality from cancer in different countries, they were struck by an odd fact: It seemed that certain countries had a much higher mortality rate than others. What was the factor that made the United States, for example, so much worse than Japan? The researchers looked for a clue. Then, they tried comparing the amount of animal protein that different nations ate and their cancer mortality.[73] The results of their study are reflected in Figure 4.1 on the next page.

There is a clear relationship between the amount of animal protein in the national diet and the incidence of certain types of cancer mortality. But this wasn't the only dietary connection. The same correlation seemed to exist between total fat consumption and cancer, animal fat consumption and cancer, and various other associated factors, as well.

But perhaps certain nations were genetically more likely to contract cancers, no matter what they ate? To examine this possibility, studies

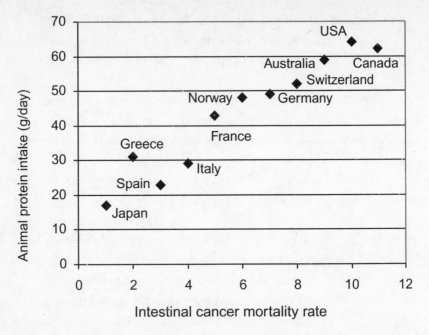

Figure 4.1. Animal protein consumption and intestinal cancer mortality.

were undertaken among immigrant populations. If the root cause of cancer was genetic, rather than environmental, the same races should have the same incidence of cancers, wherever they lived. The Japanese seemed to be a good subject, because they traditionally had low incidences of most forms of cancer. So three groups of Japanese were chosen, together with a "control" group of Caucasians.

The first group of Japanese lived in Japan, and followed a largely traditional diet. The second group was born in Japan but lived in the United States. The third group consisted of Japanese Americans—men and women born in the United States to Japanese parents. This is what they found.[74]

The results in Figure 4.2 speak for themselves. A comparison between the extreme left and right columns shows that the Japanese living in Japan (left column) have only one-quarter of the risk of contracting cancer of the colon compared with Caucasian Americans living in the States. But even more significantly, when the Japanese move to the States, their chance of contracting colon cancer increases by three—almost the same risk as a Caucasian. The place of birth didn't

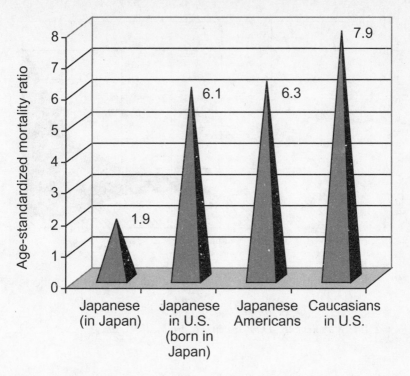

Figure 4.2. Deaths from colon cancer—East versus West.

seem to matter. This was good proof that environmental, and not genetic, factors were indeed very significant.

And now the scientific detective work really began. Because if the diet really was so important, then it should be possible to track down which specific factors related most strongly to increased cancer risk, and, hopefully, try to control them. So the focus began to shift from international comparisons, which had pointed the way, to very specific studies among very similar groups. Similar, that is, except for one or two key factors, which could be isolated, studied, and perhaps even controlled.

A group that was quickly identified as being a particular interest was the American Seventh-Day Adventist population. This group was subject to repeated studies, because the feature that distinguished them from the general American population was their differing diet. One key area of difference is dramatically demonstrated by Figure 4.3.[75]

The figure shows that Seventh-Day Adventists eat a radically differ-

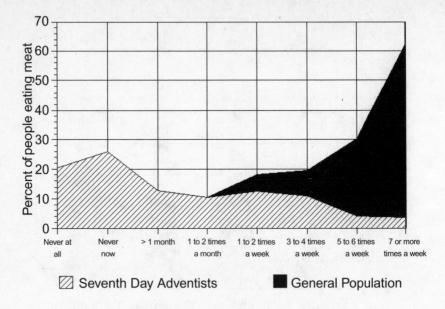

Figure 4.3. Why Seventh-Day Adventists are ideal to study.

ent diet than the average American. The vast majority of the general population consume meat or poultry products seven or more times each week, but the picture is quite the reverse for the Seventh-Day Adventist group. About half of them don't consume meat or meat products. They do not smoke or drink (although in the survey one-third of the men were previous smokers), and they tend to practice a "healthy" lifestyle that emphasizes fresh fruits, whole grains, vegetables, and nuts. So now the scientists had found a good group of people to study. A seven-year scientific study tabulated the cause of death of 35,460 Adventists. Figure 4.4 shows what they found:[76]

The death-rate from all cancers among Adventists was, amazingly, half that of the general population. The top bar on the chart shows Adventists having only 53 percent as many deaths from cancer when compared to the norm. Some of this could probably be attributed to their abstinence from smoking. Cancer of the respiratory system, for example (the bottom bar on the chart), was only 10 percent of the general population's. But other cancers, such as gastrointestinal and reproductive ones, are not causatively related to smoking. The scientists concluded, "It is quite clear that these results are supportive of the hypothesis that beef, meat, and saturated fat or fat in general are etiologically related to colon cancer."

Another study set out to check these remarkable findings, this time studying cancers of the large bowel, breast, and prostate—the three most common ones that are unrelated to smoking.[77] Twenty thousand Seventh-Day Adventists were studied, and this time, they were compared to two other population groups. First, they were checked against cancer mortality figures for all Caucasians in the U.S., and then they were compared to a special group of 113,000 people who were chosen because their lifestyles closely matched the Adventists—except, that is, for their diet. In other respects, such as place of residence, income, and socioeconomic status, the third group was very closely matched to the Adventists. Figure 4.5 on the next page shows the results.

Once again, the picture is pretty dramatic. The Adventists are compared with the general population as well as a special group whose lifestyle closely matched the Adventists—apart from the food they ate. You can see that for all three cancers, deaths among the Adventists

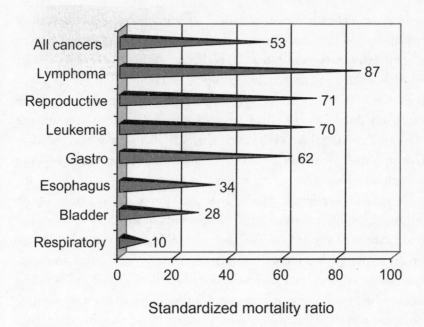

Figure 4.4. Deaths among Seventh-Day Adventists from cancer.

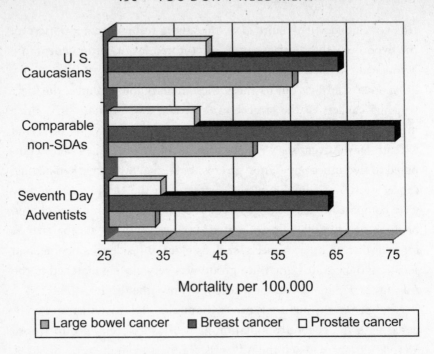

Figure 4.5. Comparison of deaths from cancer.

were lower than for the other groups. It is interesting that there does not appear to be a very great reduction in the risk of breast cancer among Adventists—until, that is, you compare the Adventists results with those of the comparable group. The comparable group has a higher risk of contracting breast cancer than the national average (probably due to local environmental factors in California, where the study was undertaken). However, the Adventists have succeeded in reducing their own risk down to below the national average—even though only half of them never consume meat.

A major correlation study analyzed the diets of thirty-seven nations, and then correlated the components of the diets to mortality from cancer of the intestines.[78] Before looking at the results, let me briefly explain what a correlation study is. It's really quite simple. A correlation ends up as a number somewhere between −1 and +1. The higher the figure, the closer the connection between the two factors. For example, if someone is paid on an hourly basis, then the more they work, the more money they earn. This is an example of a perfect correlation, and would have a figure of +1.

On the other hand, the more money you spend, the less you have in your bank account. This is a perfect negative correlation, since the connection between more expenditure and a decreasing bank balance is an inverse one: in this case, the correlation would be −1. And if any two factors, such as today's temperature and your bank balance, are not related at all, then the correlation would have a figure of zero. So the closer the figure gets to either +1 or −1, the stronger the connection, positive or negative. You can see from Figure 4.6 that all the meat factors correlate very strongly with cancer. Total calories, total protein, and total fat also correlate strongly, which is not surprising, since meat is heavy in all three. But calories and protein from vegetable sources have a negative correlation—in other words, they confer protection. The study concluded, "Animal sources of food were clearly associated with the cancer rates."

Correlation studies like this are very important, because although we may not know precisely why and how meat in the diet contributes to various cancers (this may take many years to finally prove), we can see that there is a clear relationship, and this enables us to take the necessary precautions for our own well-being.

More data, this time from an Israeli study, revealed a connection

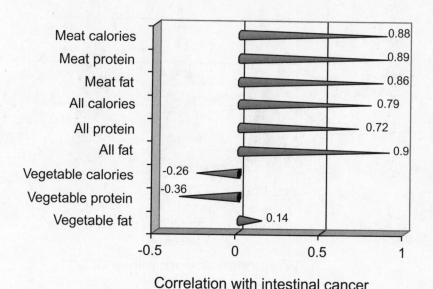

Figure 4.6. Intestinal cancer: riskier and safer diets.

between both fats from animal sources and fats from plant sources, suggesting that saturated and even unsaturated fats may be connected with increased mortality.[79] The study followed the Jewish population as it grew from 1.17 million in 1949 to 3.5 million in 1975, over which period meat consumption increased by 454 percent, and the death rate from malignant cancers doubled.

Meat and Breast Cancer

More and more evidence was starting to accumulate. In Alberta, Canada, researchers set about analyzing the diets of 577 women with breast cancer, and compared them to a similar group of women without the disease.[80] Was there any food, or type of foods, that might be linked to the development of breast cancer? Indeed there was. The results were, in the scientists' own words, "consistent with the notion that breast cancer risk is affected by certain dietary patterns, especially those related to the consumption of beef and pork." In fact, the

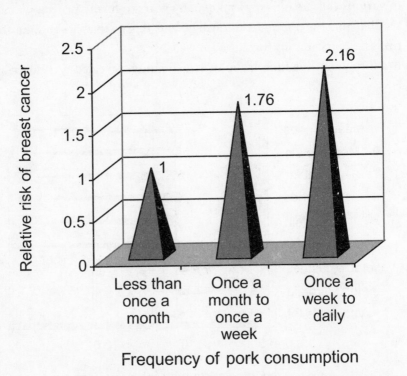

Figure 4.7. The connection between pork consumption and breast cancer.

strongest association of all was with pork consumption. Figure 4.7 illustrates how the relative risk of breast cancer rose with the frequency of eating pork. As for beef, consuming it more than once a week was also associated with an increase in relative risk of breast cancer. Yet more disturbing evidence that a meat-dominated diet might indeed be a real health risk.

In Hawaii another study showed the same pattern.[81] It concentrated on a representative sample of Hawaii's residents—Caucasians, Japanese, Chinese, Filipinos, and, of course, Hawaiians. The great variety of ethnic groups was useful, since they had a particularly wide range of food habits. Significant associations were established between

- Breast cancer and all forms of fat and animal protein
- Cancer of the uterus and all forms of fat and animal protein
- Prostate cancer and all forms of fat and animal protein.

The positive correlations between various forms of food and breast cancer are shown in Figure 4.8. The only negative correlation is between breast cancer and complex carbohydrates—which are, of course, found exclusively in plant food. Almost exactly the same relationship emerged when the same study examined cancer of the uterus.

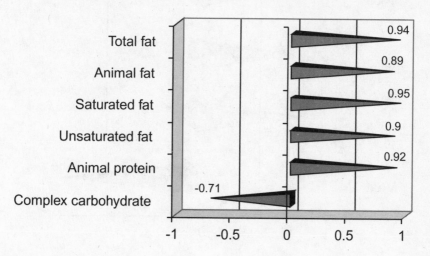

Figure 4.8. Breast cancer and diet.

More Meat Equals More Risk

In 1981 yet another massive statistical world survey of 41 countries, including the U.S. and the U.K., was completed.[82] The results confirm the connection between eating meat and the risk of certain types of cancer. And yet again, they also show that plant foods seem to confer protection. Here are two charts drawn from data that the survey produced, Figures 4.9 and 4.10.

"Less Is Better"

One of the largest studies ever undertaken on the effect of meat eating and cancer was published in 1990.[83] Over 88,000 women between the ages of 34 and 59 were recruited for the study (none of them had a history of cancer or bowel disease). Their health was tracked for six years, and it was found that women who ate beef, pork, or lamb as a main dish every day were 2½ times more likely to contract colon cancer when compared to those who ate meat less than once a month. The study clearly demonstrated beyond reasonable doubt that meat in itself was a major risk factor. It wasn't that the meat eaters were defi-

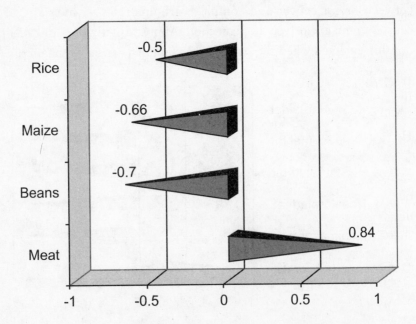

Figure 4.9. Correlation with breast cancer.

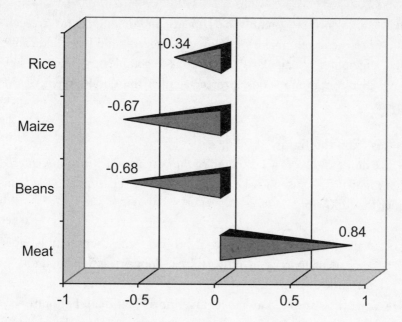

Figure 4.10. Correlation with colon cancer.

cient in other nutrients—fiber, for example. The more meat they ate, the greater the risk.

The leader of the team of scientists commented, "Reducing red meat consumption is likely to reduce the risk. There is no cut-off point so, really, less is better."[84] All by itself, this study truly puts an end to the myth that "meat is part of a healthy diet."

How the Vegetarian Diet Can Help

So what actually happens when you start to change your diet? A clue comes from an intriguing study, carried out in Greece, that set out to establish whether consuming certain types of food might be linked to the development—or prevention—of cancer.[85] The results show that eating spinach, beets, cabbage, and lettuce is associated with a reduction in the risk of colorectal cancer. However, eating beef or lamb was strongly associated with an increase in cancer risk. Figure 4.11 shows what it looks like graphically.

The study concluded the following: "The results of most of these studies appear to fall into two broad categories: those indicating

that animal protein (mainly beef meat) and/or animal fat are con-
ducive to the development of colorectal cancer—and those indicating
that vegetables (particularly cruciferous vegetables) or, more generally, fiber-containing foods, protect against the development of this
disease."

Pieces from the Jigsaw

We don't know every last detail of the way in which a meat-centered
diet predisposes one toward cancer. But we do know quite a lot. Consider the following:

- In just 2.2 pounds of charcoal-broiled steak there may be as
  much benzopyrene (a powerful carcinogen) as in the smoke
  from 600 cigarettes.[86]
- Scientists at the Lawrence Livermore National Laboratory
  have been engaged in a five-year project cooking "thousands
  of pounds of hamburgers" to see what toxic substances are

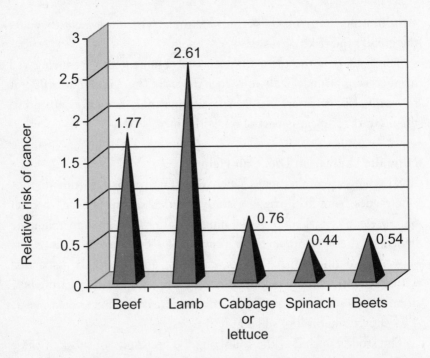

Figure 4.11. Risk of colorectal cancer when consumption of a food increases.

produced in overcooked meat.[87] They have identified at least eight chemicals that are linked to cancer and chromosome damage. "You don't get these structures if you cook tofu or cheese," commented the senior investigator.

- Nitrites may be present in meat products, which can combine with other substances in the human body to form nitrosamines— extremely powerful carcinogens.[88]

- A high-meat diet lowers the age of puberty, and early puberty is associated with an increased risk of breast cancer.[89]

- Certain drugs given to farm animals can cause cancer. One drug which had been given to young pigs for the prevention of respiratory diseases, and was used to treat pneumonia in older animals, has been shown to be carcinogenic.[90]

- Vegetarians are known to have a different composition of bile acids when compared to meat eaters, and it is thought that this may profoundly affect the development of cancer.[91]

- The immune system of vegetarians is stronger than that of meat eaters. One study has shown that although vegetarians have the same overall number of natural killer cells (the kind that are responsible for nipping cancer in the bud), they are *twice* as cytotoxic (potent) as those of meat eaters.[92]

- Vegetarians consume fewer environmental pollutants than do meat eaters. At least one study has indicated that breast milk of vegetarian women is lower in PCBs (polychlorinated biphenyls—widely dispersed industrial compounds that are highly toxic and thought to be carcinogenic) than meat eaters.[93] Organochlorines, such as DDT and the dioxin family, include some of the most poisonous and environmentally per-sistent chemicals known. One published scientific paper cau-tions that 80 percent of the organochlorines absorbed by humans comes from our food.[94] The same paper also states that the main dietary sources of organochlorines are meat, fish, dairy products, and commercial fruit. "The vegetarian diet including unsprayed fruit minimizes contamination," con-cludes the report.

- Vegetarians take in a large amount of vitamin A in the form of beta-carotene in plant foods. Beta-carotene is believed to protect people from cancers of the lungs, bladder, larynx and colon.[95]

- Vegetarians also eat diets that are rich in substances that suppress free-radical formation. Molecules of oxygen are turned into free radicals inside your body by the continual process of metabolism. During this process, more molecules are generated that have an electron missing—called "free radicals." These free radical molecules immediately start to scavenge for electrons to kidnap from other molecules, and this sets in motion a continuing chain reaction, which produces even more free radicals, in the process damaging cell membranes, proteins, carbohydrates, and deoxyribonucleic acid (DNA). Up to now, some sixty diseases have been associated with free radical activity, including Alzheimer's disease, arthritis, multiple sclerosis, and, of course, cancer. The vegetarian diet naturally contains substances (such as vitamin A, retinoids, and protease inhibitors) that have been shown to be capable of blocking this process and halting the development of cancer.[96]

Leukemia

There is another way in which contact with animal flesh might give rise to leukemia, the name used to describe a number of cancerous diseases of the blood-forming organs. The acute and chronic leukemias, together with the other types of tumors of the blood, bone cells, and lymphatic tissue, cause about 10 percent of all cancer deaths and about 50 percent of all cancer deaths in children and adults less than 30 years old.[97]

Is leukemia infectious? Such a notion is commonly dismissed as being absurd. When a cancer charity recently released a report about public myths and misconceptions surrounding cancer, they cited a survey showing that "one in ten teenagers believes that cancer is infectious," presumably with the intention of proving how bizarre our beliefs about cancer can be.

What it really revealed, however, was how out of touch that particular charity was itself. Because there is incontrovertible scientific evidence to show that cancers are, indeed, transmissible—both within species and across them.

It has taken a long time for much of the scientific community to accept that cancers could be caused and transmitted by a virus. In experiments conducted as far back as 1911, it was demonstrated that tumors taken from one chicken and implanted in another would infect the second chicken with a cancerous growth. In 1936, it was demonstrated that breast cancer could be transmitted between mice via a virus present in the milk of lactating mice. More recently, scientists at the University of Glasgow discovered feline leukemia virus in cats. Today, cancer-causing viruses (oncoviruses) are now scientifically categorized as a part of the retrovirus family. Despite this, the belief still persists that cancer somehow "ought not" to be capable of being virally induced. One pathologist commented:

"Indefinite statements are often expressed concerning identifying a certain cancer virus in humans by the antibodies produced in an animal. We show no such insecurity with other viruses: why should we do so with cancer viruses? If we find antibodies to smallpox virus or measles virus in an animal, we confidently say the animal has had the infection of smallpox or measles. But when a cancer virus stimulates an antibody response in an animal, we do not confidently state that the animal was infected by that particular virus. It is as if we are afraid to say that the virus that caused cancer in the cow or dog is the same virus that produces an identical antibody in humans."[98]

Just like human beings, the animals that we eat suffer from various forms of cancer, sometimes caused by a virus. For example:

- Bovine leukemia virus (BLV) causes cancer of the lymph tissue in cows.
- The avian leucosis viruses (ALV) cause leukemias in chickens.
- Marek's disease virus (MDV) causes a cancer of the lymph and nervous systems in chickens.

"Virtually all commercial chickens are heavily infected with leucosis virus [ALV]," one American report found. "Since the tumors induced are not grossly apparent until about 20 weeks of age, this virus is not economically as important as is the Marek's disease virus, which induces tumors by 6–8 weeks of age. Bovine leukemia virus is widespread in commercial dairy herds; more than 20 percent of dairy cows and 60 percent of herds surveyed in the USA are infected."[99]

Now the key question is this: Can eating meat, or being exposed to food animals or their produce, result in a greater likelihood of contracting leukemia or another cancer? To investigate whether these viruses can cross the species barrier and infect humans, a study was established, paid for by the U.S. National Cancer Institute.[100] "The viruses are widely distributed naturally in their respective hosts," wrote the scientists conducting the study, "and are present not only in diseased but also in healthy cattle and chickens destined for human consumption." Therefore, it seemed logical to examine the health of the people who would have maximum exposure to these animals—slaughtermen.

Accordingly, the health of 13,844 members of a meat cutters unions was checked during the period 1949 to 1980. After statistical analysis, it was found that abattoir workers were nearly three times more likely to die from Hodgkin's disease (a cancer of the lymphatic system) than the general population. The scientists concluded, "The excess risk was observed only in abattoir workers and seems to be associated with the slaughtering of cattle, pigs, and sheep. . . . Thus, the excess risk seems to be in keeping with a postulate of an infectious origin for these cases, as no other occupational exposure could adequately explain this occurrence."

By itself, this report is very significant. But now, consider the following additional evidence:

- It has been shown in laboratory experiments that bovine leukemia virus can survive and replicate itself when placed in a human cell culture.[101]
- Scientists have found a close similarity between bovine leukemia virus and HTLV-1, the first human retrovirus ever shown to cause cancer.[102]
- A study conducted in France has concluded that children of fathers who work in the meat trade are at greater risk of developing childhood cancers.[103] The study examined over 200 cases of leukemia diagnosed in the Lyons area, and found that

a significantly large number of fathers of children with leukemia worked as butchers or in slaughterhouses. The scientists suggest that bovine leukemia virus could be to blame.

- In another experiment, chimpanzees were fed from birth on milk taken from cows known to be infected with bovine leukemia virus, with the result that two out of six of them died from leukemia.[104] To defend unpleasant experiments such as these, the idea is often advanced that they are necessary in order to improve human health. One is forced to wonder, however, whether "inconvenient" results such as this are acted upon or simply swept aside.

- Statistical analyses of human deaths from leukemia and other cancers have shown that people who have close contact with food animals (vets, farmers, butchers) run a significantly higher risk of dying from certain types of cancer than the general population. For example, in a Nebraskan study, it was shown that men who had regular contact with cattle were twice as likely to die from leukemia.[105]

- In a study from Poland it has been shown that farmers, butchers, and tanners are more likely to develop leukemia than other people.[106] And another Polish study concluded, "It should be inferred that cattle affected with leukemia may, in favoring circumstances, be a factor disposing man to neoplasms [cancer] especially to the proliferation of the lymphatic system, either through longer contact with a sick animal or the longer ingestion of milk and milk products from cows with leukemia. The fact that with a rise in the incidence of leukemia in cattle there also appears an increase in proliferating diseases of the lymphatic system is particularly worthy of attention."[107]

- A study conducted in Minnesota among leukemia sufferers showed that a surprisingly high number of them were farmers who had regular contact with animals.[108] A similar study conducted in Iowa found a connection between leukemias in humans, cattle density, and the presence of bovine leukemia virus in cows.[109]

- A study of mortality from leukemia and Hodgkin's disease

among vets has shown that they run a significantly higher risk of dying from lymphoid cancer than the norm. The vets were in clinical practice, in close contact with food-producing animals, and the authors of the report suggested that a viral cause may be responsible.[110]

- A study conducted in France and Switzerland in 1990 reveals that male sufferers from breast cancer (generally rare in men) were most likely to work as butchers.[111]
- Like the French study previously mentioned, an Italian study conducted by scientists at the University of Turin has confirmed that the children of butchers are more likely to contract cancer.[112]

All this evidence should be considered very seriously, because it has extraordinarily profound implications. "The Food and Drug Administration states that many unanswered questions remain about BLV," says Dr. Virgil Hulse, a physician who spent fifteen years as a milk inspector for the state of California: "Such as transmission, infectiousness, and whether it's a threat to humans. Some of the questions fuelling the controversy are whether pasteurization, which inhibits infection, destroys the aspect of the virus capable of producing cancer. Also, how great is the risk of pasteurized milk being accidentally contaminated with raw milk? If we wipe out BLV, will we see a reduction of those cancers related to fat consumption? Might it be the viruses, and not the fat, that are linked to some human cancers?"[113]

How could an animal cancer virus induce the disease in humans? There are several possible ways. One theory suggests that a "helper virus" can form an association with another relatively harmless one, and in the process produce a virus that can induce cancer. An animal virus may not, therefore, directly precipitate the disease in humans, but it may be able to convert otherwise harmless human viruses into killers.

It will certainly be many years before every feature of the complex process of zoonotic carcinogenesis (cancers caused by or transmitted from animals) has been resolved. And there will, no doubt, be many people who will not wish to see these rather dark and disquieting fringes of medical and veterinary knowledge examined too closely.

But that, of course, is no reason not to ask questions, nor to take prudent defensive measures.

You can see from all this how difficult it is to isolate just one component of the vegetarian diet, and pin an "anticancer" label on it. Once more, it is the totality of the healthy vegetarian diet—the whole thing—which naturally works to reduce disease.

What Else Can You Do?

Vitamin A. Beta-carotene is the form of vitamin A available in plant foods, and is strongly suspected of having cancer-preventive properties (several studies are currently underway to validate this).[114] In particular, it is thought to protect people from cancers of the lungs, bladder, larynx, and colon.[115] Most researchers believe that beta-carotene offers more protection from cancer than retinol. It is unlikely to cause toxicity, is a powerful antioxidant, is taken in and used according to the body's needs, and it comes in a "packages," which includes secondary plant constituents—nonnutritive compounds that seem to inhibit the onset and growth of cancers and may be vital to beta-carotene's anticancer action. To obtain beta-carotene, eat any of the fruits and vegetables with a deep, bright green, yellow, or orange coloring. Look for carrots, pumpkin, squash, spinach, broccoli, cantaloupe, sweet potatoes, and papaya. Eat these foods lightly cooked or raw, and organically grown if possible.

Vitamin C. This vitamin helps to minimize the effects of pollutants and carcinogens in your food and environment. In particular, vitamin C seems to block the formation of nitrosamines, which are known to be powerful cancer-causing chemicals (they are particularly associated with cancers of the stomach and esophagus). The good news is that if a vitamin C–rich food is taken at the same time as foods containing nitrates or nitrites, then the production of nitrosamines is greatly reduced.[116] Women with abnormal cervical smear results often have low amounts of vitamin C in their body.[117] This may shed new light on the underlying damage caused by smoking, because it has long been established that women who smoke have higher levels of cervical cancer, and smoking impairs the absorption of vitamin C.

Vitamin E. This vitamin also has antioxidant properties, and can combat the production of free radicals in your body. It is available in cold-pressed vegetable oils, nuts, seeds, and soy beans.

Selenium. This trace mineral is essential to health, though only required in minute quantities. In America, the National Research Council has recommended a daily intake of 50 to 200 micrograms of selenium for adults (a microgram is one thousandth of a milligram, so 200 micrograms equal 0.2 milligrams). However, one authority, Gerhard Schrauzer, Ph.D., of the University of California, says that 250 to 300 micrograms can protect against most cancers, and that most people consume only about 100 micrograms daily.[118] At higher doses, selenium can be toxic to the human body. Although it is not certain at precisely what level selenium begins to cause adverse effects, it has been found that doses of 900 micrograms (0.9 milligrams) per day can make hair and nails fall out and can affect the nervous system.[119] Selenium works best in conjunction with vitamin E, since both are antioxidants and can increase the production of antibodies by up to thirty times,[120] thereby greatly enhancing your immune response. Together they help to detoxify your body and prevent the formation of free radicals. Selenium is naturally present in the soil, and the quantities available in our food relate to soil levels of selenium where the food was grown. A study undertaken at the University of Tampere, Finland, involved taking blood samples from 21,172 Finnish men. The samples were then frozen. Eleven years after the samples had been taken, 143 of the men had contracted lung cancer. The researchers found that the men who eventually developed lung cancer had less selenium in their blood than those who did not. Overall, it was found that people with the lowest selenium levels were 3.3 times more likely to develop lung cancer than those with high levels. The researchers said their results were "in accord with other studies which strongly suggest that poor selenium nutrition is a highly significant risk factor for lung cancer."[121] In West Germany, a study conducted at the University of Bonn has shown that selenium can protect against the harmful effects of ultraviolet radiation. Blood selenium levels were examined in 101 patients with malignant melanoma (a lethal form of skin cancer) and compared to a control group of healthy people. The skin cancer patients showed a significantly lower level of selenium, and the researchers concluded that their results "strongly suggest that sub-optimal selenium nutrition preceded the onset of the disease and may even have contributed to its genesis."[122]

Calcium and vitamin D. Calcium may be important in preventing both breast and colon cancer, and it has been suggested that it may reduce the risk of colon cancer by two-thirds when taken with vitamin D.[123] Vitamin D is necessary for the proper absorption of calcium. Your body manufactures this vitamin when sunlight reacts with dehydro-cholesterol, a substance in your skin. Obtain vitamin D either from fortified foods or by ensuring that you have ten minutes of daylight on your face and hands each day. Calcium is available in tofu; dark green, leafy vegetables, such as, spinach, watercress, and parsley; sea-weeds; nuts and seeds; dairy foods; molasses, and dried fruits.

Calories. A high-calorie diet may increase your risk of cancer. Cancer seems to be more common in obese people, especially those who are more than 40 percent over their ideal weight.[124] Do your best to keep your weight within recommended limits.

Cabbage. Cruciferous vegetables include cabbage, broccoli, cauliflower, brussels sprouts, and kale, all of which contain secondary plant con-stituents.[125] These compounds, (i.e., indoles, phenols, flavones) are present in many plant foods, but are particularly abundant in crucifer-ous vegetables. They are not available in supplement form. Eat a serv-ing of cruciferous vegetables at least three times per week.

CONSTIPATION

What Is It?

Approximately four people out of every ten in Western countries are constipated. In two out of ten, constipation is so severe that laxa-tives are used regularly. Here's another startling fact: 77 percent of the population only excrete between five and seven stools per week. That's over three-quarters of the total population! On top of that, a further 8 percent of people only pass three to four stools a week. That makes 85 percent with sluggish bowel movements.[126] Although constipation, and its unwilling products, are subjects to talk or write jokingly about, there is a serious side, too. As you will see, constipation is a very clear sign that the body is functioning poorly. And when that happens, many serious diseases can follow.

Chronic constipation occurs when you retain your stools in the colon and rectum so that the water they naturally contain is reabsorbed by the body. The stools then harden even more, making defecation more and more difficult. Eventually, your bowel will lose its muscle tone and constipation becomes a way of life. Conventional medicine treats the symptom of constipation and brings about short-term purgative relief through the use of laxatives, most of which fall into these categories:

Bulk laxatives. These substances increase the size of stools and stimulate bowel motion. They include ingredients such as bran and methylcellulose. They are generally safe, if somewhat slow to take effect, although internal obstruction may be caused if insufficient water is taken or if excessive amounts of the substances are consumed.

Irritant laxatives. This group includes such substances as danthron, senna, aloes, rhubarb, and cascara (known as "anthraquinone laxatives") and phenolphthalein and castor oil. They are thought to work by stimulating the intestinal smooth muscle, creating contractions and motion that lead to the passing of a movement, but they also may increase the amount of fluid in the intestines. As with all laxatives, overly frequent use can damage natural bowel functions.

Saline or osmotic laxatives. These substances, which include magnesium sulphate, potassium sodium tartrate, sodium sulphate, lactulose, and magnesium hydroxide, work by attracting water to the bowel and so increase the bulk of its contents, leading to a watery evacuation.

Lubricant laxatives. Lubricant laxatives soften and lubricate the stools, making them easier to pass. Liquid paraffin and sodium dioctyl sulphosuccinate are two examples of lubricant laxatives and fecal softeners. Liquid paraffin can dissolve fat-soluble vitamins, and if inhaled it may cause a type of pneumonia.

As you can see, conventional medicine offers us a veritable armory of cathartics with which to goad our sluggish bowels into action. However, you should know that the continuing use/abuse of laxatives can make you dependent on them, thus precipitating further health problems. Although some types of constipation are not diet related (such as drug-induced constipation), most are. It is, therefore, much better to treat the underlying cause, rather than the eventual symptom.

How the Vegetarian Diet Can Help

Dr. Denis Burkitt, a famous advocate of dietary fiber, performed a classic experiment that revealed just how effective the vegetarian diet can be at preventing constipation.[127] He carefully collected information from various populations concerning the size of their stools, the average time it took food to pass all the way through their bodies, and the types of diets they ate. You can see some of his results in Figure 4.12.

His findings were extremely revealing. From left to right on the chart, the first group, with the shortest stool transit time, were schoolchildren living in rural Africa, who ate an unrefined diet. Their food positively shot through their insides, taking on average less than a day and a half from one end to the other. Next came another group of Africans, this time adults living in villages in Uganda. Once again, their food hardly touched the sides on the way down.

But it is the next group that is so interesting from our point of view. This consisted of ordinary vegetarians living in the United Kingdom. Despite enormous differences in environment and food availability, the Western vegetarians' diet came close to equaling the African results.

The next group on the chart consisted of nurses living and working in southern India. Once again, their diet tended to be meat-free, and their transit times were only slightly longer than the U.K. vegetarians.

The really big jump comes with the next group on the graph—labeled schoolchildren—with nearly *twice as long* a transit time as any

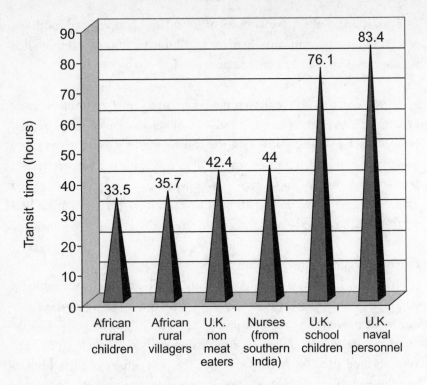

Figure 4.12. The Western way of toilet straining.

of the preceding ones. This group was drawn from children at a boarding school in the U.K., who ate a refined diet typical of institutionalized catering—greasy, meat dominated, and low in natural fiber. And the next group is even worse—naval ratings and their wives, all shore based in the U.K. This group had a mean transit time of 83.4 hours, and the longest time was 144 hours! That's 6 whole days for the food to hang around someone's intestines!

This study revealed something else, too. You might suppose that small stools would whiz through the system quickly, but you'd be wrong. For Dr. Burkitt found that the larger the stool, the faster it was processed. So, for example, the mean weight of stools passed by naval ratings was a mere 104 grams. On the other hand, the mean weight for rural Ugandan villagers was more than four times as heavy. This is also very significant, because stool weights of below 150 grams a day denote an increased risk of bowel cancer.[128] Somewhere in the middle came the U.K. vegetarians, with a mean weight of 225 grams, who compare very favorably with South African schoolchildren (275 grams) and Indian nurses (155 grams).

This information is crucial to our understanding of the importance of a diet high in natural fiber. Further evidence has shown that, without exception, countries that have a refined diet in which meat is predominant face a whole range of diseases that the so-called "less developed" countries rarely see. Some of these western plagues are:

- Appendicitis. The commonest abdominal emergency in the West. Over 300,000 appendixes are removed every year in the United States alone. It has now been shown that a low-fiber diet makes the risk of suffering appendicitis much greater.
- Diverticular disease. Thirty percent of all people over forty-five years have symptoms of this.
- Cancer of the large bowel. One of the commonest causes of death from cancer in the West.

All these diseases were comparatively rare in the West until the beginning of the twentieth century. Then the amount of animal fat in the diet began to steadily increase, and the amount of natural fiber began to decrease. Figure 4.13 shows how the American diet has changed in less than 100 years.

One hundred years ago, meat, fat, and sugar between them contributed only 15 percent of the total number of calories in an average diet. Today, the figure is nearer 60 percent. Perhaps the biggest change in the diet has been the tremendous fall in the quantity of cereal fiber, which dropped by 90 percent. Most scientists now accept that there is a definite connection between the increase in modern diseases and the radical change in our eating patterns. Dr. Burkitt explained:

There are basically two types of fiber, insoluble fiber and water-soluble fiber. The classic insoluble fiber is wheat fiber, with bran and all the bran products. That is highly effective for combating constipation, increasing stool weight, and preventing things like

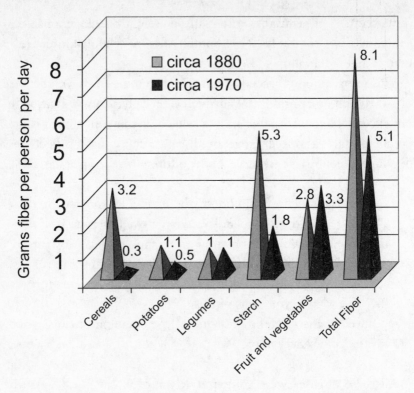

Figure 4.13. How fiber fell from favor.

hemorrhoids and diverticular diseases. It's very good for the guts. But it does almost nothing for what we call the "metabolic diseases" associated with lack of fiber, particularly diabetes and coronary heart disease. Now soluble fiber, on the other hand, does have an effect on combating constipation, but it also has an effect on lowering raised serum lipid [i.e. fats in your blood] levels, and also on glucose tolerance, so that it has a profoundly beneficial effect on diabetes. Now, as to how this fiber works in lowering the blood lipids, there are many suggestions. It affects bile acids and so on, but the main way in which soluble fiber is beneficial for diabetes is that it enormously slows down the absorption of energy from the gut. So instead of all the energy being absorbed, a high-fiber product makes the intestinal content into a sort of a gel, so that the energy is only absorbed into the circulation very slowly, and so you don't have great and sudden demands on insulin, and so on.

The scope of diseases that Dr. Burkitt mentions is quite breathtaking. Suddenly, instead of merely being a useful preventive measure to ward off constipation, it seems as if fiber (in all its many natural forms) lies at the heart of healthy living. Once regarded as revolutionary, Dr. Burkitt's views on the importance of fiber are now universally accepted. Actually, it is almost impossible to overstate the huge range of diseases to which our drastic change in eating patterns has contributed. Colon cancer, for example, appears to be due to carcinogens created in the colon itself[129]—which can be negatively influenced by consuming a high level of saturated fat in the diet, and positively influenced by a good consumption of dietary fiber. High-fiber diets have also been shown to reduce the incidence of breast, uterine, and ovarian cancer. Experts at the U.S. Department of Health and Human Services estimate that if Americans ate more fiber and less fat, 20,000 deaths from cancer could be avoided every year.[130]

It is *barely* possible to be vegetarian and not eat a diet high in natural forms of fiber. But you'd have to work very hard to do so. You'd have to eat a diet composed exclusively of junk food—chocolate, ice cream, sweets, and so on—and you'd have to punctiliously avoid contact with anything remotely plantlike. In reality, both vegetarians and vegans *can't help* but get lashings of dietary fiber in their everyday diets, which accounts for their lack of constipation. By the same token, it is barely possible to be a meat eater and have the same high intake of fiber as vegetarians. But again, you'd have to work very hard at it. Meat is a dense food and fills you up quickly (scientists term this "satiety"), and so meat eaters have neither the room nor the appetite to eat significant quantities of food with fiber (meat, of course, contains none). Figure 4.14 shows how, in the real world, various diets compare in fiber intake.

Studies confirm what common sense suggests. In Britain, scientists measured the actual fiber content of daily food intake for meat eaters, vegetarians, and vegans, and found that the meat eaters did worst of all (a meager 23 grams a day). Next came the vegetarians (37 grams) and at the top of the league came the vegans (47 grams)—twice as much as meat eaters.[131]

Fiber intake varies from one country to another, depending on the supply of fruit and vegetables, and on the time of year, and methods

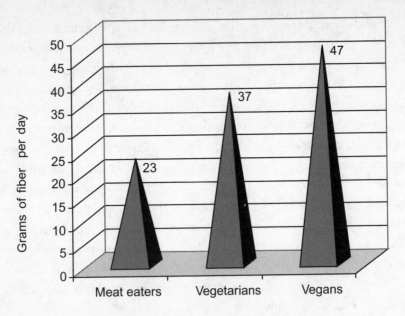

Figure 4.14. Vegans get high on fiber: fiber intake compared.

of analyzing fiber intake vary as well. But the all-important difference between the fiber intake of vegetarians and meat eaters is usually constant. In America, another study found that meat eaters were consuming just 12 grams of dietary fiber per day, compared to 28 grams for vegetarians.[132] In Sweden, a similar experiment found that vegans consume *three times* as much fiber as meat eaters.[133]

One question that is sometimes asked is: Can you consume too much fiber? It has been suggested that fiber may have undesirable nutritional effects—that the phytate it contains, for example, may prevent other nutrients from being absorbed. Although this may be demonstrated in the laboratory, in practice it looks as if this should be the least of our worries. Eating a good, nutritious, plant-based diet, as described on page 288–89, provides a naturally high level of both fiber and other nutrients. This is confirmed by a careful analysis of vegetarians' diets performed in Israel.[134] The scientists found that the intake of iron and magnesium was significantly higher in vegetarians compared to meat eaters, and they concluded that a long-term vegetarian diet does not lead to mineral deficiencies. Another scientific paper examined the benefits of dietary fiber in 1987, and pointed out that "vegetarians routinely consume 40 to 50 grams dietary fiber daily without ill effect."[135] A painstaking examination of the effect of dietary fiber confirms these same findings. In this study, the participants were divided into three categories: a group of 68 people who regularly supplemented their diet with an average of 3 tablespoons of bran a day for a year, 43 "controls" who didn't consume bran supplements, and 20 vegetarians who had a very high fiber consumption for many years. Then the scientists carefully measured the blood level of nutrients in all three groups, including serum iron, total iron binding capacity, calcium, phosphorus, zinc, and magnesium. In their own words: "We evaluated the hypothesis that a healthy population taking a high-fiber diet may develop deficiencies of various minerals and nutrients. . . . There was no correlation between the amount of bran consumed and the blood level of nutrients. The fiber consumption of the vegetarians was very high, more than three times that of the controls. Our study indicates that a moderately or even extremely high consumption of fiber for a long time does not by itself cause mineral or nutrient deficiencies in a western type population."[136]

These findings have since been confirmed by an American study, which also concluded, "The higher level of fiber intake did not appear to affect mineral utilization by the vegetarians."[137] If any group were to be vulnerable to this effect, it would probably be infants. Comments Dr. Gill Langley, "It has been speculated . . . that a vegan diet may not be suitable for infants and small children. In fact it is easy to ensure that infants eat enough suitably prepared high-energy foods such as beans, grains and nuts."[138]

What Else Can You Do?

Here are a few further suggestions for the natural relief of constipation:

Beet juice. Either bottled or freshly juiced, it is a very useful, short-term natural stool softener and laxative.

High-Fiber Salad. This salad really has get up and go! Ingredients: Canned kidney beans, carrots, beets, cabbage, watercress, broccoli, potatoes, tofu, sunflower seeds, almonds, pumpkin seeds; plus any seasonal vegetables, including winter roots. Pick any six from these twelve! There's no need for lettuce, but make it a romaine if you want it: it's got some flavor and it won't go limp. Next, get a really large bowl. Cube the potatoes and lightly steam them and the broccoli. Roast the pumpkin seeds. Cube the tofu. Grate the raw carrots and beets (don't slice). Thinly shred the cabbage. Finely chop the watercress. Wash and roughly chop the lettuce, don't forget the sunflower seeds and almonds. All this is quick to do, but get a food processor if you want to speed it up even more. Now prepare your favorite dressing. Two suggestions: olive oil, cider vinegar, and French mustard (real French mustard, please—no appalling English substitutes). Or, for the most unusual dressing you've ever tasted—try this and you'll never use anything else—buy some powdered black salt from an Indian market. Add 2 teaspoonfuls to oil and cider vinegar, and shake thoroughly until dissolved. Finally, place the lettuce in the bottom and round the side of the bowl, if desired. Mix the other ingredients together and put them on top. Pour on the dressing. One serving of a salad like this will give you a third of your total daily requirement of protein, almost twice your vitamin A requirement, all your vitamin C, and half your iron and fiber. It's so good you'll want to eat it every day! Tofu and, even nicer, marinated tofu are available in health food stores.

Take your time. Set aside half an hour a day to do your business—yes, literally: you can take a phone in there with you if you want, or at least read the paper. Never suppress an urge to go—this is giving your body entirely the wrong message. If you can do some simple exercise just before going—stretching or yoga is good—this will help.

Colonic irrigation. This can provide you with an internal spring cleaning, and set up your bowels so that you're starting all over again with a nice, clean intestinal passage. Much more natural and pleasant than an enema, colonic irrigation is nothing more complicated or sinister than an internal bath to remove poisons, gases, fecal matter, and mucus deposits. Sterilized equipment with an inlet and outlet attachment is used to flush filtered water through the rectum, into the colon and out again, taking the waste products with it. Unlike regular use of laxatives, it is not habit forming!

DIABETES

What Is It?

Diabetes mellitus is a disorder in which the body is unable to control the amount of sugar in the blood, because the mechanism that converts sugar to energy is no longer functioning properly.[139] It is a disease of the Western world, brought about by both genetic and environmental factors. An estimated 30 million people are thought to suffer from it worldwide.

Normally, the food you eat is gradually broken down and converted to glucose (blood sugar), the source of energy for all your body's functions. The conversion of glucose into energy requires insulin, a hormone produced in the pancreas. Insulin is released into your system in order to control the level of glucose in your blood, especially to prevent your blood sugar level from climbing too high. However, in diabetics, there is either a shortage of insulin or the available insulin does not function as it should. The result is that glucose is not converted into energy, but builds up in the blood and eventually spills over into your urine. This is often one of the first signs of diabetes.

Though there is an abundance of glucose in your blood, the body is still deprived of the energy it needs (because the glucose has not been converted to energy), and so the liver begins to produce yet more glucose to meet demands. Shortly, your body's stores of fat and protein begin to break down in another attempt to supply more glucose. The resulting weight loss is often another sign of diabetes. Thus begins a chain of events within your body that can eventually cause severe health problems, even death. In the U.K. alone, approximately 20,000 people die prematurely each year from diabetes-related problems.[140] There are two main classifications:

Maturity-onset diabetes; non–insulin dependent. "Overfed, overweight and underactive." That is a common description of many, but not all, adults who develop diabetes in their middle years. Maturity-onset diabetics experience the basic symptoms of thirst, fatigue, hunger, and frequent urination. However, their health may improve by losing weight, increasing their level of exercise, and monitoring their food intake to avoid foods high in calories, fats, and sugar. In some people, diabetic symptoms can actually disappear following a strict regime of dietary control and exercise. Others must live the rest of their lives with the precautions, medications, and attention to diet that have for so long been associated with the disorder. In maturity-onset diabetes, the adult need not become insulin dependent.

Juvenile-onset diabetes; insulin dependent. Although a person of any age may develop diabetes, those who develop it under the age of forty years are most likely to suffer the more severe, insulin-dependent form. Children who develop diabetes are almost always insulin dependent. The insulin-dependent diabetic produces very little or no insulin and so relies on insulin injections. Without a supply of insulin, he would not survive. Before the discovery of insulin, diabetes was considered to be invariably fatal, and most patients died within a short time of its diagnosis. Diabetes can be treated effectively today, although it does increase the risk of suffering other serious illnesses, such as cardiovascular disease, eye disorders, gangrene and other circulatory problems, nerve and muscle problems, and an increased susceptibility to ordinary infections.

Diabetes is a serious disorder, and unfortunately, its incidence is increasing. The number of children diagnosed as diabetic has doubled in the past twenty years, and this appears to be a worldwide trend. Yet there are simple, effective steps that may prevent the onset of diabetes or minimize its erosion of your health if you already have it.

How the Vegetarian Diet Can Help

According to a report submitted by Diabetes Epidemiology Research International (DERI) to the *British Medical Journal*, between 60 and 95 percent of cases of insulin-dependent diabetes can be prevented.[141] The DERI scientists believe that environmental factors are largely responsible for the increase in diabetes, claiming that genetic factors could not account for such great increases over such a very short period of time. Of the possible environmental causes, diet is perhaps the most significant and certainly one over which we have control.

We also know that diabetics can benefit from a high-fiber vegetarian diet. A study carried out at the Veterans Administration Medical Center in Lexington, Kentucky, compared two diets for the treatment of nonobese diabetic men, all of whom required insulin therapy.[142] The "control" diet provided 20 grams per day of plant fiber—an average amount in a Western meat-centered diet. The other diet included over three times as much fiber—65 grams per day. The researchers found that the men on high fiber, high carbohydrate diets needed 73 percent *less* insulin therapy than those on ordinary diets—quite a remarkable reduction.

Further, it seems that the same dietary measures used in prevention of diabetes can be used with great success in treatment. There have been several clues pointing to this possibility. For instance, Nauru, a remote island in the Pacific, had never had any cases of diabetes until it suddenly became rich and began to import American-style fast food. Now, more than 40 percent of its population over the age of twenty have diabetes! Similarly, diabetes is noticeably rare in parts of Africa and China where the traditional diet is intact and free of Western influence. So what are the dietary influences that can prevent or treat diabetes?

The American Diabetes Association suggests that diabetics eat a diet in which carbohydrates make up about 60 percent of total calorie intake, these carbohydrates to be mostly unrefined, complex and high in fiber.[143] Fat intake should total less than 30 percent of calories consumed, with an emphasis on reducing saturated fats and cholesterol, replacing them with monounsaturated fats such as olive oil. Protein intake should be moderate.

The fact is, diabetes is more common among meat-eating people than non–meat eaters. Meat eating increases consumption of saturated fats, which may affect insulin sensitivity. Also, the N-nitroso compounds in meat may actually be a trigger to the development of diabetes.

Some very significant research from the School of Public Health at the University of Minnesota reveals how we can reduce our risk of contracting diabetes.[144] They started a massive study of the subject in 1960, which lasted for twenty-one years and involved 25,698 adult Americans. They belonged to the Seventh-Day Adventist church, a group of people who are often used by scientists investigating the vegetarian diet, because half of them never eat meat.

The results of this investigation showed that people on meat-free diets had a substantially reduced risk (45 percent) of contracting diabetes when compared to the population as a whole. They also found that people who consumed meat ran over twice the risk of dying from a diabetes-related cause. The correlation between meat consumption and diabetes was found to be particularly strong in males. The study was carefully designed to eliminate confusion arising from confounding factors, such as over- or underweight, other dietary habits, or amount of physical activity. The results are summarized in Figure 4.15.

You can see that there is, of course, a striking difference between

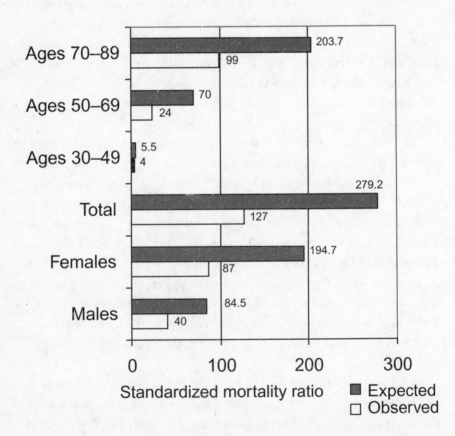

Figure 4.15. Deaths from diabetes among Seventh-Day Adventists: what was expected and what really happened.

the number of people who were expected to die ("Expected") and the number of people who actually died ("Observed"). But the study went even further than this: By analyzing death certificates over the period under study, it was possible to assess the increased risk of dying from a diabetic illness for those who consumed meat. Figure 4.16 shows how it looks graphically.

This shows that including *any* meat in the diet increases the risk, on average, by 1.8 times. For light meat eaters (people who eat meat only once or twice per week), the relative risk compared to a non–meat eater is 1.4 times. But for heavy meat eaters—those who consume it six or more times a week—the risk rises steeply to 3.8 times.

Why should this be so? One explanation may be that diabetics are particularly vulnerable to high levels of fat in their blood, and meat is a prime source of saturated fat. There may be an associated problem with excess protein consumption, too. Several clinical studies have shown that a low-protein diet along with good blood glucose control can help slow the decline in kidney function that diabetics may experience.[145]

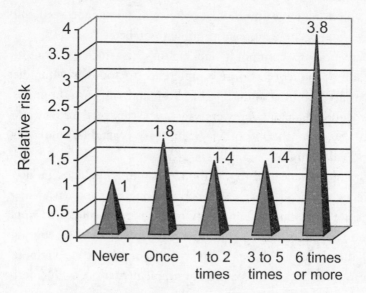

Figure 4.16. Frequency of meat consumption and the risk of diabetes mortality.

What Else Can You Do?

- It seems that babies who are breastfed early in life may be less prone to developing diabetes, whereas children given cow's milk appear to be more likely to suffer from it in later life.[146] A recent study examined international milk consumption patterns, and found a strong correlation with the incidence of insulin-dependent diabetes. "The study raises the possibility that when diabetes runs in families, parents may be able to protect their children by eliminating dairy products during the formative first nine months or so after birth," reported The Associated Press. "If true, we should be able to do something to prevent diabetes altogether," commented Dr. Hans-Michael Dosch, senior author of the study at the Hospital for Sick Children in Toronto. This study suggests that milk proteins cause an autoimmune reaction in which the body mistakenly attacks its own insulin-producing cells.

- Coffee raises the concentration of sugar in the blood. As this is the major symptom of diabetes, coffee consumption may have serious implications for diabetics and potential diabetics alike. If you drink large amounts of coffee while pregnant, your children will become more susceptible to diabetes.[147]

- Diabetics are commonly lacking in B_6, which is vital for insulin production. So give preference to foods in your diet that are rich in vitamin B_6—oat bran and oat germ, hummus, avocados, bananas, brewers yeast, yeast extract, brown rice, parsley, spinach, and other green, leafy vegetables, molasses, and whole grains.

- Vitamin C is needed to metabolize insulin and glucose; a deficiency can lead to cell degeneration in the pancreas, where insulin is produced. Eat plenty of citrus fruit, alfalfa sprouts, and vegetables such as potato, green pepper, and broccoli.

- Diabetics often have a deficiency of the trace mineral chromium and can benefit from supplementation, with elderly and non–insulin dependent diabetics responding particularly well. Chromium acts with insulin to transport glucose through cell walls. Highly processed foods always have reduced levels of chromium, and years of eating such foods can invite the onset of maturity-onset diabetes. A diet rich in chromium may prevent this. Eat plenty of wheat germ, brewer's yeast, whole grains, and corn oil.

- Zinc plays a crucial role in the synthesis and storage of insulin in the pancreas. It is a mineral that many of us, not just diabetics, are continually short of. Eat mushrooms, sunflower and pumpkin seeds, brewer's yeast, and soy beans to boost your zinc intake.

- Foods rich in magnesium may help to prevent retinopathy, a deterioration of the retina that is a real threat to diabetics. Foods rich in magnesium include nuts, whole grains, dark green vegetables, and molasses.

- Although there may be a genetic component in diabetes, obesity is very strongly implicated in its development. In Japan almost all sumo wrestlers become diabetic before they are thirty-five years old, and it is strongly suspected that this is induced by the amazingly high-fat diet they are given.

ECZEMA AND PSORIASIS

What Are They?

Most of us are familiar with the red, scaly, often painful skin that typifies psoriasis and eczema. Both are chronic, noncontagious skin disorders that affect people of all ages. The joints, scalp, back, chest, bottom, hands and legs, and in acute cases, virtually the whole body, can all be affected. Both conditions can be brought on by allergy, stress, anxiety, viruses, flu, exhaustion, or injury—especially if you have a history of either disorder in the family. Rather than accept the problem as inevitable, however, there are dietary changes that can help to minimize or solve these skin problems.

How the Vegetarian Diet Can Help

A poorly functioning digestive system results in the proliferation of various toxins within the gut, some of which may contribute to the development of psoriasis and eczema.[148] Adopting a dairy- and gluten-free diet for at least two to three weeks is certainly worth trying to determine whether your skin problem is aggravated by these food groups. In addition, there are several other dietary steps you may take to improve digestion and therefore prevent or minimize your skin problem.

What Else Can You Do?

- Adopt a low-sugar or even a sugar-free diet to prevent an overgrowth of the candida albicans yeast in your gut. This yeast is normally present in a healthy person, but when present to excess, can cause disease or reduced immunity. Psoriasis is particularly responsive to a reduction in your sugar intake, and a few days or weeks on a sugar-free diet (sometimes called an antifungal diet) may improve your condition.[149] Remember, sugar includes honey, molasses, concentrated fruit juices, and syrups.

- In some people, a deficiency in the B complex of vitamins can hinder the proper metabolism of fats and proteins and problems such as psoriasis and eczema can result. To correct a deficiency, you may take a B complex supplement daily. Simply ensure that your supplement includes the whole range of B vitamins because they work best when taken as a group. The B vitamins are essential to the health of skin, mucous membranes, and nerves. In fact, as stress is so often a trigger for eczema and psoriasis, a sufficiency of the B complex may help prevent an attack by reducing the initial effects of stress on your body. Foods especially rich in the B complex are yeasts, such as brewer's or nutritional yeast, and whole grains. Legumes (peas, beans, lentils) and seeds are also useful sources. Ensure that you have a serving of each of these foods in your diet each day.

- Gamma-linolenic acid is a substance that we produce in our bodies. Some people, however, do not produce enough and are more likely to suffer from eczema as a result. A bowl of porridge each day is a good source of gamma-linolenic acid,[150] as is a supplement in the form of evening primrose oil.[151]

- Omega-3 fatty acids reduce the itching and scaling of eczema and psoriasis in many people.[152] Sources of omega-3 fatty acids include flaxseed and soy oils.

- Selenium and vitamin E are both antioxidants and work together to preserve and promote healthy metabolic processes. Of particular importance to sufferers of eczema and psoriasis, this combination can retard the oxidation of essential fatty acids, which are so crucial to healthy skin. Selenium is a mineral found in whole grains, especially the bran and germ, and vegetables such as onions, celery, cabbage, and broccoli. Vitamin E is abundant in the cold-pressed vegetable oils, in soybeans and in all raw nuts and seeds. Supplements are also available.

- Increase your intake of dietary fiber. Start by altering your diet to include an abundance of fresh fruit and vegetables as well as 2 to 3 servings daily of whole, unprocessed grains.

- Boost your intake of folic acid as some psoriasis sufferers have been shown to have low blood levels of folic acid.[153] Folic acid is found in green, leafy vegetables and brewer's yeast. Supplements are also available.

- Zinc is essential for the production of hydrochloric acid in your stomach, a shortage of which produces digestive problems that can lead to eczema or psoriasis. Zinc is found in whole grains, pumpkin seeds, and brewer's yeast. It may also be taken in supplement form.

- Vitamin A is necessary for the health of all body tissue, especially the skin and mucous membranes. Skin problems such as eczema and psoriasis can be one sign of deficiency and may respond well to increased intakes of vitamin A or carotene, the vegetable substance that your body converts to vitamin A. To boost your intake of vitamin A, eat plenty of carotene-rich foods, including dark green, leafy vegetables, such as spinach, and vegetables of a dark orange color, such as carrots and pumpkin.

- Some people's eczema or psoriasis is an allergic response. If you suspect this might be true for you, try amending your diet in these ways: Eat only fresh, organic produce to avoid chemical residues and unnecessary additives. Eliminate the foods that most commonly cause an allergic response. These include dairy products, eggs, fish, peanuts and soybeans, chicken, citrus, tomato, and corn.[154]

- Moderately high alcohol consumption can aggravate psoriasis. A Finnish study concluded that men who consumed 5 or more units of alcohol per day were likely to suffer a worsening of their condition.[155] Try keeping your alcohol intake to the recommended 21 units per week for men, 14 units per week for women.

GALLSTONES

What Are They?

Gallstones are more common among women than men—25 percent of all women and 10 percent of all men will develop gallstones before they are sixty years old. This is how they occur: the liver secretes bile, a substance that is high in cholesterol (which literally means "solid bile" in Greek), and is stored in the gallbladder. Lecithin (found in soybeans and corn) and bile salts together help to keep the cholesterol dissolved in the bile. However, if the level of cholesterol becomes so high that no more can be dissolved, then it begins to precipitate, and gallstones are the result. Stones vary considerably in size. The largest reported stone was almost seven inches in diameter, but that is very rare. Most are between one-eighth and three-quarters of an inch. When the gallbladder contracts to release bile, a stone may shoot up and plug the opening of the cystic duct. Then, no matter how hard the gallbladder tries to empty itself, bile cannot flow out. The result is intense pain in the upper abdomen, which increases until, after several hours, the stone falls back into the gallbladder, ending the attack. About half of all those people with gallstones feel no symptoms. But for those who do, the suffering can be intense. It's like "being kicked in the guts by a horse—all the time," as one sufferer has described it. Gallstones can also lead to infection, resulting in inflammation of the gallbladder, colic, peritonitis, gangrene of the gallbladder, and jaundice. As an indication of the prevalence of this condition, it is surprising to discover that over one million Americans are diagnosed with gallstones every year, and in half of these cases, the symptoms are so severe that their gallbladders are surgically removed.[156]

As the Western diet has changed, so has the incidence of gallstones, quadrupling since 1940 in many areas. Significantly, Asians and rural

Africans, who traditionally consume a low-fat, high-fiber diet, suffer very little from them, and *only* humans and domesticated animals experience them—wild animals do not. All this strongly suggests that the problem is connected with our modern, Western way of eating.

How the Vegetarian Diet Can Help

In an experiment carried out in Oxford, England, two groups of women were compared to see if their diets might have any influence on the occurrence of gallstones.[157] The first group, consisting of 632 meat-eating women, were selected at random. The second group consisted of 130 women who did not eat meat, and had a diet naturally higher in fiber. All the women were thoroughly examined, using ultrasound detection techniques, for gallstones. The experimenters found that the meat eaters were *two and a half times* more likely to develop gallstones than the non–meat eaters. The scientists concluded that the low-fat, high-fiber diet of the vegetarian women gave them protection.

Building on this study, the scientists then undertook a further investigation of 121 nonvegetarian women suffering from gallstones, who were then age-matched with other nonvegetarian women without gallstones.[158] The aim was to find out if there was any particular factor in the diets of the women with gallstones that made them more prone to suffer—for example, did they eat more fat? After analyzing the diets of both groups, the scientists found out that there was actually very little difference between the groups in terms of their nutrient intake. They concluded, "This may indicate the existence of a threshold effect where virtually all non-vegetarian women in affluent societies have a diet high in saturated fat, animal protein, and simple sugar to the extent that it is not possible to distinguish between cases and controls." In other words, only vegetarian (and vegan) diets are sufficiently low in saturated fat, and high in fiber, to result in a lower incidence of gallstones.

What Else Can You Do?

- If you are obese you are four times more likely to suffer from stones. But a word of warning—rapid weight loss can actually increase your risk of suffering from gallstones. Obese people who lose a lot of weight on very low-calorie diets are quite likely to form stones. Once the weight has been lost, however, and relatively normal eating patterns are restored, the stones may dissolve of their own accord. This, and all other treatments, should naturally be supervised by a doctor.

- Fatty foods are known to stimulate gallbladder contractions, which can cause a painful gallstone attack. So consider trying a reduced-fat diet. Also, consuming smaller, more frequent meals may help limit gallbladder contractions and gallstone attacks.

- Research suggests that aspirin can inhibit substances that may cause cholesterol to crystallize into stones.[159] It could therefore prevent gallstones in obese people during weight loss; or halt the recurrence in people who had their stones dissolved with drugs.

- Taking estrogen or oral contraceptives can increase the amount of cholesterol in your bile fluid and thus the chances of having gallstones.[160] At least three studies have found an increased risk of gall bladder disease among women who use oral contraceptives.

- Recently, there has been speculation that a diet high in soluble fiber might increase the solubility of cholesterol in the bile, and so prevent, and perhaps even reverse, the formation of gallstones. Good sources of soluble fiber include oat bran, pectin, and beans.

- And finally, a word of warning: the so-called olive-oil cure, which involves fasting for three days and then drinking a mug of olive oil and lemon juice to make the gallbladder contract and push through extremely small stones, can be dangerous. If larger stones are ejected in this way, they could stick in the bile duct, causing jaundice, infection, and a possible medical emergency.

HEART DISEASE

The Size of the Problem

You may be shocked to learn that the first clinical account of someone suffering a heart attack was only recorded as recently as 1912. Until then, it seems that heart attacks were so rare they just weren't written about or recorded. Today, heart disease is the commonest cause of death in the Western world. Within the past century, an ominous change has occurred in our lifestyles—a change that has made a once rare and unusual form of death the most common.

What Makes You Tick?

Every living cell in your body has a specific job to do, and in order that each cell may do its job well, it must somehow take in essential products and put out waste material. To meet this requirement, the cells of your body need a reliable transport system that will perform both deliveries and removals. The circulation of blood is such a system. It is called the cardiovascular system because it is structured around the heart ("cardio") and the blood vessels ("vascular") and all the functions included in the relationship between them. With almost unbelievable speed and efficiency, your blood is able to maintain the health of every living cell in your body by supplying it with nutrients and oxygen specific to its needs, and then removing waste material and carbon dioxide as the nutrients and oxygen are utilized.

Blood is composed of red cells, white cells, and platelets suspended in plasma. If you've ever made a salad dressing from vinegar, oil, and a few herbs you'll understand the idea of suspension. When you stir the mixture vigorously, it changes in consistency and, temporarily at least, the oil, vinegar, and herbs are evenly distributed, making a smooth emulsion. Blood is, for the sake of analogy only, a similar mixture. All four components—plasma, platelets, and red and white cells—are present in measured and changing proportions to make healthy blood.

Plasma. If any substance on earth could be called "primordial soup," it would have to be plasma. To make it, take several liters of water and add microscopic portions of several dozen compounds, such as amino acids, hormones, antibodies, "tissue salts" (e.g., sodium, potassium, calcium, and chloride), and proteins (e.g., albumin, globulin, and fibrinogen). These nutrients are transferred to your needy cells in exchange for waste material for eventual excretion. Here's how: Every cell in your body is surrounded by a plasmalike liquid called "tissue fluid." This fluid gets right up next to the cell, every cell, and removes any waste material that the cell generates as it functions. This waste is transferred through the tissue fluid to the plasma and, at this point, is exchanged for whichever of the compounds in the plasma the needy cell requires. These compounds are again transferred from the plasma, through the tissue fluid, to the waiting body cell. This whole cycle happens about 100 times faster than it took you to read about it!

Red Blood Cells. These cells (also called "erythrocytes") are suspended in your plasma. They are red because they contain a red pigment, called hemoglobin, which has a little bit of iron in its center. However, hemoglobin does more than color your blood red: it is the aspect of each red blood cell that enables that cell to carry oxygen and transfer it, eventually, to your body tissues. In environments where there is a high concentration of oxygen, such as in your lungs, hemoglobin actually combines with oxygen. Then, when that red blood cell moves into an area where the concentration of oxygen is low, such as tissue in your limbs, it releases its oxygen. In other words, the oxygen is transferred from the red blood cell to the needy tissues.

White Blood Cells. Also called "leucocytes," these cells are much larger in size than the red blood cells, but there is only one white cell to every 500 or 600 red, depending on where they are measured in your body. The white blood cells come in three forms, each with its distinct function; their collective purpose is to destroy or protect you from foreign organisms such as viruses and bacteria. So next time you cut your finger, give a special thought to those white blood cells that are rapidly gathering at the site to carry off dead tissue and destroy invading bacteria. And during the next cold or bout of flu you fall victim to, trust your white blood cells to do battle. It's what they are there for.

Platelets. These are tiny cells that are present to help in the process of clotting. They are necessary in order for fibrinogen (a protein in your plasma) to convert to fibrin. Fibrin forms fine threads, which surround the blood cells and then contract to form them into an ever more solid mass—a blood clot.

The average man has 5 to 6 liters of blood in his body at any one time; the average woman has 4 to 5 liters. In order for this wonderful liquid to do its work, however, it needs to move around the body, to circulate. Your body achieves circulation of the blood in a fairly mechanical way using a pump, a network of channels or conduits, and a variety of valves. Using this equipment, your blood is circulated to all of the organs and tissues of your body. Let's look at each aspect of this circulation.

The heart. Your heart is a small, muscular sac about the size of your clenched fist. It is located in a fairly central position in your body—just behind and slightly to the left of your breastbone—so that its pumping action can be performed efficiently. Your heart pumps blood to every part of your body between sixty and ninety times each minute, every day of your life, just by contracting its muscles. Let's look inside the heart to see how it is made and precisely what is happening as it pumps. A thick wall divides the inside of your heart into two completely separate halves, left and right. Within each of these halves are two further divisions—the top chambers, called "atria," and the bottom chambers, called "ventricles." That is four chambers in total: the top chamber on each side communicates with the chamber beneath it, but the left chambers do not communicate with the right chambers.

The top chambers, the atria, have thin walls of muscle, and these chambers act as "waiting rooms" for the blood that enters them. Once the blood enters the atrium, it cannot leave except by passing through a valve, a sort of one-way door, into the lower chamber. This door only opens when it is forced: the muscular walls of the atrium contract and push the blood against the valve, causing it to open, and allowing the blood to flow through into the lower chamber.

The lower chamber in each half of your heart is called a "ventricle." The ventricles have thick walls of muscle because they have to work harder than the atria. Once blood is pushed out of the atria and into the ventricles, it cannot return to the upper chamber (remember, that valve was one-way). Instead, it will be pushed out of the ventricle, through another one-way valve, into a narrow conduit. This conduit will channel the blood to a number of destinations in your body—your toes, fingertips, lungs, and brain. Wherever it is traveling, it will need a very strong push to keep it going. The initial push given to that blood occurs when the muscles of each ventricle contract. Now you can see why the muscle walls of these chambers are thicker than those of the atria.

This transfer of blood from the atria to the ventricles takes place in a rhythmic cycle every moment of your life. By and large, one remains unaware of this cycle but, after exertion or by putting a stethoscope or your ear to another person's heart, you may listen to its rhythmic workings. The characteristic "lubb dupp" sound of the heartbeat is caused by the valves closing: the "lubb" indicates the closing of the valves between the atria and the ventricles, while the "dupp" indicates the closing of the valves between the ventricles and the conduits, or arteries.

The arteries. Arteries are the conduits that channel blood away from your heart to your limbs and organs. Arteries are round tubes constructed in three layers: The outer layer is tough and fibrous, to protect the artery and give it strength. The middle layer is predominantly muscle tissue, with a small number of elastic fibers. This combination gives the artery flexibility as well as the ability to adjust its internal diameter (caliber) to increase or decrease both the amount and the pressure of blood flowing through it. The third and inner layer is in two parts: a lining, which is in contact with the circulating blood, and an elastic layer between the lining and the muscular, middle layer of the artery. Arteries vary in size considerably—the aorta and the pulmonary artery are quite large as they leave the heart but gradually branch off into smaller and smaller arteries. Most arteries have specific names, which help doctors and other interested persons locate their position in the body. When arteries become very small they are called "arterioles." Arterioles link up with the capillaries, the smallest form of conduit, to supply blood to all the body tissues.

The Capillaries. Capillaries are tiny channels whose walls are only one cell thick. They are loosely formed to allow cells to pass through them. Capillaries form a very dense network throughout the body to ensure that all the body tissues are supplied with blood. As the blood passes through the capillary walls, it transfers oxygen and nutrients to the tissue cells and collects waste material and carbon dioxide from them. Because the capillary walls are permeable, this transfer is able to take place instantly without the flow of blood being impaired. The permeable nature of the capillaries also accounts for the speed with which white blood cells accumulate at the site of a wound or infection. Once the blood cells have exchanged oxygen and nutrients for waste products, they must move away from the tissues in order to excrete that waste. The flow of blood continues, but now it is flowing toward the heart. To accomplish this return circulation, the capillaries gradually join up to form venules (small veins), and these, in turn, join and thicken to become veins.

The Veins. Veins are, externally, slightly narrower than arteries but with larger interior diameters. Their walls are constructed of the same three layers of tissue that arteries have, but each layer is much thinner because the pressure of blood within a vein is much less than the pressure within an artery. Veins are also less elastic than arteries, so there are valves within some veins to prevent the backflow of blood. These two factors, reduced pressure and reduced elasticity, mean that the veins in your body function at their best when your overall muscle tone is good. Your muscles support the veins and help to prevent collapse of the vein or backflow of blood, which happens in varicose veins. The veins always carry blood back to the heart. Blood returning to the heart from the lungs enters the left side of the heart through the pulmonary veins. Blood returning from the head and arms enters the right atrium through the superior vena cava; blood from the heart, through the coronary sinus; blood from the middle and lower body through the inferior vena cava. Each of these main veins are the result of many smaller veins and venules merging together.

When Things Go Wrong

This beautiful system works with remarkable efficiency and, unlike circulatory systems constructed by humans (for example, your central heating system), it is capable of decades of faultless use without any obvious maintenance. The truth is, of course, the human circulatory system is busy repairing itself all the time. Unfortunately, while this repair work is going on, many of us seem determined to inflict as much damage on our precious life-support system as possible. Some of the main ways we choose to self-destruct are:

- Smoking
- High blood pressure
- Obesity
- High cholesterol
- Lack of exercise

Sometimes, you hear about a genetic factor in heart disease—that people with a history of heart disease in the family are more likely to contract heart disease themselves. Scientific evidence shows that this is true, and doctors have termed this inherited high level of blood cholesterol as "familial hypercholesterolemia," or FH for short. However, it would be a great mistake to assume that either you are "doomed" to suffer from heart disease simply because one member of your family has suffered from it, or, alternatively, that you will miraculously escape it because no close relative has succumbed. Here are some important points to bear in mind:

- FH is not a diagnosis you can make for yourself. Just because a relative died from heart disease doesn't mean that you have FH.
- Only 1 in 500 people has FH, whereas 1 in every 5 adults has an excessively high level of blood cholesterol.
- If you do have a history of heart disease in your family, it is even more important that you take preventive measures.

Arteriosclerosis is the name given to three distinct disease processes that cause a gradual and significant hardening and narrowing of the arteries. In one form, the arteries are hardened by a gradual deposition of calcium in the middle muscle layer of the artery walls. In a second form, the small arteries, or arterioles, become hardened and thick. And in the third, most familiar, form, the large and medium arteries acquire a buildup of cholesterol, fats, blood cells, and calcium on their inner layers. This last form is called atherosclerosis.

It is thought that hypertension may be one cause or contributing factor in the development of atherosclerosis. Certainly, once either disease is apparent, the other is usually not long in manifesting. Whichever disease comes first, the resulting loss of arterial flexibility increases the likelihood of further damage being done to the lining of the arteries and eventually to the heart itself. Here is the process described:

When the artery lining is weakened or damaged, muscle tissue from the middle layer of the artery wall multiply and grow into the artery. Then fat molecules already in the blood begin to collect at the site of the damage. Blood normally carries fat molecules, so that it may transfer them to body tissues. But when the concentration of fat in the blood is too high, or when the artery wall is damaged, these molecules begin to form into plaques, which adhere to the artery walls. A buildup of fat at specific places along the lining of an already weak and damaged artery increases the stress placed on the artery and it bleeds into the fatty deposits. The white cells in the blood try to fight off bacteria and inflammation while the red cells combine with the platelets in the blood and begin a clotting process. This combination of fatty deposit and clotting blood is called "atheroma." No one can *feel* atheroma accumulate. Even when an artery becomes more than half blocked by this fatty, cholesterol-rich sludge, you still may not be aware of any warning signs to tell you that something is badly wrong. In fact, an artery usually has to be more than 75 percent blocked before blood flow is seriously impeded. But by this stage, time is definitely running out. When a deposit eventually blocks an artery, the blood flow is stopped and, with it, the supply of oxygen to tissue cells. This causes death to the deprived tissues and, if occurring in the heart muscle, a heart attack follows (see below).

Once the buildup of fat and blood begins, calcium deposits begin to harden the atheroma—especially in people entering late middle age. As the atheroma hardens and becomes brittle, it, too, can break from the artery wall and float away in the blood where, further along, it may block the artery. This form of blockage is called an "embolism." The place in your artery where the brittle atheroma broke away is left raw and bleeding and a blood clot soon forms, called a "thrombus." That clot may either block the artery there and then, or it too may break away and block the artery further along.

When an embolism and/or thrombosis occur, there is further damage done to the artery. More important, both create an obstruction of the blood flow through the artery. Loss of blood flow means loss of essential oxygen and nutrients; therefore, an obstruction such as this usually means the subsequent death of the affected tissue. If the obstruction occurs in or near the heart, a heart attack occurs. If in the brain, a stroke occurs. If this obstruction occurs in the eye, a degree of blindness may ensue, and if in the extremities, death of tissue may cause gangrene and require amputation of the affected part.

Strokes

There are two basic types of stroke. The first is an aneurysm or hemorrhage. This is the rupture of a blood vessel, such as an arteriole or capillary, that has been weakened by consistently high blood pressure. The second type is an obstruction of a blood vessel by an atheroma (embolism) or by a blood clot (thrombus). Both types of stroke have the result of killing nerve cells in the brain, leaving the area of the body controlled by those nerve cells unable to function. Typically, a stroke victim may suffer paralysis, impaired speech, loss of memory, confusion, or death. Those who experience a mild stroke have a chance of good recovery through the many therapeutic methods currently employed, such as physiotherapy, speech therapy, and correction of diet and lifestyle habits.

Ischemic Heart Disease

During exercise, stress, or when you are cold, your heart needs to pump harder to maintain a sufficient supply of blood to your tissues. In a healthy person, this occurs without any problem, though you may become slightly flushed or breathless. However, when the arteries and arterioles are constricted, as in atherosclerosis, hypertension, or through a nervous reaction, your heart must work even harder to supply adequate blood to your body tissues. Sometimes it doesn't succeed.

"Ischemic" means "an insufficient supply of blood." Therefore ischemic heart disease is an insufficient supply of blood to the myocardium, or heart muscle. There are three forms of this disease: angina pectoris, myocardial infarction, and sudden death.

Angina Pectoris. In angina pectoris the heart itself becomes deprived of the blood needed to supply its own muscle tissues. This may be due to atheroma, which narrows the coronary arteries, or it may occur when the arteries are constricted by a nervous reaction from stress or the cold. In either case, the result is a strong, distinctive pain in the region of the heart. This pain is often described as "vicelike, aching, tight, heavy, or dull" and is usually felt in the chest. In some angina sufferers, the pain may radiate to the neck, arms (especially the left arm), or even the back. The pain of angina pectoris is usually eased with rest (unlike a heart attack, where the pain is prolonged and does not disappear with rest). Additionally, the underlying cause of angina may be treated in several ways so that the symptoms are minimized or disappear altogether. Drug treatment is an obvious means of affecting the course of angina pectoris, which can disable or cause death if left to progress. However, improving one's level of fitness and finding ways of coping with all forms of stress in everyday life are measures that may be taken immediately to prevent or relieve the threat of angina. Diet and lifestyle are, once again, important factors in both the cause and the prevention of angina pectoris.

Myocardial Infarction. The myocardium is the muscular wall of the heart and, like all muscle tissue, it is supplied with oxygenated blood that circulates through the arteries. The coronary arteries that supply the myocardium may become obstructed in the same way as other arteries in the body. When obstruction is only partial, some blood gets through and the heart only suffers when it is challenged—as with angina pectoris. When the obstruction is total, however, the area of myocardium that is completely deprived of blood dies. This area of dead tissue is called an "infarct." the process of obstruction, pain, and death of tissue is called a "myocardial infarction," or heart attack. Heart attacks may be caused by obstruction of the coronary arteries due to atherosclerosis, embolism, or a blood clot (thrombus). In some cases, atheroma and coronary thrombosis are both present and together contribute to the heart attack. The area of myocardium affected by the obstruction stops contracting, or pumping, when it is deprived of blood, and that area of tissue dies shortly after, usually within hours. This period of time is very painful for the victim. If the victim survives the heart attack, the myocardium in the region of the obstruction becomes scar tissue. Scar is dead tissue, which the body cannot replace. If the obstructed artery supplied a small area of myocardium, then the infarct, or scar, will be relatively small also. If, however, a larger coronary artery is obstructed, the infarct will be larger. A large infarct is more likely to cause a loss of heart rhythm and, in some people, the sudden loss of heart rhythm due to infarct causes immediate death. In other victims the area of muscle tissue affected is so small that no symptoms are felt. This is called a "silent infarct." A number of "silent infarcts" may occur before a major heart attack is experienced. During a heart attack, the victim suffers from persistent pains similar to those described for angina. That is, vicelike, tight, crushing pains that radiate to the neck, jaw, arms, and sometimes the back. These pains may last for hours or even days, and do not disappear with rest or by altering the victim's position. In addition, the victim may have symptoms such as profuse sweating, vomiting, nausea, chills, and a sense of doom. In the event any of these symptoms appears in someone close to you, get hospital treatment immediately to prevent death.

Sudden Death. Sadly, this is often the first sign of any cardiovascular disease. Although it may be caused by injury, it is more often due to atherosclerosis and ischemia (deficiency of blood supply), which acts swiftly and profoundly on the victim. Such people are often said to die "instantly." There is no treatment for this form of heart attack, and no way of predicting it. The causes, which are the same as those for all other forms of cardiovascular disease, provide the only insight as to how it may be prevented.

For the majority of heart attack victims, their attack was the first they knew of any cardiovascular problems. Only one in every four or five victims were known to have had symptoms of hypertension or angina prior to their heart attack. Yet, undoubtedly, hypertension and its companion, atherosclerosis, are the basic disorders underlying myocardial infarction. Therefore, it is important that we consider how to prevent or minimize these conditions if we wish to reduce the incidence of stroke, angina pectoris, heart attack, and sudden death. Make no mistake—this is one epidemic we can prevent.

How the Vegetarian Diet Can Help

In 1990, the editor in chief of *The American Journal of Cardiology* wrote these telling words in an editorial:

"Although human beings eat meat, we are not natural carnivores. We were intended to eat plants, fruits and starches! No matter how much fat carnivores eat, they do not develop atherosclerosis. It's virtually impossible, for example, to produce atherosclerosis in the dog even when 100 grams of cholesterol and 120 grams of butter fat are added to its meat ration (This amount of cholesterol is approximately 200 times the average amount that human beings in the USA eat each day!). In contrast, herbivores rapidly develop atherosclerosis if they are fed foods, namely fat and cholesterol, intended for natural carnivores. . . .

"Thus, although we think we are one and we act as if we are one, human beings are not natural carnivores. When we kill animals to eat them, they end up killing us because their flesh, which contains cholesterol and saturated fat, was never intended for human beings, who are natural herbivores."[161]

It was an astonishing editorial, because most doctors rarely use such clear and forthright language in support of vegetarianism. But the evidence has been clear for decades.

The Big Picture

In the first chapter, we examined a major Japanese study that tracked the health of 122,261 people over sixteen years (see pages 12–14).[162] Apart from showing that vegetarians cut their risk of all kinds of cancer by more than one half, this study also provided a large volume of high-quality data on deaths from heart disease. Remember, the scientists were particularly interested to discover the effects of four lifestyle components on mortality:

- Smoking
- Drinking alcohol
- Eating meat
- Eating green and yellow vegetables.

The findings confirmed previous studies, and are shown graphically in Figure 4.17. The lowest-risk lifestyle was found to be people who don't smoke, drink, or eat meat, but who do eat green and yellow vegetables. The next group up the "ladder of risk" were people who lived the same lifestyle except for smoking. Among this group, the risk of dying from ischemic heart disease was nearly 1.5 times that of the lowest-risk group. Further up again are people who also drink; for

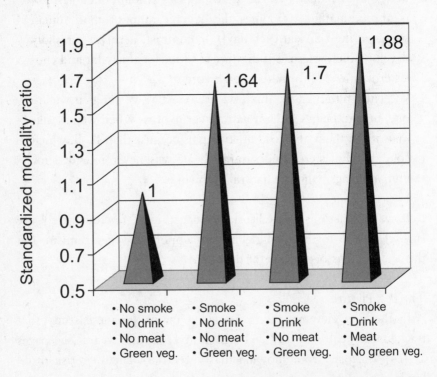

Figure 4.17. How the odds are stacked against meat eaters: comparison of the risks of ischemic heart disease.

them, the risk is increased 1.7 times. Finally, at greatest risk of all of heart disease are those who smoke, drink, eat meat, and don't eat vegetables. Compared to the lowest-risk group, they are nearly twice as likely to die from ischemic heart disease.

Another interesting result of this study was the scientists' ability to quantify the extra risk that eating meat confers upon an otherwise low-risk lifestyle. By computer analyzing all the causes of death, it was possible to calculate that the effect of meat consumption on a non-smoking, nondrinking, plenty-of-green-vegetables lifestyle was to increase the risk of dying from heart disease by nearly 30 percent.

These findings are corroborated by various other studies, described below:

- British scientists recruited over 1,000 vegetarians and 1,000 meat eaters and compared their health. The meat eaters served as the "control" group, and were chosen from the family and friends of the vegetarians, so that other lifestyle factors would be as close as possible between the two groups. Blood was taken from each person in the study, and analyzed. The researchers found that the meat eaters had the highest level of cholesterol in their blood, followed by the vegetarians, and then the vegans. "Our data confirm the findings of several other studies," the scientists wrote, "that lower concentrations of . . . cholesterol are found in vegetarians than in meat eaters." By comparing cholesterol levels in the two groups measured, the researchers calculated the relative risks of heart disease, and concluded, "Our data suggest that in Britain the incidence of coronary heart disease may be 20 percent lower in lifelong vegetarians and 57 percent lower in lifelong vegans than in meat eaters."[163]
- The German Cancer Research Center investigation cited on page 14 also recorded deaths from heart disease.[164] They found that out of the group of nearly 2,000 vegetarians, 25 of them would have been expected to die from ischemic heart disease—if they had the same mortality rate as equivalent nonvegetarian Germans. In reality, only 5 had died, meaning that the vegetarians had reduced their death rate to just 20 percent of the meat eaters' rate.

- From Norway, a study was published in 1992 that had tracked the health and cause of death of vegetarian Seventh-Day Adventists from 1962 to 1986—an impressive 24 years.[165] It confirmed that their lifestyle was protective against heart disease—death rates were significantly lower than the general population's: men had only 44 percent of general population's risk of heart disease, and women, 52 percent. The scientists found that the earlier in life the vegetarian diet was adopted, the lower the subsequent risk became.

The scientific and medical communities have generally responded to these and similar studies by asking the simple question, Why? This has, in turn, spurred more research undertaken with the intention of pinpointing the precise reason for the considerably reduced risk of heart disease conferred on vegetarians and vegans. Many possible explanations have been put forward, but none of them are universally accepted or proven beyond doubt. Suggested factors include lower consumption of saturated fat, higher intake of fiber, and greater intake of protective nutritional factors such as beta-carotene, vitamin C, and vitamin E.

One really has to question the ethical basis of some of this type of work. If it is established that a certain lifestyle considerably reduces the incidence of the Western world's major cause of death, surely the correct medical response should be to advocate those dietary changes at once, and start saving lives? Undertaking yet more research into every last detail of the process by which the meat-free lifestyle bestows protection is at best perfectionist, and at worst downright immoral. Countless lives could have been saved if our medical masters had not been so reticent to recommend vegetarianism to their patients.

Luckily for some people, a few scientists haven't been quite so reactionary.

The Best News Of All

In recent years, irrefutable scientific evidence has emerged that a vegan diet can actually heal the damage inflicted on our clogged-up arteries. It sounds too good to be true, but here is the proof. It's worth reading closely, because the science is so neat and tidy.

In 1985, a very significant paper was published in the *New England Journal of Medicine*.[166] A team of scientists from the University of Leiden in the Netherlands studied a group of 39 patients, all of whom suffered from angina, and all of whom had at least one blood vessel with 50 percent blockage, as revealed by coronary arteriography. Then they put the patients on a vegetarian diet.

After two years, the scientists took further measurements. In 21 of the 39 patients, the blockages had gotten worse. However, in 18 patients things hadn't deteriorated. What was more, it was clear that the coronary lesion growth correlated with the ratio of total cholesterol to HDL cholesterol in the blood—the higher the ratio, the more the disease had progressed. By contrast, in those patients where the ratio was low, there was no progression. This evidence opened up a whole new line of tackling heart disease. First, Dr. David Blankenhorn of the University of Southern California and Dr. Greg Brown at the University of Washington both performed scientific trials that showed that the buildup of arterial plaque could be reversed in some people by a combination of drugs and a low-fat diet.[167]

Then, in 1990, a landmark paper was published in *The Lancet*. For the first time, scientists irrefutably proved that a vegetarian diet—without the assistance of medication or drugs—could be used to regress coronary heart disease.[168] The science was impeccable. The study was both randomized and controlled (meaning that patients were randomly assigned to either the experimental group, or to a control group that was used for comparison). Patients in both groups had their coronary artery lesions carefully measured at the start of the study, and after one year.

Members of the experimental group were asked to eat a low-fat vegetarian diet, consisting of fruits, vegetables, grains, legumes, and soybean products. Remarkably, they were allowed to eat as much as they wanted to—no calorie counting was required. Now, that's not even "dieting" by most people's standards!

No animal products were allowed except for egg white and a maximum of 1 serving per day of low-fat milk or yogurt. The diet contained 10 percent of its calories as fat, 15 to 20 percent as protein, and 70 to 75 percent as complex carbohydrates. No caffeine, very little alcohol. Relaxation was encouraged, and patients were asked to exercise for a total of 3 hours a week, even though at the beginning of the study, many participants suffered from such severe chest pain that they could barely walk across a room without resting.

Now for the results: After 1 year, blockages in the arteries of two-thirds of the control group (the group that hadn't followed the vegetarian diet) had worsened. But for 18 of the 22 in the experimental group, the blockages had reduced in size, resulting in an increased blood flow to the heart. And the more severe blockages showed the most improvement.

So was this regression entirely due to a lowering of cholesterol? Dr. Dean Ornish, leader of the team, doesn't think so. "If lowering cholesterol were the primary factor in causing reversal of heart disease," he believes, "most of the patients in the studies by Dr. Blankenhorn and Dr. Brown who were taking cholesterol-lowering drugs should have shown reversal, since almost all of these patients had substantial decreases in blood-cholesterol levels. Yet only a minority showed reversal."[169]

Once again, it strongly suggests that it is the totality of the vegan diet that can work this miraculous effect. "Nutritional factors other than fat and cholesterol play a role in heart disease," asserts Dr. Ornish. And one such may be beta-carotene (vitamin A). "People who consume a low-fat vegetarian diet naturally consume not only beta-carotene," he explains, "but other anti-oxidants that may play a role in preventing and reversing heart disease."[170]

This pioneering work has since been confirmed by similar studies published in *The Lancet* and *The American Journal of Cardiology* in 1992.[171,172] If you, or a loved one, might benefit from this research, make sure you bring these studies to your doctor's attention.

HIGH BLOOD PRESSURE

What is It?

Hypertension is the medical name for high blood pressure, one of the key risk factors in the development of heart and cerebrovascular disease. Thirty-three percent—one third—of all deaths that occur in people under sixty-five are attributable to hypertensive causes.

Blood pressure is measured by the height in millimeters of a column of mercury that can be raised inside a vacuum. The more pressure there is, the higher the column will rise. Since blood pressure varies with every heartbeat, two readings are taken—one measures the pressure of the beat itself (called "systolic blood pressure") and the other measures the pressure in between beats, when the heart is resting (this is called "diastolic blood pressure." These two figures are written with the systolic figure first followed by the diastolic figure, like this— 120:80.

When we're born, our systolic blood pressure is about 40; then it doubles to about 80 within the first month. Thereafter, the increase is slower, but inexorable, for the rest of our life. Many people do not realize they suffer from hypertension. There may be no symptoms, and it may only be discovered during a visit to the doctor's office for another complaint. In its later stages symptoms may include headache, dizziness, fatigue, and insomnia.

A pressure of 150:90 would be considered above average in a young person, and 160:95 would be abnormally high. In older people, systolic pressure could be 140 at age sixty, and 160 at age eighty years. Comparatively small changes in the pressure of those people who are in the "at risk" category could have very worthwhile results. This was emphasized by a government report, which stated:

"It has been estimated that a relatively small reduction (2–3mm) in mean blood pressure in the population, if the distribution were to remain similar to the present distribution of blood pressures, would result in a major benefit in terms of mortality, and that a shift of this magnitude would be comparable to the benefit currently achieved by antihypertensive therapy. This estimated benefit seems applicable to mild as well as severe hypertension."[173]

If a small change in the population's blood pressure could be as beneficial as all the drugs that people are now taking, then what are we waiting for?

How the Vegetarian Diet Can Help
Scientists have known for a long time that some populations are apparently "immune" to hypertension, and do not display the rise in blood pressure that is associated in the West with getting older. These populations generally tend to have a high level of physical activity, are

not overweight, have a low level of animal fat in their diet, and don't take much salt (sodium) in their food. In other words, hypertension seems to be an illness of our Western way of life.

As long ago as 1926, it was experimentally shown that certain dietary components could be connected to hypertension. In that year, a pioneering Californian study had showed that the blood pressure of vegetarians could be raised—by as much as 10 percent—in just two weeks of eating a diet that centered around meat.[174] Subsequent experiments have confirmed this effect. One was undertaken in Australia, where two groups of people were selected, one of which regularly ate meat in their diets, and the other didn't.[175] The results were extremely significant, and are summarized for you in Figure 4.18.

The top line charts the blood pressure of the meat eaters. The bottom line shows the non–meat eaters, and the bottom axis shows the five age groups that were surveyed. You can see that, at all ages, blood pressure is significantly lower among the vegetarians. Among the meat eaters, there is a steady rise in blood pressure with advancing age. But among the vegetarians, there is very little increase—and, in fact, a surprising drop in blood pressure in the oldest age group. These results

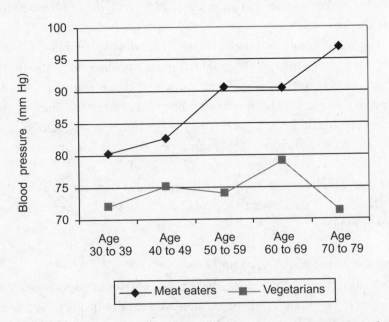

Figure 4.18. Diastolic blood pressure of vegetarians compared to that of meat eaters.

were adjusted to exclude other factors such as exercise, tea, coffee, or alcohol consumption.

Another study was carried out in Britain, and again compared the blood pressure levels in people who didn't eat meat to those who did.[176] The results showed exactly the same pattern. This was true in men as well as women. Figure 4.19 shows the mean results that were obtained.

The difference in the "underlying" blood pressure (diastolic), which is generally thought to be a better guide to the real health of the individual, is considerable. On average, diastolic blood pressure was 15 percent less in the vegetarians compared to the meat eaters.

In another study, a group of 115 vegetarians were compared to a similar group of 115 meat eaters, who were closely matched to the vegetarians apart from diet.[177] The results demonstrated that systolic blood pressure of the vegetarians was 9.3 percent lower than the meat eaters, and diastolic pressure a massive 18.2 percent lower.

In America, in another case, a vegetarian diet was devised that included much fiber from whole-grain cereals, bran cereals, whole-grain breads, vegetables, beans, lentils, and peas.[178] Interestingly,

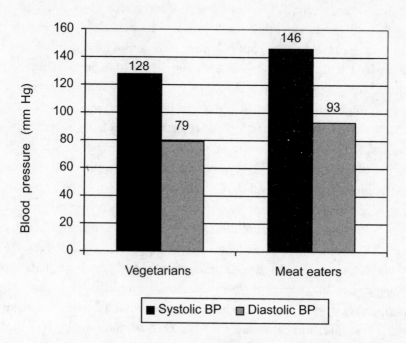

Figure 4.19. Meat eaters compared with vegetarians—blood pressure.

members of the group put on this diet were allowed to use as much salt in their food as they wanted. This group was then compared to a standard "control" group, who carried on eating normally. The average blood pressure of the men on the plant fiber diet was 10 percent lower than the control group.

A recent "crossover" trial has confirmed the results of the original 1926 study (see page 244).[179] Fifty-eight patients aged between thirty and sixty-four with mild untreated hypertension were put onto an ovo-lacto-vegetarian diet (including dairy products and eggs). Within a few weeks, the average systolic blood pressure dropped by 5 mm. When they started to eat meat again, it rose by the same amount—very clear evidence that the meat element of the diet was responsible for the improvement.

We know from studies such as those mentioned above that vegetarians generally exhibit lower blood pressure than meat eaters. But can a vegetarian diet also be used to treat high blood pressure? The evidence clearly shows it can.

Scientists at the Royal Perth Hospital in Australia found that people with high blood pressure could indeed reduce it on a vegetarian diet.[180] They wrote, "If the usual aim of treatment of mild hypertensives is to reduce systolic blood pressure to below 140mmHg then thirty per cent of those eating a meat-free diet achieved this criteria compared with only eight per cent on their usual diet." They concluded by suggesting that if drug therapy was required by a hypertensive, it might also be worthwhile to consider modifying the diet.

Another persuasive case for a vegetarian diet to help hypertensives comes from a year-long study in Sweden, where there is a strong tradition of using dietary means to prevent or cure a number of diseases, including hypertension. All the 26 subjects had a history of high blood pressure, on average for 8 years. They were all receiving medication, but even so, 8 of the group had excessively high readings (more than 165:95). Many of the patients complained of such symptoms as headache, dizziness, tiredness, and chest pains, symptoms that were either due to the disease or the medication the patients happened to be taking. They were put on a vegan diet, from which coffee, tea, sugar, salt, chocolate, and chlorinated tap water were eliminated. Their fresh fruit and vegetables were organic, when possible. When their diets were analyzed, it was found that they were higher in vitamins and minerals than most people on a meat diet!

"With the exception of a few essential medicines (for example, insulin)," wrote the scientists, "patients were encouraged to give up medicines when they felt that these were no longer needed. Thus, analgesics were dispensed with in the absence of pain, tranquillizers when anxiety was not experienced and sleep was sound, and antihypertensive medication when the blood pressure was normal."[181]

The results were certainly impressive. First of all, the patients simply felt much healthier. None of them said that the treatment had left them unchanged or made them feel worse, and 15 percent said they felt "better." Over 50 percent of them said they felt "much better," and 30 percent said they felt "completely recovered." Reductions in blood pressure ranged from 7 to 9 mm, systolic, and 5 to 10 mm diastolic. "When the decrease in blood pressure was considered for the entire group," the scientists wrote, "it was found that it occurred at the time when most of the medicines were withdrawn. Of the twenty-six patients, twenty had given up their medication completely after one year while six still took some medicine, although the dose was lower, usually halved." Several other sorts of benefits were found as well. Their serum cholesterol levels were found to have dropped an average of 15 percent. And the health authorities computed that they had saved £1,000 ($1,500) per patient over the year, by reducing the costs of drugs and hospitalization.

Many studies have tried to identify the one, single factor that makes the vegetarian diet beneficial for blood pressure, but the evidence so far shows that neither polyunsaturated fat, saturated fat, cholesterol, potassium, magnesium, sodium, or total protein intake are independently responsible for this effect.[182] Again, we are forced to come back to the position that it is the *totality* of the vegetarian diet that is beneficial, and no single component. Hypertension is sometimes preceded by the word "essential," which rather confusingly means that the cause of it is not known. The studies above, and many others, give us convincing proof that a vegetarian diet can offer vital assistance in preventing, and treating, this modern silent killer.

What Else You Can Do

A diagnosis of high blood pressure is not a death sentence. There is a lot you can do to bring it down—providing you are willing to try seriously. Much research now clearly shows that many "hypertensives" can lower their blood pressure by amending their lifestyle and dietary habits.

- Get to understand your own blood pressure. The common device that measures blood pressure, called a "sphygmomanometer," consists of an inflatable cuff that is wrapped around the arm, and is connected via a tube to the measuring device. Simple sphygmomanometers are quite cheap, and it might be worth buying one and tracking your blood pressure as it rises and falls over a period of time. Blood pressure fluctuates considerably even in normal individuals—the reading taken at the doctor's office won't be the same as the one taken at home later in the day. Physical activity, excitement, fear, or emotional stress can all send it shooting up. When you understand how your blood pressure changes, you're on the way to controlling it.

  One recent study has found that as many as 20 percent of patients treated for hypertension could be receiving unnecessary medication, simply because their blood pressure rises in the presence of a doctor. They coined the term "white coat hypertension" for this phenomenon.[183] With your own sphygmomanometer, you'll be able to rule this out.

- Normalize your weight. Most hypertensives are overweight, and a 20-pound reduction in weight can result in a blood pressure reduction of 20 mm systolic and 10 mm diastolic.[184]

- Reduce or avoid alcohol consumption. Most long-term studies have shown that blood pressure can be significantly reduced by cutting out or cutting down on the amount of alcohol consumed. For example, one study shows that among women taking more than 2 alcoholic drinks per day, one-third of all cases of hypertension are caused by alcohol consumption. This suggests that hypertension in these women may be treatable by restriction of alcohol intake.[185]

- Stop smoking. Nicotine stimulates the heart and at the same time constricts the blood vessels, making it difficult for your blood pressure not to rise! If you are a man with high blood pressure and you smoke you are 3.5 times more likely to develop cardiovascular disease than if you were a healthy non-smoker.

- Learn to relax and to exercise. Both of these activities help you to feel more in control of your body and your life.

- Consider a drastic change at work. People in demanding jobs with little freedom to make decisions have three times the risk of developing high blood pressure compared to others who have either a less-demanding job or more decision-making latitude.[186]

- Adjust your sodium and potassium intake. Both of these minerals are salts (sodium is table salt), which regulate the balance of fluid in your body. An excess of sodium increases the volume of blood, which puts more strain on the circulatory system, causing high blood pressure. Thus, sodium has been blamed for many cases of hypertension. However, it is now shown that potassium can protect the body from hypertension because it balances the effects of sodium.[187]

- You can reduce your intake of sodium and increase your intake of potassium by limiting the amount of processed foods you eat, which are high in sodium and low in potassium. Instead, eat potassium-rich foods such as avocado, banana, broccoli, brussels sprouts, dates, prunes, and raisins. Potatoes with their skins on and cantaloupes are also good sources.

- Increase your intake of magnesium. This mineral is lost when you take diuretics—often prescribed for hypertensives. Yet 50 percent of magnesium deficient patients have high blood pressure, usually normalizing when this deficiency is rectified. Foods rich in magnesium include green vegetables, nuts, whole grains and yeast extracts.[188]

- Boost your calcium intake. It has been found that people with high blood pressure often have low levels of calcium.[189] In one study, researchers demonstrated a 23 percent decrease in hypertension risk among women receiving 800 milligrams a day of calcium, compared with women consuming just 400 milligrams a day.[190] Foods rich in calcium include tofu, spinach, figs, molasses, seaweeds, nuts and seeds, watercress, and parsley.

- Consider taking a selenium supplement. Although its role is not yet fully known, selenium may act to prevent hypertension caused by cadmium. Cadmium is a heavy metal that raises blood pressure; it comes from some water pipes, car exhaust, and other pollution, and smoking. Dr. Raymond Shamberger and Dr. Charles E. Willis, of the Cleveland Clinic, in Ohio, conducted an epidemiological study that has shown that people living in an area where the soil has a low concentration of selenium are three times more likely to die from hypertension-related diseases than people who live where the selenium level in the soil (and hence in the food they eat) is higher. "We don't known selenium's precise action concerning high blood pressure," said Dr. Shamberger, "but our study strongly suggests that it has a beneficial effect on high blood pressure problems in man."[191]

MULTIPLE SCLEROSIS

What is It?

Multiple sclerosis (MS) is a degenerative disease of the central nervous system. In the course of the disease, myelin (a white, fatty substance that acts as an electrical insulator for the nerves) is progressively destroyed. The resulting formation of hard scar tissue on the protective myelin sheath that surrounds nerves stops the nerve cells from working. This scarring results in permanent loss of nervous control to areas of the body. MS is a crippling disease that attacks every body function. With time it can be fatal. It affects both men and women, and usually is first diagnosed between the ages of twenty and forty.

The cause of multiple sclerosis remains problematic. Literally dozens of explanations have been suggested over the years. A great deal of research has gone into investigating the possibility that MS is caused by a virus, although to date, it has not proved possible to pinpoint precisely which one. Similarly, it has long been suspected that MS is an autoimmune disease, a sort of allergic reaction in which the body responds to an antigen by acting against itself. Again, pinpointing the antigen in question has proved difficult. Yet another theory proposes that giving cow's milk to infants predisposes them to nervous system injury later in life, because cow's milk has only a fifth as much linoleic acid (an essential fatty acid) as human breast milk, and linoleic acid makes up the building blocks for nervous tissues.[192] The list could go on and on, but while waiting for conclusive proof of cause, it is possible to deal with multiple sclerosis so as to minimize its crippling effect and, perhaps, prolong life.

How the Vegetarian Diet Can Help

Most health professionals have traditionally dismissed the idea that multiple sclerosis might be linked to diet. However, Dr. Roy Swank, former professor of Neurology at the University of Oregon, was intrigued by some wartime research. During World War II, the consumption of animal fat decreased in Western Europe. Meat and dairy products were rationed, and instead the consumption of grains and vegetables increased to replace them. It was noticed at this time that patients with MS had 2 to 2.5 times fewer hospitalizations during the war years, when saturated fat consumption was low.[193] Greatly excited by the possible implication of these findings, Dr. Swank began treating his own patients with a low-fat diet. Over the next thirty-five years, he treated thousands of MS patients in this way. By any medical standard, his results have been remarkable. Many of his success stories were told in a book published in 1977.[194] Patients generally fared better if the condition was detected early, but even longtime MS sufferers experienced a slowing of the disease's progression. The basics of Dr. Swank's diet are

- No more than 10 grams of saturated fat per day
- 40 to 50 grams of polyunsaturated fat (but *not* margarine or other hydrogenated fats)
- At least 1 teaspoon of cod liver oil daily
- No animal food (although fish was consumed 3 times a week).[195]

Protein intake should be kept up with a good supply of mixed vegetable proteins. The long-term results of the Swank diet show that of those who ate less than 20 grams of fat per day, only 31 percent have died (close to normal) and the condition of the rest has deteriorated only slightly. Of those who ate more than 20 grams, 81 percent have died.[196] However, many orthodox medical practitioners are still very wary of accepting such evidence. An editorial in the medical magazine *The Lancet* stated, "there are still no firm answers as to whether a relationship (between MS and dietary fats) does indeed exist and if so, what its mechanism might be. . . . more work is needed at the biochemical level. . . . Until such studies are undertaken, the role of lipids in MS cannot be said to be proven."[197] Yet in the words of another doctor who uses the Swank diet to treat patients, "I've been very gratified by the results of this dietary treatment, not only because the progress of most of my MS patients' disease has been halted, but also because their overall health has unquestionably improved."[198]

OSTEOPOROSIS

What is It?

"Osteoporosis" literally means "porous bones." If you are a woman, by the time you are sixty, there is a 1 in 4 chance that osteoporosis will have caused you to break a bone.[199] And more than 10 percent of people who suffer a hip fracture caused by osteoporosis will die.[200] Both men and women *can* suffer from osteoporosis, but it is rarer in men (one estimate is that only 1 in 40 men are ever diagnosed with it.[201] Oriental and Caucasian women are most at risk, due to their tendency to have thinner, lighter bones. Women of African, Mediterranean, or Aboriginal extraction are less likely to suffer from it. You may not even realize that you have osteoporosis until you suddenly break a bone, by which time, the harm has been done. Other telltale signs can include severe back pain, loss of height, or deformities such as a curvature of the spine. It is estimated that more than 50,000 women fracture a hip each year due to osteoporosis.[202] And the number of deaths from fractured hips is greater than the number of deaths from cancers of the cervix, uterus, and breast combined,[203] which makes osteoporosis one of the major killers of our time.

Osteoporosis is caused by a slow loss of bone mass. By the age of thirty-five or so, your bones will be as strong as they're ever likely to be. Hormones in our bodies are responsible for continuously balancing the growth of new bone with the reabsorption of old bone. When levels of these hormones fall significantly, as happens in menopause, this balance is lost and a gradual loss of bone mass occurs. Eventually, the bones can become very brittle and break easily. In some women this process is sufficiently slow to avoid fractures, pain, and loss of height. In others, however, the loss is rapid—some women can lose up to half of their bone mass within ten or so years of menopause, leaving them very vulnerable to fractures. Since it is clear that estrogen, the female sex hormone, plays a protective role in the maintenance of bone mass, one current treatment for women suffering from osteoporosis is hormone replacement therapy (HRT). HRT provides your body with a supplement of several hormones, including the female hormone estrogen. HRT has a number of very worthwhile advantages:

- It slows down the loss of bone mineral content, decreasing the likelihood of fractures of the spine, hips, and wrists.
- It prevents loss of height.
- It lowers LDL cholesterol in your blood and increases HDL cholesterol, thus prolonging life expectancy by decreasing the risk of heart disease.
- It decreases hot flashes, increases sex drive, and prevents vaginal dryness.
- It decreases the risk of ovarian cancer.[204]

On the other hand, concerns have been expressed about its long-term safety (as they have for the estrogen-based contraceptive pill). Although many women—and some doctors—are concerned about an increased risk of cancer from HRT, most of the scientific evidence does not confirm these worries. While some studies do indeed show that estrogen therapy may increase the risk of developing cancer,[205] today's HRT includes other hormones (progestogens) that studies show can actually reduce the cancer risk quite appreciably.[206]This is an area of ongoing research, and it is worth keeping up to date with the latest findings. There are, however some problems associated with HRT, as with all drugs. These can sometimes include breast soreness, gallstones, weight gain, return of periods, and with them, break-through bleeding.

Is Milk the Answer?

Osteoporosis first hit the headlines in 1984, when the U.S. National Institutes of Health issued an advisory paper stating that women should increase their intake of calcium to prevent osteoporosis. The demand for calcium supplements suddenly hit the roof. And the dairy industry wasn't slow to appreciate the potential for increased sales. Since milk contains plenty of calcium (just the right amount for a fast-growing calf, not necessarily so right for humans), they clearly had a hit on their hands. So, with the help of the vast promotional resources of the dairy industry, the public quickly perceived that:

1. Osteoporosis is caused by a lack of calcium in the diet.
2. Milk contains oodles of calcium.
3. Therefore you should gulp gallons of milk to avoid osteo-porosis.

On the face of it, it all sounds very plausible. Since osteoporosis is caused by a slow loss of bone mass, a heavy dose of calcium should put things right again, shouldn't it? The answer is no. Although the theory "has an intuitive appeal," an article in the *British Medical Journal* stated, "the logic is similar to that which might lead doctors to give ground-up brains for dementia."[207]

Nevertheless, many people now seem to believe that a large intake of dairy products will safeguard them against this crippling condition. And the myths abound, as plentifully as ever, for example, take this piece of advice from a recent article in a health food magazine: "Veg-etarians who do not use dairy products or take supplements are espe-cially at risk in developing osteoporosis, either because they do not get sufficient amounts of nutrients from their diet or do not absorb the nutrients properly."[208]

Meanwhile, the recommended intakes for calcium continue to sky-rocket—up to 3,000 milligrams (3 grams) a day, in some cases.[209]

Now to get this amount of calcium from dairy produce, you'd have to drink 10 glasses of milk a day, which—even assuming you drank low-fat milk—would also give you a very unhealthy 180 milligrams of cholesterol and 30 grams of saturated fat.[210] Alternatively, you could munch your way through one pound of cheddar cheese, which would also give you a whacking 150 grams of fat, most of it saturated![211]

The fact is, you don't need to drink milk to prevent osteoporosis. For example, most Chinese consume no dairy products at all and instead get all their calcium from vegetables. While the Chinese consume only half the dietary calcium Westerners do, osteoporosis is uncommon in China despite an average life expectancy of seventy years. "Osteoporosis tends to occur in countries where calcium intake is highest and most of it comes from protein-rich dairy products," says Dr. T. Colin Campbell, a nutritional biochemist from Cornell University and the American authority behind the famous China study. He said, in conclusion, "The Chinese data indicate that people need less calcium than we think and can get adequate amounts from vegetables."[212]

At the other end of the scale, the Eskimo population is known to have the highest dietary calcium intake in the world (over 2,000 milligrams a day, mainly from fish bones), yet they also have one of the highest rates of osteoporosis in the world.[213]

Clearly, we haven't been given the full picture.

How the Vegetarian Diet Can Help

Says dietary reformer Nathan Pritikin, "African Bantu women take in only 350 milligrams of calcium per day. They bear nine children during their lifetime and breast feed them for two years. They never have calcium deficiency, seldom break a bone, rarely lose a tooth. Their children grow up nice and strong. How can they do that on 350 milligrams of calcium a day when the recommendation is 1,200 milligrams? It's very simple. They're on a low-protein diet that doesn't kick the calcium out of the body . . . In our country (America), those who can afford it are eating 20 percent of their total calories in protein, which guarantees negative mineral balance, not only of calcium, but of magnesium, zinc, and iron. It's all directly related to the amount of protein you eat."[214]

Now we're getting to the truth of the matter. In fact, the difference in bone loss between vegetarians and meat eaters can be explained by several factors:

As Pritikin says, the more protein you consume, the more it "kicks the calcium out of the body." Since the 1920s, scientists have known that diets that are high in protein cause calcium to be lost through the urine.[215] In one typical study, young men were fed experimental diets whose protein content ranged from 48 grams a day right up to 141 grams a day. It was found that the higher level of protein consumption doubled the urinary excretion of calcium.[216] And a diet that is high in animal protein—as opposed to vegetable proteins—particularly increases this effect.[217] Scientists believe that flesh foods cause an acid load in the body, which must be neutralized by a release of calcium stored in bones.[218]

It has recently been found that boron—a trace mineral—helps to prevent calcium loss and subsequent loss of bone mass. It is also thought to help in the manufacture of vitamin D in the body. The first study to look at the nutritional effects of boron in humans took place in 1987.[219] Twelve postmenopausal women were fed a diet very low in boron for 17 weeks, after which they were given a daily supplement of 3 milligrams for another 7 weeks. The addition of boron had a dramatic effect: the women lost 40 percent less calcium and 30 percent less magnesium through their urine. The study therefore concluded that boron can reduce bodily losses of elements necessary to maintain bone integrity and prevent osteoporosis. Nutritionist Forrest Nielsen, director of the U.S. Department of Agriculture's Human Nutrition Research Center, called it "a remarkable effect."[220]

Even more extraordinary was the discovery that boron could double the most active form of estrogen (estradiol 17B) in the women's blood. Their estradiol levels actually equaled those of women on estrogen replacement therapy. Curtiss Hunt, of the U.S. Human Nutrition Research Center, said he "suspects the body needs boron to synthesize estrogen, vitamin D and other steroid hormones. And it may protect these hormones against rapid breakdown." He also suggested that boron could be important in treating many other diseases of "unknown cause including some forms of arthritis." And where can you get boron from? Why, by eating apples, pears, grapes, nuts, leafy vegetables, and legumes—in other words, a healthy vegetarian diet (one medium apple contains approximately 1 milligram of boron; researchers suggest our boron requirement is in the region of 1 or 2 milligrams a day).[221]

These two important facts, and probably more yet to be discovered, are reflected in the results of a recent study performed by scientists from Andrews University, in Michigan.[222] They used a sophisticated technique called direct photon absorptiometry to compare the bone mass of vegetarians to meat eaters. After studying a group of 1,600 women, they found that by the time they reached 80, women who had eaten a vegetarian diet for at least 20 years had only lost an average of 18 percent of their bone mineral. On the other hand, women who did not eat a vegetarian diet had lost an average of 35 percent of their bone mineral. Interestingly, there was no statistical difference in the nutrient intakes between the two groups—in other words, the vegetarian's advantage was *not* due to increased calcium intake.

Just a word to the wise.

What Else Can You Do?

Get enough exercise. Especially important are weight-bearing exercises such as walking, dancing, running, and many sports. (Swimming and chess playing, are *not* weight-bearing exercises.) Proper exercise exerts the muscles around your bones, stimulating them to maintain bone density. Leading a sedentary life will increase the likelihood of osteoporosis developing later in your life.

Avoid smoking, caffeine, and excess alcohol. All of these can increase your risk of suffering from osteoporosis.[223] A study of women aged 36 to 45 found that those who drank two cups of coffee a day suffered a net calcium loss of 22 milligrams daily. The authors concluded that a negative calcium balance of 40 milligrams a day (i.e. about 4 cups of coffee) was enough to explain the 1 to 1.5 percent loss in skeletal mass in post-menopausal women each year.[224]

Get regular doses of sunlight. Sunlight reacts with a substance in your skin—dehydrocholesterol—to produce vitamin D. This vitamin is essential to the proper absorption of calcium, and a deficiency will cause you to lose bone mass. Most people get enough vitamin D just by being outside for part of the day with their face, hands, and arms exposed.[225]

Avoid aluminum-containing antacids. If antacids containing aluminum are used for prolonged periods of time, they may produce bone abnormalities by interfering with calcium and phosphorous metabolism, and so contribute to the development of osteoporosis.[226] So if you must use an antacid, choose one that does not include aluminum.

Eat food rich in vitamin B complex, vitamin K, and magnesium. These are all believed to play a role in the prevention of osteoporosis. The B group is available in brewer's yeast, whole grains, molasses, nuts and seeds, and dark green, leafy vegetables. Vitamin K is present in cauliflower, soybeans, molasses, safflowers oil and, again, dark green leafy vegetables. Magnesium is a constituent of chlorophyll and so is abundant in green vegetables. Other excellent sources are whole grains, wheat germ, molasses, seeds and nuts, apples and figs.

Consider calcium carbonate. If you want to take a calcium supplement, it has a high content of calcium and a low price.

SALMONELLA

According to information that Britain's Meat and Livestock Commission gives to schoolchildren, "Meat itself doesn't cause disease or ill-health—it is only unprofessional or unhygienic handling and preparation which can bring about a problem."[227]

This is a scandalous statement, because it neatly shifts the blame for food poisoning from the supplier onto the "handler"—usually, the poor beleaguered cook. Now if meat is smeared with animal feces because intestines are commonly ruptured during slaughter; if knives used for cutting meat in slaughterhouses are inadequately sterilized; and if the lesions and tumors on condemned meat literally spill out of waste bins—now, who's fault is that?[228] When I interviewed a slaughterhouse vet for the original *You Don't Need Meat,* he told me:

"We hear a lot about food poisoning cases these days, and in just about every case there's meat or poultry as the root cause. Now who gets the blame when patients in hospital die from it? It's almost always the cook, who's blamed for not cooking the beef long enough or for leaving it out in the open. But that's only partly true, because if the meat wasn't grossly infected with salmonella organisms to start with, there'd be no problem."[229]

More than 1,500 types of salmonella have now been identified, usually isolated from the intestinal tract of humans and animals. Salmonella organisms are responsible for a variety of human diseases, ranging from typhoid fever to food poisoning, but it is salmonella typhimurium that has accounted for most cases of food infection. In 1988 a new strain—salmonella enteritidis phage type 4—emerged, and it is apparently more virulent than others and can cause a systemic infection in chickens, invading the ovary and oviducts, not just the gut. Consequently, the bacteria can end up deep inside the egg.[230]

It is difficult to estimate how many animal carcasses are contaminated with salmonella, although, in the case of chicken, estimates have ranged from 25 percent to 80 percent.[231] When you learn that cases of salmonella poisoning rose by 25 percent in 1992 compared to 1991, it is clear that we are living in the midst of an epidemic.[232] In America, there are approximately 2.5 million cases of salmonella poisoning a year, 500,000 hospitalizations, and 9,000 deaths.[233] Rather than force the industry to clean up its act, the U.S. Agriculture Department announced that poultry processors would be allowed to zap chickens, turkeys, and game hens with gamma rays, in an attempt to destroy disease-causing bacteria.[234]

The headline stories have become so commonplace that many of us seem to have become thoroughly inured to them. A cow with anthrax is slaughtered and left in the abattoir for twenty-four hours before being discovered, and even then, the slaughterhouse is allowed to continue killing and processing animals for human consumption.[235] Complacent officials allow pigs from a farm hit by the largest outbreak of anthrax for half a century to continue to be slaughtered for human consumption.[236] Beef officially stamped as fit for human consumption is later found to be riddled with arthritis and septicemia.[237] Things have got so bad that schoolchildren visiting farms should now be given an official health warning.[238] And incredibly, officials recommend that animal "rejects" from failed genetic engineering experiments should be sold for human consumption, to allow the experimenters to recoup some of their costs (the failure rate is colossal—for every 1,000 animals experimented on, 999 are rejected).[239]

But these are merely the public scandals. It is only when you get a glimpse of the ordinarily unseen aspects of the meat business that you really begin to appreciate the enormity of the situation. A few years ago (the meat trade will undoubtedly say the situation has now improved—in which case, the onus is on them to prove it) I received an anonymous bundle of photocopied documents in the mail. No doubt I committed some heinous crime against the state by merely opening the envelope; in which case, I hope you will send me some food in prison. It contained copies of correspondence between the Ministry of Agriculture and a major operator of slaughterhouses. As I read, my jaw literally dropped. The papers revealed that

- Sheep were being killed in full sight of each other.
- Cattle were being shot in the head two or three times before they were stunned; many were shot in the wrong place.
- Pigs were damaged in transit or dead on arrival at the slaughterhouse.
- Electric tongs were used to goad pigs.
- Men's work wear and gloves were encrusted with fat, rarely cleaned.
- Knife sterilizers were contaminated with foul blood and were fat encrusted.
- No soap, nail brushes, or paper towels were in the washroom.
- Kosher carcasses were allowed to drag along the floor.
- The kosher butcher was not cleaning his hands and arms before inserting them into the animal's chest.
- A pithing rod (stuck into the animal's brain) was unsterilized.
- Green algae were growing on the walls.
- There were "unsatisfactory procedures and a complete lack of regard for sanitation of the product and equipment."

All these points, and many more besides, were made in the official reports of inspection. And in an internal memorandum, one of the employees had written the most telling comment of all: "Frankly I am amazed that we are not already under heavy pressure to change things."

If you think about it, there is a kind of logic to all this. An industry that treats its raw material—sentient animals—with such contempt and cruelty while they are alive is hardly likely to treat them any better when they're dead. And that means, of course, that consumers suffer too, which gives another meaning to the phrase "meat is murder." Apart from not eating the foodstuffs most likely to give you food poisoning, here are some further measures to consider:

- If you live in a household where some people eat meat, insist that it be kept scrupulously away from vegetarian food. A plate of chicken or beef, for example, on an upper shelf in a refrigerator can easily splash its nasty secretions onto vegetables further down.
- Store raw and cooked foods separately. Never leave leftover canned food in its tin. Buy salads and vegetables that are unprepared and unprocessed—nature's own packaging is usually the best.
- Wash food before you eat it—even if you've grown it yourself. Vegetables and fruit can occasionally harbor bacteria from the soil.
- Never reheat food more than once. Make sure it's not underheated.
- Don't take chances. If your food smells "off," throw it away.
- Be certain that frozen food is thoroughly defrosted before cooking.
- Be sure all kitchen towels, sponges, surfaces, food equipment, and cutting boards are kept clean. When you're preparing a meal, it's also prudent to wash utensils and countertops between stages. Don't allow the same knife or chopping board to be used for raw meat and then for cooked food and fresh vegetables.
- Put all rubbish and scraps of food straight into the waste bin— and always keep the lid on securely, so that flies can't get in and germs can't get out.

X, Y, Z . . . for the Unknown

When AIDS was discovered in cows, I admit I had a hard time believing it. There are, after all, just about as many theories about the origin of the human immunodeficiency virus (HIV) as there are about the assassination of President Kennedy. To add one more initially seemed to me to be way past credibility.

Then I thought again. If someone had told me, just a decade ago, that a disease as bizarre and mystifying as BSE would reach epidemic proportions in the cattle population, I would have disbelieved that, too. The plain fact is, there *are* lots of new diseases out there. But they're not *staying* out there.

The evidence shows that many new viral diseases are emerging at this point in our history—over a dozen previously undescribed viral diseases in humans and other animals have been discovered in the last decade.[240] There are many reasons why this should be so. The exploding populations of cities in newly industrialized nations creates unique breeding conditions for new diseases. Air travel around the globe provides an incredibly rapid and effective vector. And humanity's constant erosion of the world's last remaining wilderness areas may expose viruses that have been undisturbed for millennia—a kind of Gaia's revenge.

"Suddenly, it seems we are besieged with new diseases," writes Edwin D. Kilbourne in a thoughtful article published in the *Journal of the American Medical Association*. "The acquired immunodeficiency syndrome (AIDS), legionnaires' disease, Lyme disease, and others alien to these pages only a decade ago."[241] Kilbourne believes that the most frequent causes of "new" viral infections are "old" viruses, which are transmitted to us from other species. And viruses whose genetic material is contained in RNA, rather than DNA, are particularly worrying, because they mutate faster and can insert themselves directly into human genes.

"I certainly do think we should set aside resources and recognize that viral evolution is proceeding more rapidly," Nobel laureate Joshua Lederberg told a meeting of the National Institutes of Health, in Washington. "I'm just saying there is a faint possibility that the world will fall apart tomorrow."[242]

So as soon as I heard the "Cow AIDS" story, I started to do some checking. And what I found made me feel very uneasy.

NEW VIRUSES

Vector or Virus	Target	Carrier
Canine parvovirus	Dogs	Fecal material
Rocio encephalitis	Humans	Mosquitoes
Necrotic hepatitis	Rabbits	Rabbit blood
Rev-T	Birds	Bird droppings
Marburg disease	Humans	Human blood, monkeys
Seal plague	Seal	Unknown
HIV-1 (AIDS)	Humans	Blood and semen
HIV-2 (AIDS)	Humans	Blood and semen
HTLV-1	Humans	Blood and semen
HTLV-2	Humans	Blood and semen
Ebola virus	Humans	Blood
O'nyong-nyong	Humans	Mosquitoes
Delta virus	Humans	Blood and semen

OLD VIRUSES FOUND IN A NEW LOCALE OR USING A NEW VECTOR

Vector or Virus	Target	Carrier
Lassa fever	Humans	Mice, human blood
Hemorrhagic fever	Humans	Mice
Seoul Hantaan	Humans	Rats
Dengue fever	Humans	Mosquitoes
Rift Valley fever	Humans	Insects

Vector or Virus	Target	Carrier
Human monkey pox	Humans	Monkeys
Kyasanur Forest disease	Humans	Mosquitoes
Oropuche fever	Humans	Mosquitoes

There are certainly ominous similarities with the BSE story. A disease called "visna" was first diagnosed in sheep and goats in Iceland in 1938–39.[243] *Visna* is Icelandic for "shrinkage" or "wasting," which pretty much describes the symptoms. The disease seemed to take two rather different forms: visna would be characterized by an infection of the brain and spinal cord, but the term *maedi* ("difficult breathing") would be used if the infected animal was also suffering from pneumonia-type symptoms. Thus, the lentivirus that caused this disease was sometimes known as "visna-maedi," or "maedi/visna." The symptoms are actually not unlike scrapie, without the persistent scratching.[244]

The discovery of visna virus in cows was only of passing, academic interest to most scientists.[245] However, with the emergence of AIDS as a serious health threat in the 1980s, scientists began to look around for other similar animal viruses, and visna came under greater scrutiny. In 1987, the name "bovine immunodeficiency-like virus" (BIV) was proposed by researchers, "to reflect its genetic relationship and biological similarity to HIV."[246] A year later, a disturbing letter appeared in the pages of the *Journal of the Royal Society of Medicine*.[247] It made several key connections:

- Considerable doubt had already been cast on the "African green monkey" theory for the origin of HIV.
- HIV demonstrates great genetic similarity to visna found in sheep.
- Now that visna virus has been found in cattle (BIV), the worrying possibility emerged that humans could also have been contaminated with BIV.

One way humans might have been contaminated is as follows: To manufacture human vaccines, viruses are cultured in fetal calf serum.

Although this serum is screened for "contaminants," it is entirely possible that not all such infections—such as BIV—would be detected. Consequently, humans might have been injected with BIV. The letter concluded, "It seems absolutely vital that all vaccines are screened for HIV prior to use and that BVV [BIV] is further investigated as to its relationship to HIV and its possible causal role in progression towards AIDS."[248]

Subsequently, the *Journal* published a reply to these points from two British government scientists, who concluded, "As far as we are aware there has been no report of the isolation of bovine visna virus [BIV] from fetal calf serum."[249]

But this is hardly reassuring, in view of the fact that BIV is far more widespread than was first thought. Originally, it was presumed to be restricted to just one cow in Louisiana. Yet in a recent study in Mississippi, 50 percent of cattle examined were found to be infected.[250]

There is enough here to make me feel uneasy. Although officials claim that "the potential for human infection from BIV is zero," my own natural caution and the Precautionary Principle suggest that discretion is the better part of valor.[251] Under the circumstances, we should be cautious and humble. Nature is more than capable of taking our species down a peg or two, and although we may delude ourselves into believing that we now control the very secrets of life itself, a nasty surprise could be just around the next corner. What, for example, would happen if the human immunodeficiency virus suddenly learned the tricks of airborne transmission? Recent studies suggest that this concern is not without foundation.[252] The outcome might be much the same as the devastation that myxomatosis wrought on rabbits.

What it comes down to is this: as long as we choose to ingest animals, we must also be prepared to ingest their diseases, and to cope with the consequences. To pretend otherwise is to indulge in pure self-deception, of the most dangerous kind.

Of course, there is another way, a better way. As the years go by, I believe that the consumption of animal flesh will increasingly be perceived as a barbaric relic from our distant past, much in the same way as public lynchings and slavery are viewed today. Instead of trying to win a losing battle with the consequences of a meat-based diet, science and technology will provide us with healthier, more logical foodstuffs. Many are already on sale today.

So there you have it. Eating a meat-free diet is kinder, cheaper, far more healthy, and indeed better for the health of our entire planet. So how do you do it? We'll cover that in the next chapter.

5

HOW TO GO VEGETARIAN

"What can I eat if I don't eat meat?"

That's the most daunting question of all for new or would-be vegetarians, and I'm going to answer it for you in this chapter. We'll look at the way you should structure a healthy vegetarian diet, and I'll give you some of my personal favorite recipes to try. But first, let's spend a moment examining how our food preferences are actually created.

One of life's biggest deceptions is the belief that we choose the food we eat for ourselves. Nothing could be further from the truth. You may *think* that your taste preferences reflect your own likes and dislikes, but in all probability they owe more to your parents than they really do to you. As human infants, we are more dependent upon our parents and more vulnerable over a far greater period of time than the young of any other species on the face of the Earth. It takes us years to achieve the same degree of control over even the most basic activities, which the young of other species manage to achieve in a matter of months, or even weeks.

Year after year, we rely upon adults to take most of our simple, everyday decisions for us. Now, biologically speaking, this works out very well because we have a lot more growing to do than most other species do, and while we're doing all this growing, we need the protection that parents can give us.

But parents give you more than just protection. They pass on to you their own values and beliefs, so that by the time you're old enough to take informed decisions for yourself, you've acquired a whole set of inherited likes, dislikes, and habits that, by sheer force of repetition, you've grown to regard as your own. Habits such as what you eat, the way you eat, and indeed, what you think about what you eat. All these habits have been largely predetermined for you. Other people made these decisions, because you weren't able to at the time. But you *are* able to now.

MEAT HOOKED?

The difficult thing with meat is that, just like tobacco and some other drugs, although you may not enjoy it at the beginning, your taste buds get hooked on its fatty, salty flavor quite quickly. Humans are not the only animals to respond like this. Gorillas are naturally gentle vegetarians, but when captive ones in zoos have been forcibly fed a meat diet they, too, develop carnivorous appetites—the more they eat, the more they must have. These behavioral changes are also accompanied by physical changes in their digestive system, whereby the ciliate protozoa (useful microorganisms we all need) in their intestines, which would normally help to digest the fiber in their natural diet, disappear. So returning to plant food isn't very easy for them.

It isn't so strange, then, that when young humans are fed animal flesh, they also become accustomed to the taste of it, and grow up believing that large quantities of flesh are an indispensable part of their diet. However, what has really happened is that we have been "taught" to eat meat, taught to regard its taste as palatable, and taught to consider it (if, indeed, we think about it at all) as a perfectly normal part of our diet. Many young children instinctively resist eating meat—I did, and perhaps you did, too. But by the time you were old enough to think objectively about the issue, you may already have been hooked.

The only chance to break this cycle is to do precisely what you're doing now: examine the evidence, and make an informed decision, based on your own personal feelings. I seriously believe that this may be the most important decision that you'll ever make. It may be the first time that you've ever had the chance to consciously and rationally reclaim control of a crucial area of your daily activity, that has, until now, been preprogrammed by a pattern of behavior that someone else decided upon decades ago. It's a great opportunity to get things right!

YOUR FIRST STEPS

Eating a vegetarian or vegan diet is not like taking holy orders, running for sainthood, or canvassing for the presidency. In fact, perfectly normal people do it all the time. The very phrase "becoming a vegetarian" can be off-putting, because it carries overtones of withdrawing from the world, even moral smugness. So let's remind ourselves that the only common ground that all vegetarians and vegans have is the fact that we *don't* do something—in this case, eat animal flesh. If that's all you want it to be, fine. It's your decision.

So do whatever you feel comfortable with. There's one thing, however, that you must never do. And that's apologize. Saying "I'm sorry, I don't eat meat" is demeaning to you, to other vegetarians and vegans, and to a healthy and deeply principled way of living. Subconsciously, it reinforces the prejudice that a few still have toward vegetarianism. It implies that vegetarianism is so freaky that it's "followers" have to apologize for it.

Words carry multitudes of meanings. When you say, "Don't cook any meat for me," you're often putting yourself into a minority. But turn it around, and say, "If you're going to eat animal flesh today, count me out." Then you're making people think about what they're really putting into their mouths. And they often squirm.

It's all a matter of perception. Here's something else that's a question of perception—the question that frequently baffles many would-be vegetarians and vegans: just *how* do you do it? When you live in a society that for the time being—views the eating of dead animals as the norm, how do you make the break? This can puzzle many people. If you're used to thinking of a meal as "meat and two veg," and you take away the meat, what are you left with? Just how long can you live on boiled potatoes and cabbage?

There's one group of people who are not puzzled by this question, however. And that's vegetarians and vegans. Now I have to tell you that—good as I hope this book is—the very best source of help and advice about the flesh-free way of living is actually other vegetarians and vegans. They can, and will, help you—in the same way you will help others, I hope, in the months and years ahead. However, I've noticed one strange circumstance in which vegetarians and vegans don't seem able to offer much in the way of assistance—and that's in the transition to vegetarianism. Here's why: Meat eaters find it difficult to imagine what vegetarians live on, but vegetarians find it equally difficult to imagine why that should be so. For many vegetarians and vegans, their lifestyles are so easy, and so natural, that they simply can't conceive of it ever appearing to be the least bit difficult or intimidating. I've frequently seen vegetarians look genuinely perplexed when asked, by an inquiring meat eater, "What do you eat?"

So be patient with your vegetarians friends and acquaintances if you ask them, "What's the best way to start?" and they respond by giving you an amazed look. Not long ago, that question probably bothered them, too. But now, they genuinely can't see what the problem is. Pretty soon, you won't either.

Making the Break

So what happens? Do you come home at six o'clock one Friday evening and have a nut cutlet instead of a lamb cutlet? Do you have to sign a pledge that meat will never pass your lips again? Or do you just do it in private, with consenting adults? Here are some ideas for making the break that I know have worked very well for other people. But do remember that fundamentally it's *your* decision—you're trying to find what genuinely suits you. So you should take everything that follows as suggestions, not as firm rules.

Cut Back

This method is a gradual transition from meat eating to vegetarianism. Aim to reduce your meat intake by about 50 percent per week. For example, if you now eat meat two meals a day, cut this back during the first week to just one meal a day. Then, for the second week, cut it back again to one meal every other day. The third week you probably won't eat more than a couple of meat meals in total. And the fourth week, you'll be free. This gradual process of cutting back gives you the chance to spread the transition over several weeks, and allows you to experiment with lots of new meat-free recipes. It also creates some thinking space in your life—something that is in very short supply for most of us these days. When you're eating meat, just think about what you're *really* eating—where it came from, what it really tastes like.

Other cultures are fundamentally different from us in the way they encourage an awareness—and respect for—food. In the West, fast food is king. Most of us don't judge food by its qualities and subtleties—for us, the fastest food is the best. We barely have time to bite the food as we shovel it down, before we bulldoze the next mouthful in. Once you start to become aware of what sort of food you're really putting inside your body, you may be rather shocked. For example, try chewing your food rather longer, and leave it in your mouth a few more seconds to experience the full range of tastes it offers. You'll find that a mouthful of dead flesh is really rather repugnant to hold there for more than a second or so. And you'll find that much of the processed food now sold to us tastes truly awful after the first "hit"—chemicals in the food give you an initial sensation of flavor, which produces maximum salivation, thus deceiving your senses into thinking that the food is appetizing. The first bite is then followed by a bitter, synthetic disintegration of unwholesome tastes. When you allow your mind and body to guide you in your food choices, you will, quite naturally, stop eating flesh.

Cut Out

Here's another technique that many have used as a successful transition to vegetarianism. It creates a clearly defined moment in your life when you take charge of your food intake; it represents a kind of personal watershed.

What you do is to eat a completely raw diet for seven to ten days. Nothing—absolutely nothing—that has been cooked, processed, or preserved is allowed down! Meat, of course, is automatically excluded. Similarly, bread, biscuits, jams, butter, tea, coffee, alcohol, and canned food are all absolutely out. However, the diet *must* contain lots of fresh fruit and vegetables—there is no limit to the quantity, eat as much as you can take. Aim to buy only organic vegetables.

Don't overlook nuts and seeds, and try making salad dressings using only cold-pressed oils and lemon juice.

You'll find it very difficult to overeat on raw food. Although you'll be taking in lots of vitamins from all this fresh food, it might be a good idea to supplement your diet with a good multivitamin and mineral pill, as well. During this period all sorts of things may start to happen. You may feel wonderfully elated or (very rarely) rather depressed. Your body may start to feel lighter and younger. On the other hand, you may very well have some kind of "deferred reaction"—you may get spots and pimples, and a bad headache is quite common as your body detoxifies. After seven to ten days, you can start to add some cooked food. In this short but intense period, your tastes will have changed for good. You will have developed an appreciation for fresh food, and a lasting desire to eat something fresh at least once a day. And then you won't look back! You will have made the break, given your body a thorough detoxification, and started to set the pattern for a better, healthier life.

And Replace!

Without doubt, this is the easiest method of all. A few years ago, it wasn't possible to find meat replacement or meat substitute products anywhere. Then a host of new products came along, and times changed for good. Today, the easiest way of going meat-free is simply to replace meat with any one of these convenience products (they're nutritionally superior to animal flesh, too). You can find them in all health food stores (as dry mixes and also fresh in the frozen foods section). Increasingly, supermarkets sell them, too. Products such as these are real lifesavers in many circumstances.

If there's just one vegetarian in the family (a younger son or daughter, for example) then this may be the way to go. It seems that what frequently happens is that the rest of the family come to the conclusion that the vegetarian option is actually much better than meat (and cheaper), and very often they'll go vegetarian, too.

A few brief words of advice: If you or your family like a "meaty" taste and texture, remember that TVP (textured vegetable protein) can be bought in all health food stores. Remember, also, that contrary to most people's expectations, ordinary gravy mixture is often totally vegan (check the label). Please *don't* just replace meat with mountains of hard cheese—it's far too high in fat. Also, consider expanding your culinary repertoire. Many of the world's finest cuisines don't require meat or dairy products; it's only in the West that our diet has become so unhealthily meat dominated. Now, start enjoying it! As the instruction booklets that accompany all those Japanese high-tech gadgets always begin by saying, "Congratulations! You've made the right decision!"

SURVIVING AND THRIVING WITH YOUR FAMILY

It's not difficult to stop eating animal flesh—people do it all the time! But sometimes, the hardest part is coping with the unpredictable, and occasionally hostile, reactions of friends or family. In my own case, it was quite easy. In common with many other children, I refused point blank to swallow dead animals from the age of two. I even persuaded my parents to go vegetarian some years later. This, by the way, isn't unusual: I've met many children who've done the same thing.

Sadly, some people seem to have more opposition than I had. The lone vegetarian in a large family can be teased to the point of persecution; and when one partner in a relationship decides to stop eating meat, but the other one insists on continuing, then the strain can sometimes be considerable. Although there is no simple answer to cover every possible situation, the combined experiences of many vegetarians and vegans do suggest that there are techniques and approaches you can use that usually work successfully. Here, in their own words, a variety of vegetarians describe how they've coped, and what's worked for them.

The Hard Way

David Hobbs,[1] a senior sociology major in New York, has been vegetarian for two years, and he's the first to admit they've been two difficult years.

I've been subject to plenty of criticism. Being the only one in my family, it took them a long time to accept my decision, and I had to really stand by my position before they gave up trying to make me eat meat. My father still continues to tell me there's no room in this world for my ideas about animal rights. . . . My maternal grandmother says I should be more flexible in my diet since when I go out to eat with friends, they might want to eat at a restaurant that only serves meat. But why should I be expected to eat something that makes me nauseous and is bad for me? This is terribly unfair to my sense of ethics.

The event that originally compelled me to abandon eating dead animals was in a biology lab, when I had to dissect the brain of a pig fetus! This sounds insane and it is—even the lab instructor told us he'd rather use computer models if the school had the funds. Anyway, after this depraved lab activity, I went to the delicatessen for lunch, where I bought my usual turkey sandwich on a hard roll. The color and texture of the meat reminded me exactly of the pig's brain, and I vowed to myself I'd never eat another animal for the rest of my life. I was literally about to vomit while eating it!

The only time I've eaten meat since then was on one Father's Day, when my maternal grandparents insisted on going to a restaurant where the only entrées were fish. When I looked at the menu before we were seated and realized this, my father sarcastically asked me if I intended to order ten portions of the carrot soufflé (a side dish). I ultimately reluctantly ordered a piece of dead salmon, but I hated every bit of it. My grandmother was satisfied that I was flexible enough to compromise my ideals. My whole family, including my younger sister, who claims to love animals, was paranoid that I would humiliate them and "make a scene," as my mother would put it. I truly resented them for making me do something that contradicted my entire set of values. They all think I am too opinionated, and as my mother would say, if I don't watch what I say, "someone might take out a knife!"

Eventually, my parents caught on and reluctantly gave in to my refusal to eat dead beings. I've also discovered a local group of vegetarians, where I can meet like-minded people and hopefully develop close friendships.

It took my family a long time to accept my "radical" decision to go veggie, but eventually my mother started buying me prepared dinners. I wish I could figure out a way to convince them to kick the meat habit for their own benefit, without being told not to give them a "lecture," as my mother and sister would say. I want to enjoy family get-togethers without being seen as a kook. As far as other people who want to become vegetarians, I advise them to stand up for what they believe in, no matter what may stand in the way. People who want to stop eating animals should not be afraid to openly defy the status quo. What makes any country great is the ability and desire of its people to stand up for what they believe in. It is better not to conform to accepted standards if you see an injustice being committed as a consequence of that norm.

Enlightenment by Degrees

Happily, the transition to a flesh-free way of living doesn't always have to be so painful or as fraught with conflict. Jo Ann Davis, a library assistant in Pennsylvania, was much luckier with her family and, in the process, converted most of them to vegetarianism.

My transition to vegetarianism was quite easily accomplished because of the ethical position my parents always have taken regarding animal life and kindness. Eighteen years ago, I decided to become a vegetarian "temporarily" because of deer-hunting season in Pennsylvania. Being opposed to hunting, I found it difficult to refute the hunters' statements about my consumption of meat. So that year, I became a vegetarian for a few weeks, just so I could say that I don't eat any meat. My parents supported me because they, too, believed as I did. At the end of hunting season, I had found it was so easy being a vegetarian, that I decided to stay meatless for awhile longer. I prepared my own meals, separate from my parents, so there was no conflict in that respect. After about a year, my mother saw that I didn't wither and die, so she decided to try vegetarianism herself. Her hardest struggle was in social situations—she felt that it wasn't polite to refuse the meat passed to her when visiting friends, so she still sometimes ate meat. Since my parents are both excellent cooks, my father would make his own meat, my mother would usually make the rest of the meal.

Several years later, my brother and sister-in-law, also for ethical and moral reasons, became vegetarians. Whenever my father eats at their house, he eats vegetarian along with the rest of us—and has no problem with it. Although he sometimes mulls over the idea of joining our side, he can't quite give up meat. After seventy-four years of eating it, it is a hard habit to break. I occasionally try to coax him to turn veggie, but he can't make the commitment. That's okay, though, because we all are happy with our chosen diets and don't feel the need to nag him. At least there are four out of five of us that animals aren't dying for.

I think the main opposition most parents have to vegetarianism is their fear of the unknown—they have been raised in a system that taught them that "meat is might," and without meat, a person will whither away to nothing. A visit to the local library should offer sources of support, too. I work in an academic library, and we have a number of books on meatless diets, ethics of vegetarianism, and recipes for veggies. I suppose the main thing is enlightenment. The more that family members are educated, the better the chance of their acceptance of the dietary change. I'm an avid canoeist, and when people ask if I'm weak because of being a veggie, I just point to my solo canoe and tell them the tales of my wilderness adventures!

Jane Evans, currently a university student, is another who sees her chosen lifestyle gradually having its effect on those around her.

I was fifteen when I decided to become a vegetarian. My motivation to become a vegetarian was pretty simple. I wasn't able to rationalize the reason that human beings think they are given the power to end another living creature's life. I believe that every living creature is given one thing—life—and no one is allowed to take that from them. That's where my family and I differ the most; they can understand the health aspect of vegetarianism, but they have always had the mentality that animals were put on this Earth for our use. Even if they were, I still can't rationalize how they deserve to be tortured and made miserable during their keep before slaughtering!

My parents and family were very much against this way of life. My family believed that meat was an essential part of everyone's diet. So I made an agreement with my mother; I told her I would do it for a summer, and if I showed any signs of being unhealthy I would stop. So I did my research and was on a mission to prove to everyone that my choice was a good one. It was, and since then I have remained a vegan. I also don't use any animal products, or wear leather. The criticism from my family was pretty minimal once they understood that this was a major decision on my part. It was something that I truly believe in, and they have grown to respect it. As for peers and new acquaintances, I still get the meat waved in my face, the comments asking if I want a big, fat, juicy burger, and so on. I have been able to conclude that these rude comments are not directed to me out of dislike, but rather, they are ways in which people are unconsciously defending their meat-eating habits. Some individuals are put into an uncomfortable position around me and are trying to deal with their own insecurities about their own ways of life.

Today, my immediate family has taken my new lifestyle to heart, and they rarely consume red meat. It's a step for them. I am living proof that a teenager can grow and develop without consuming meat!

For Sarah LaPorte, a computer programmer in Cupertino, California, the process was also one of gradual change.

I became vegetarian in college, so when I went home for Thanksgiving vacation, I was the only vegetarian. Initially I was not successful in coping with it. My mother was concerned about my nutrition, and had made a tuna fish casserole, with the tuna shredded into microscopic pieces. I didn't have the heart to turn it down, and I regretfully ate it.

I must say that she was correct in assuming that I hadn't learned enough about nutrition. However, I was correct in my gut feeling that my diet was already terrible, even though I was eating meat. You know the comeback you get when you tell a family member you're a new vegetarian—"But how can you get a balanced diet?" As if meat is the answer!

The truth is that my mother didn't know too much about nutrition, either! The next time I went home, in February, I had learned a bit more. They were dubious, but could not get me to eat meat, so we had a truce.

Now I am married. I have learned a lot more in the last sixteen years. Through his own reading, and my influence, my husband has become convinced to eat vegetarian at home, and to raise the children vegetarian.

Persistence Pays!

Student Steve Keen was seventeen years old when he decided to become a vegetarian.

At first, my mother kept saying that "that's nice." But when she started realizing that I wasn't going to eat any kind of animal flesh, she got upset. She thought that I couldn't grow up healthy without eating meat. She would say things like "You're still going to eat turkey and fish, right?" When I convinced her that I could get all the protein and vitamins even without meat, she tried a different approach. She started to tell me that I couldn't be a vegetarian because it was too much trouble for her. So I said that I would take care of all my cooking. Well, I started cooking for myself and was pleased with what I was coming up with. She would occasionally try some of the things I made, such as tofu loaf and tofu chili, and she began to realize that it is possible to be healthy and happy while being a vegetarian. After the first three months, she stopped pestering me about eating meat and finally accepted it. Now she fully understands and accepts my lifestyle and is much less ignorant. I am still the only vegetarian in my family, but the rest of them are a bit more aware now of the great joys of being a vegetarian.

A Change of Heart

An experience common to many vegetarians is a "paradigm shift" of awareness after regular meat-eating has ceased. For a time, new vegetarians are often content to tolerate the habits of their meat-eating friends or family—even, sometimes, to prepare meat for them. Then, things change. This was the experience of Ann Mason, another student. When she first went vegetarian, it didn't bother her to see others eating meat.

In fact, I even prepared meat at a cafe I worked in. Things have changed a lot over the last year. I just cannot bear watching people consume a dead animal. It sometimes brings tears to my eyes. I've had problems with my mom over this, because she thinks that I've become too radical. She wants me to come to family gatherings, but I refuse if I know there is going to be a carcass present. I spent Thanksgiving with vegan friends rather than going home to my family. I think my mom understands that the way I feel is not going to change, so she avoids eating meat when I am at home. She's close to being vegetarian herself, but does not seem to want to completely disclaim her "God-given right" to eat meat. Problems only arise when other people are involved in the situation—my mom will do without for me, but my other relatives won't. I think the best way to get loved ones to do without meat when you are with them is to let them know exactly how it makes you feel—the pain, disgust, whatever. If someone really loves you, they will not do something that brings you pain.

Step by Step

Jane Green, an administrative assistant from St. Paul, Minnesota, went vegetarian together with her husband in gradual stages, as part of a conscious program to improve the quality of their diets.

When I married my husband, he was very health conscious, but I was a meat and junk food consumer. As we began our life together, we both agreed to eliminate red meat and endeavor to have a healthy food program. I, being a compulsive overeater, ate good healthy food at mealtimes, but continued to sneak my atrocious snacks on the fly.

Gradually, we eliminated more and more animal flesh, enjoying vegetarian meals several times a week. I made the decision to become an ovo-lacto vegetarian about three years ago. My husband continued eating chicken and fish. I cooked vegetarian meals, but very occasionally, I would make tuna sandwiches for my spouse or cook him some fish or chicken. Eventually that stopped; he didn't want it as much, and felt concerned asking me to do that for him, as well. He did often have chicken at restaurants. For the past year or so, he has wanted fowl or fish less and less; now he can't recall the last time he ate it. He also considers himself ovo-lacto vegetarian. I, now, am on the verge of making a commitment to veganism.

This was very much the strategy of Helen Littlewood, a systems analyst, who initially faced some resistance from her spouse.

He thought it was passing stage. He initially supported the idea, then became a little exasperated when it became obvious how much of an impact it was going to have on the life we were living. He believed that we had a good life and did not really want to see it disturbed. There were all the standard problems with going out to friends. Even when I made no criticism of the restaurants chosen, it would upset him that I didn't eat (sometimes there was nothing I could eat), but I would go for the community only. However, occasions like that did convince him that I wasn't undertaking a fad. There were a few harsh conversations about what I perceived as his inability to accept change, and in the end, his eyes were opened. It's interesting. While he continues along his own way, it is he that constructs the better arguments in favor of vegetarianism when it comes up in conversations with others. He has told me that although it is not for him at this stage, he admires people who have consciously chosen vegetarianism in the kinds of societies most of us find ourselves living in. I suppose if I had more of a tendency to preach and press the issues, I might have converted him by now, but I guess I'd rather that he came to vegetarianism not out of pressure from me, but by his own free will.

Tolerance Triumphs

Stephanie Stevens, a Washington-based management consultant, went vegetarian in her student days seven years ago, mainly because she simply couldn't afford to eat meat.

After quitting meat, I noticed that I lost fifteen pounds without even trying, and I felt great! I was a college athlete (volleyball, basketball), and I also felt that quitting meat helped me have more endurance and better performance. Now that I've thought more about my family's heart disease, high cholesterol, high blood pressure, and arteriosclerosis, I would never change my dietary habits, even though I can afford to eat meat if I want to.

I'd say that I'm one of the lucky ones when it comes to veggie-compatible significant others! I don't get grossed out if other people in my life want to eat meat. I see vegetarianism as a healthy, sane alternative to the average American diet. I met my husband-to-be at a vegetarian restaurant, so at least I could see that he was open-minded enough to be there! As I got to know him, I discovered that he was not a vegetarian, but wasn't opposed to trying the foods I would make and exploring foods he hadn't tried before. He had noticed problems with his digestive-excretory health before, and when we started living together, he didn't drop meat altogether, but he said (without me asking) that he felt more energetic and his digestive discomforts disappeared almost completely when he cut down on the amount of meat he ate. He still eats meat every so often (probably about once a month), but he'll go out and get a hamburger, or make it when I'm not home, and then he'll confess when I come home from work. So, we've reached a sort of compromise, that when we eat together we eat vegetarian style, but he doesn't get any negative feedback from me when he occasionally decides to eat meat. I figure that it's healthier than eating meat all of the time. The best part is that we've agreed to bring up our children as vegetarians, and we're hoping to promote the idea that meat is an *alternative* to being vegetarian, the way people now think of vegetarianism as being alternative to meat.

Tell Them the Truth

Women who are responsible for feeding a family can have a particularly difficult time. Often feeling under an obligation to cook the sort of food her family demands to eat, a woman can find herself at odds with her own conscience—ultimately, an impossible situation. Sometimes, the problem can be simply overcome by resolving to have a frank discussion with all family members about the ugly truth of meat production. Serita Bricklin, a secretary, succeeded in converting her family to the meat-free way of living, motivated in part by the staunch refusal of her eight-year-old son to eat animal flesh since birth.

> He really helped put me on the right track, since I had to find something for the kid to eat! At first my husband complained. I quietly told him how much healthier he would be and he began losing weight. Now he prides himself on the fact that he no longer eats meat. My daughter was easy. She's only five so I just explained to her that hamburger came from cows, bacon from pigs, and so on. She grossed out and doesn't complain at all now. She says all animals are her friends.

Sometimes it's not possible to eliminate meat from a family's diet at a single step. But even then, there is still plenty you can do. Robbie Dennis, a senior New York banker, is married with a seventeen-year-old daughter, and is the only vegetarian in the household.

> I respect the rights of people to make these choices for themselves. However, because I am the only cook at home, I have established boundaries for myself. I don't cook meat, and I only buy it for the family members if we go out to eat and I am buying. I expect that my husband and daughter will purchase and cook meat for themselves if they choose to eat it. I like to cook, so I serve a lot of delicious food that everyone likes. They seldom bother going out of their way to eat meat.

My family have actually moved more and more toward a veg-etarian lifestyle. I suspect that someday they will go all the way. We are all animal lovers. When we hear stories of animals being mistreated so humans can eat them, it gives my family more of a resolve to continue in the direction of complete vegetarianism.

I think you win converts by showing people the positive bene-fits of the desired action, not by shaming, preaching, or moraliz-ing! Share great vegetarian foods with those whom you would like to convert, give them little facts to think about, and give them lots of good suggestions for making the change—after all, chang-ing can be very difficult for some people. The best way to convert a person is to find recipes and restaurants that offer delicious alternatives. Cheer like hell when people try new things, and respect their choices otherwise. Also, if you can't get support from the family, find it elsewhere! I started a vegetarian group at work. It really helps.

Marcia Singer, a marketing manager from Los Angeles, adopts a similar "ween-them-off-it" approach, with the difference that she is prepared to serve some meat to her family. This is how she explains it:

I go to my local grocery store, which sells pesticide- and hor-mone-free meat products, and buy chicken breasts in bulk. I wrap them separately in freeze-lock bags and put them in the freezer. When I make dinner, I typically serve rice, beans, and lots of veg-etables and fruit, and I'll quick-fry slices of tofu for myself in soy and top with shredded ginger and daikon; the same with the chicken breasts for my husband and daughter. I began by cooking one completely vegetarian meal a week for everyone, and serving chicken or fish the other six days. I am now cooking four com-pletely vegetarian meals a week and serving chicken or fish on three. My family hardly notices because I have gradually gained more expertise in cooking vegetarian dishes—with the help of a lot of *wonderful* vegetarian cookbooks that I bought at my local bookstore! My college daughter thinks it's really cool that her mom is a vegetarian. Last weekend she brought a new boyfriend home (he is also a vegetarian), but she called ahead to discuss the menu with me, requesting several of her favorite vegetarian dishes! Next year at this time, I hope to have everyone off meat altogether!

Aiming for Excellence

Although women still unfairly bear the brunt of food preparation in our society—and therefore most often face the moral dilemma of whether they should cook to please their families or to salve their own consciences—times are slowly changing. When Daniel Sharon, an engineer, met his partner, he was vegetarian (more lately, vegan)—but she wasn't. This is how he resolved the situation:

When my current spouse and I met, she was an omnivore, but not a big meat eater (although a very serious cheese user). Her son was a complete omnivore (he would eat anything that doesn't move, and even some things that do!).

Upon our very first "encounter," I made it clear to this girl that she was getting into a different experience: we didn't meet at a restaurant or any such "neutral" ground, but rather, I invited her over to my place for dinner. I went all out and made an excellent gourmet dinner (broccoli salad, pad Thai, fresh bread, vegetable stir-fry, black forest chocolate cake with coffee-butter icing, Spanish coffee). This trend has kept up. I must state (in a humble manner) that I am a very good cook, and I have used an approach of making excellent food in order to convince and convert people.

We dated, and eventually got engaged, and bought a house together last year. Right from the start, I made it well known that there was no way any meat products would get cooked in the house. This was a condition, which was stated initially, and has held (and is nonnegotiable). I let the kids eat whatever they want (the more you try to prevent them, the more they will—and I'd rather have them understand the health and ecological issues, and do as they will with them). However, they can *not* cook meat in the house.

When we have a meal together, I cook it and we all eat the same vegan food. I make it good in order to convince everyone.

Occasionally, the three kids get together and cook a gourmet vegan dinner for us (with a little bit of my help and many of my recipes). My spouse cannot stand even the sight or smell of meat anymore. She still uses cheese, but at a much lower rate. She simply loves the food we cook together, and I would claim that she is now fully converted. Her conversion, however, is her own choice—she liked what she ate, she switched slowly, and now claims she couldn't go back. So in a nutshell, omnivores can be converted by following these three major guidelines:

- Use positive reinforcement to do it—good vegan food is a lot more convincing than an entire book full of facts.
- Lay down the ground rules right from the start—I don't think I could get meat out of the house today if I'd ever allowed it in.
- Disperse a little bit of information at a time—too much and you sound like an activist, too little, and you're not making your point. I do want my kids and my wife to understand why, not just how good it can taste.

The Breaking Point

Not every case is such a gradual transition from meat eating to vegetarianism. Janet Benson, a publisher, found that there came a crucial moment in her relationship when she found she could no longer prepare her partner's meat-based meals. This is how she successfully handled it:

After a lifetime of meat eating, I decided to become a vegetarian about six months ago. I didn't feel I had the right to insist that my partner make the same decision, because his being a vegetarian was not a requirement before we were married. I didn't feel that it was fair to change the rules after already making a lifetime commitment. In our relationship, I am almost always home earlier than he, and I love to cook, while he detests it. So I do all the cooking, and he always cleans up the kitchen (which I hate!). As I was making my adjustment early on, I would prepare vegetarian meals, but then cook a small portion of meat for him, such as grilling a chicken breast. With time, I became more and more uncomfortable with this, and actually became more grossed out by it! My diet was also evolving more and more toward veganism, until the only dairy or eggs that I ever ate were in baked goods that were purchased outside our home. I finally told him that what he chooses to eat is his decision, but I will not have any part of preparing meat for him anymore. If he wants to eat it in our home, he will have to purchase it, prepare it, and clean it up himself. Since I do most of the grocery shopping also, this has proved to be more trouble for him than it's worth, so he joins me in eating vegan meals at home. However, he still eats meat when we eat out, and will occasionally stop at fast-food places for some of their horrible concoctions.

The important thing, I think, is that in all of the discussions we have had about eating, I have made a very strong effort to be nonjudgmental and respectful of him, and his right to make his own decisions. At first, I pulled the "righteous indignation" trip when he would eat a hamburger, but this only served to irritate him and make him defensive, especially since I had joined him in eating the same thing only weeks before. So we had a long talk, and I promised to be more supportive, even though I don't agree with what he eats sometimes. The result of all of this is that he has been much more receptive to my veganism, has shown more of an interest in my cooking (our running joke is that I'm making tofu-lentil surprise), and has significantly cut down on his meat consumption. He may never become a vegetarian himself, but he does realize (even if he does only grudgingly admit) that my diet is healthier, and he is open to eating the vegetarian things I prepare.

We are still young (twenty-four and twenty-six), and don't have any kids yet. I will insist that our children be raised vegetarian or vegan, and will hold my ground on that one, because the health evidence is very convincing to me. I suspect that all of this would have been much more difficult if we had been married a long time, or already had kids, but I think it is important in marriage (or any lifetime commitment) to respect both your partner's right to change, and his right to make his own decisions.

In Conclusion: The Golden Rules of Vegetarian Family Life

- Make sure your family and friends clearly understand the reasons why you've adopted the meat-free way of living. Be assertive if necessary, but not aggressive. You are entitled to have your views respected by everyone, even if they don't agree with you.
- Aim to be an expert cook yourself, even if your repertoire consists of just a handful of dishes, prepared excellently. Good food changes minds.
- If you don't normally get involved in the kitchen, now is the time to pull your weight! Don't expect someone else to have to learn a new way of cooking just to please you.
- If you normally prepare the food for your family, and there is initial resistance to your desire to go meat-free, plan to achieve a three-stage transition: (1) Explain that buying and preparing animal flesh is a task that you find increasingly unpleasant, and ask those who wish to eat meat to cook it for themselves. (2) After a time, all the additional inconvenience involved in meat preparation will almost certainly mean that it is only eaten outside the home. Consolidate this and make it known that you would rather meat were not brought into the house. (3) Once in a while, take a few moments to educate the rest of your family about the truth of meat production, and about the many advantages of the meat-free way of living.
- If you have little or no support from within your family, find it elsewhere from like-minded people. There are lots of us around!

THE WELL-NOURISHED VEGETARIAN

The table below shows what you should eat if you want to be a very well-nourished vegetarian. I hope your mouth waters just looking at it! Devised by Dr. Michael Klaper, one of America's foremost experts on achieving optimum health through pure vegetarian nutrition, this table shows you how easy it is to eat well on a vegetarian diet.[2] Actually, if you look closely, you'll see that it includes *no animal products whatever*—it's a "pure vegetarian," or vegan, diet. Personally, I prefer a vegan diet, but it took me some years to realize that.

Group	Provides	Examples	Quantity
Whole grains and potatoes	Energy, protein, oils, vitamins, fiber	Brown rice, corn, millet, barley, bulgur, buckwheat, oats, muesli, bread, pasta, flour	2–4 servings daily
Legumes	Protein, oils	Green peas, lentils, chickpeas, kidney beans, baked beans, soy products (milk, tofu, tempeh, textured vegetable protein)	1–2 servings daily
Green and yellow vegetables	Vitamins, minerals, protein	Broccoli, brussels sprouts, spinach, cabbage, carrots, squash, sweet potatoes, pumpkins, parsnips	1–3 servings daily

Group	Provides	Examples	Quantity
Nuts and seeds	Protein, oils, calcium, trace minerals	Almonds, pumpkin seeds, walnuts, peanuts, sesame seeds, nut butters, tahini, sunflower seeds	1–3 servings daily
Fruit	Energy, vitamins, minerals	All kinds	3–6 pieces daily
Vitamin and mineral foods	Trace minerals and vitamin B_{12}	(a) Sea vegetables. (b) B_{12}-fortified foods such as soy milk, TVP, breakfast cereals, soy "meat" products	1 serving each of (a) and (b) 3 times a week

BREAKING THE NEWS

Sometimes, people worry about how they're going to tell other people that they don't indulge in quasi-cannibalism any more. Let's look at a few situations.

Parents

Depending on your relationship with them (and this depends not only on your real age, but also on how old they *think* you are), you may or may not have problems. As humans get older, they generally become less concerned about freedom, justice, and morality and more concerned with mortgages, pensions, and prosthodontics. They also tend to lose things more often, forget what they were saying in mid-sentence, and, er, where was I? Oh, yes. What this all means is they're worried about the practicalities—the details. They've spent a lot of time and money to help you become the sort of person you are today (yes, they really do think like that), and they don't want to see their genetic investment starve itself to death. Basically, there seem to be two sorts of problems. One is the "Oh-My-God-How-Are-You-Going-To-Survive" reaction, and the other is the "Oh-My-God-What-Am-I-Going-to-Cook" reaction. Both can verge on the hysterical, so try to disarm them early on.

If we take the first reaction, which mainly comes from family or friends, as basically being a sign of well-meaning concern, then it shouldn't upset you too much. Maybe they can't imagine what you're going to live on, and they're obviously expecting you to shrivel up and die at any moment. In a word, they're ignorant. So enlighten them! Lend them this book, talk to them about it ad nauseum, try to get them interested and involved. Tell them about famous people such as Leonardo da Vinci, Voltaire, George Bernard Shaw, and the many others who did pretty well for themselves without eating flesh. If there's a good natural food restaurant near by, suggest that you all go out and have a meal together. Don't try to sell them the idea if they're not ready for it, but do try to reassure them, which is all that's really needed.

The second reaction is usually found among mothers who find they've suddenly got to cope with a meat-free menu. Not surprisingly, they feel as if they've been dropped in the deep end. The best advice here is to discuss the situation with them as early as you can. Tell your mother that more and more people are finding a better, healthier way of eating, and for a variety of reasons you'd like to try it, too. You'll probably have to lead the way by obtaining a few recipe books, and also by doing your fair share of kitchen work. Providing you take it slowly and don't panic her, you'll probably find that she is extremely interested in what you're doing, and may try it as well.

The Spouse

If you're in a relationship, and one of you is going to go vegetarian, the most important thing is to talk it through, together. Don't underestimate the impact this change will have on your lifestyles. Eating is one of the most fundamental of all human activities, and any major change is bound to have considerable repercussions. By talking it through and planning it together, you'll ensure that all the consequences of your choice are good ones.

The couples who seem to have the most problems at this time are the ones who don't normally share other things together—when the wife always does the cooking, for example, and the husband always does the eating. Conversely, the couples who share the food preparation are invariably the ones who get the most pleasure out of it—and there's at least as much pleasure in making food as in eating it. It's easy to forget that, with so much instant and fast food around these days. So try rediscovering this special sort of togetherness for yourselves. If that sounds like a tall order, have a go at some of the suggestions that follow. A useful trick to involve males in the kitchen (who may have been badly spoiled by their mothers) is to appeal to their vanity. Certain aspects of cooking are more "technical" than others, and these can be presented as an intellectual challenge for the more dim-witted of the species. Here are some ideas:

- Give him a book about making soy milk and soybean curd. This is a fascinating process, and will provide him with many happy hours. Hopefully, it will even produce some food!
- Some dishes have an arbitrary cultural association with masculinity (you know, in the same way that going down to the neighborhood bar with his friends is alleged to be male bonding at its most profound. By the way, did you know that men who drink excessively grow breasts?). Use this image, if you have to, in order to get him involved in food preparation. For example, try all the many different forms of curry (there are thousands), try barbecued foods, get him to make some bread (it's very physical), or anything with alcohol in it.
- Tell him that he should think about opening a restaurant. Again, this seems to cut straight to the quick of the pathetically easy-to-flatter sense of male vanity. Most men seem to have their own distinct ideas about this, and you never know, he might just end up doing it! Even if he doesn't, he'll have learned something useful in the kitchen, like how to turn the light on.
- Try creating recipes together. You can start by asking him to suggest "improvements" to standard recipes, and then ask him to show you what he means. It'll set you both thinking!

- When you're feeling reasonably confident, throw a small party at which he can show off his newly acquired skills. Remember that men always respond well to positive reinforcement, so make sure that everyone is primed with suitable words of praise and appreciation.

In a way, I'm sorry to have to suggest ruses like these to you, but the fact is, they've worked for many couples. Well, to tell you the truth, there was *one* couple whom I could do nothing for, at all. She called when I was on a radio program, and told me the problem.

"I've gone vegetarian," she said, "but my husband's refusing to follow."

"Have you told him that it's healthier, cheaper, kinder to the environment—that he'll feel fitter, lose weight, look ten years younger, and will be smoldering with passion all night long?" I asked.

"Oh yes," she said, "he knows all that. The trouble is, he owns a butcher's shop."

"Then my dear," I said, "you'll just have to leave him."

"I'm going to," she said. And I think she did.

KNOW WHY YOU'RE DOING IT

When they know that you've "gone green," people will immediately ask you, "Why?" You may get fed up with this, but please think very carefully about this situation, which I guarantee will be repeated hundreds, or even thousands, of times throughout your life. Vegetarianism is a very attractive, even fashionable, way of living, and most people are keenly interested.

I want to put a little idea into your head, which goes like this:

"Merely to content oneself with personal abstention is to become part of the problem, rather than part of the solution."[3]

When I read those words a few years ago, they immediately stuck in my mind—I hope they stick in yours, too. What they're really telling us is that time is too short not to seize every chance you get to tell people about this saner way of living. I can explain this by telling you about one of my many encounters with meat trade spokespeople. This one happened in a debate in a radio studio a few years ago.

Sometimes, I only half listen to them, because I know their well-worn arguments so well. And this one was running true to form.

"There is no evidence," he was saying, "*absolutely* no evidence that meat is in any way bad for you." Before I could make a reply, he cut me off.

"Now look here," he said, affecting an avuncular manner. "I don't mind you people at all. Not in the slightest. Live and let live, that's what I say. But for heaven's sake, let people eat what they want to. Why don't you live and let live like I do?"

I was momentarily stunned, then the irony of the situation struck me, and I burst out laughing. A butcher just told me to live and let live. And that's precisely what's wrong with those words "live and let live." It's all too easy to use them as an excuse for inaction. And if you're not actively part of the solution, then you're actually part of the problem.

So when someone next asks you why you've chosen to go vegetarian, please tell them honestly. Don't argue, don't be provoked, and don't hesitate to seize the opportunity to spread the word a little bit more.

EATING WITH FRIENDS

If you're invited for a meal at a friend's house, it's probably best to tell him in advance that your food preferences have changed, and so avoid any problems. Usually a phone call something like this is all that it takes:

"I thought I'd give you a call just to let you know in advance that I've (we've) given up eating meat. I hope it won't be a problem for you?" Usually, your friend will thank you for being so thoughtful and letting him know. Just occasionally, he will be stumped for an answer, in which case you have various possibilities. You could offer to drop by beforehand for a chat with a few recipe books, which could be another enjoyable social occasion in its own right. Or, if you're feeling brave, you could offer to cook something yourself, and bring it for everyone to try (be warned—cook enough, or you won't get any yourself!). Whatever you and your friend decide, it's likely to be the conversational and culinary centerpiece of the evening, and will almost certainly make you the party's expert, who everyone will want to talk to!

EATING OUT

Most restaurants offer a selection of meat-free meals, and many offer vegan meals, too. Most restaurateurs know a good thing when they see one, and a meatless meal is actually more profitable for them to prepare and serve than all the fuss and waste involved in cooking meat. So more and more restaurants are quickly realizing that what's good for their customers is also good for their bank account. Most Indian, Chinese, Italian, Mexican, Greek, Jewish, Middle Eastern, and of course health food restaurants will prove particularly easy to eat in. If you don't see anything you fancy on the menu, speak to the owner or the head chef, who, in my experience, will be only too delighted to try and expand his culinary repertoire. You may even get to try some unique ethnic dish that is usually reserved for "the regulars" (that's how I first got to try tofu in a Chinese restaurant).

Speaking of food, would you like to try some?

WELCOME TO THE KITCHEN

I thought long and hard about the sort of recipes that you'd like to see here, and came to the conclusion that the best thing is to show you how my own family eats most of the time. All these recipes are very user-friendly, and will tolerate a wide margin of error. Although most cookbooks still seem to think that we all sit down to three full meals every day, very few of us actually live like that any more. Most of us "graze"—we feed when we can, not necessarily always eating together. These recipes are ideal for grazing—they'll keep for a day or more, and some of them actually improve their flavor if kept longer (the marinades, for example). And, of course, they're all horribly healthy. Most of them are low in fat, yet still provide important amounts of protein and other nutrients.[4] So, enjoy!

EASY FIVE-BEA

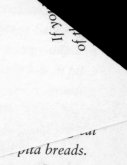

Most of us still think of salads as anem
slice of tomato and a limp lettuce leaf. V
back, and this time it's personal. Although
you can see from the per-portion analysis, it
well under 30 percent of its calories come fro
calories, just eat a smaller portion). It keeps
an excellent snack, lunch or main meal accom
favorite with children. Serve it with dry toast or pita breads.

1 (1-pound) can kidney beans, partly drained
1 (1-pound) can green beans, drained
1 (1-pound) can chickpeas, partly drained
1 (1-pound) can lima beans, partly drained
1 (1-pound) can borlotti or pinto beans, drained
5 scallions, thinly sliced
1 apple, grated
3 cloves garlic, crushed
2 teaspoons grated fresh ginger
1 tablespoon brown sugar
2 teaspoons freshly ground black pepper
Juice of 1 lemon
1 cup cider vinegar
½ cup plus 2 tablespoons olive oil

Measure all the ingredients into a nonreactive saucepan and stir well. Place over medium heat, cover, and bring to a slow boil. Reduce the heat and simmer, covered, for 10 minutes.

Leave the pan covered and remove from the heat. Allow to cool and spoon into a serving dish. Chill in the refrigerator. This salad improves as it cools and may be kept, chilled, for up to 3 days.

Allow 30 minutes, excluding cooling and chilling time.

Servings: 8; Calories per serving, 530; Protein (g) 16; Total fat (g) 16; Saturated fat (g) 2; Percent calories from fat, 26%.

LENTIL PÂTÉ

re used to thinking of pâtés as sheer heart-attack food (most
em are 80 percent fat, or more), this is going to blow your mind,
but not your arteries. No, there's no mistake—it really is just 5 per-
cent calories from fat. This is the basic pâté, delicious and attractive as
it stands. You can, however, adjust it to suit your own tastes: make it
more spicy, add finely chopped red and green pepper, slice some olives
into it, or add your own blend of herbs. Over to you!

1¼ cups dried red lentils, washed and drained
2 cups water
Pinch of salt
1 teaspoon ground turmeric
⅔ cup rolled oats
⅔ cup rice flakes (available in natural food stores)
1 teaspoon freshly ground black pepper
1 teaspoon ground ginger

In a medium saucepan, combine the lentils, water, salt, and turmeric and bring to a gentle boil over medium heat. Cover, reduce the heat, and simmer for 30 minutes, stirring often. Add the remaining ingredients, stir well, and simmer for another 5 to 10 minutes.

Remove from the heat, stir very well, and spoon into a serving dish, pressing down as you fill the dish. Allow the pâté to cool; then chill or serve immediately on bread or crackers.

Allow 45 minutes, excluding time to chill.

Servings: 8; Calories per serving, 110; Protein (g) 8; Total fat (g) 0.5; Saturated fat (g) 0.1; Percent calories from fat, 5%.

NINE-TO-FIVE STEW

Most of us dream of eating luscious stews, but think they're impossible for all but rural folk with wood-burning stoves. A hearty stew is warming, wholesome, full of flavor, and has an aroma that turns a house into a home. Make this in the morning and go to work knowing you can tuck in as soon as you get home.

> 1 pound rutabaga, cubed
> 1 pound carrots, chopped
> 1 pound parsnips, cubed
> 1 pound turnips, cubed
> 1 pound potatoes, cubed
> 1 pound very small onions
> 1 teaspoon whole cloves
> 12 whole peppercorns
> 1 (1-pound) can chestnut purée
> 8 cups water

Preheat the oven to 275°F, or a very low temperature of your choice.

Mix together the rutabaga, carrots, parsnips, turnips, and potatoes in a large bowl or pan.

Peel the onions and press 1 whole clove into each end of each onion. Add the onions, and peppercorns to the vegetables, toss, and turn into a large stew pot.

Blend the chestnut puree and water together in a bowl or pitcher and pour over the vegetable mixture. Cover the pot tightly and place in the oven for 6 to 8 hours. Don't lift the lid! At the end of this time, serve the stew hot with lots of fresh bread.

Allow 1 whole day.

Servings: 6; Calories per serving, 322; Protein (g) 7; Total fat (g) 2; Saturated fat (g) 0.4; Percent calories from fat, 6%.

PEA AND CORIANDER SOUP

*For those who thought pea soup had to have a bone. This soup
makes the most of the pea: it's nutritious, colorful, and a perfect com-
plement to the coriander.*

1 tablespoon olive oil
3 cloves garlic, finely chopped
1 medium onion, finely chopped
1¼ cups dried green split peas, washed and drained
4 cups vegetable stock or water
2 teaspoons yeast extract
1 bunch fresh cilantro, finely chopped
2 teaspoons finely ground black pepper

Heat the oil in a deep saucepan over medium heat. Add the garlic
and onion and sauté until tender, about 5 minutes, stirring frequently.

Add the peas, stock, and yeast extract to the sauté and stir the mixture well. Cover the pan, increase the heat, and bring the soup to a
boil.

When the soup begins to foam, reduce the heat and simmer, covered, for about 45 minutes, or until the peas are very tender. Stir occasionally and add a little extra water if necessary.

When the peas are very tender, add the cilantro and the black pepper to the soup. Stir well and simmer for 5 minutes more. Serve hot
with fresh bread or croutons.

Allow 1 hour.

Servings: 4; Calories per serving, 220; Protein (g) 16; Total fat (g) 4; Saturated fat (g) 0.6; Percent calories from fat, 15%.

POMMES ANNABELLE

This dish has the richness, heady flavors and the aroma of its buttery sister, Anna, but without the animal products or fat content. Don't skimp on the garlic, though!

2 pounds potatoes, peeled and thinly sliced
1 bulb garlic, broken apart and finely chopped
2 teaspoons freshly ground black pepper

SAUCE
1 tablespoon olive oil
1 tablespoon corn flour
1½ cups vegetable stock
2 teaspoons yeast extract

Preheat the oven to 350°F
Layer the potatoes, garlic, and pepper in a casserole dish.
To make the sauce, heat the oil in a saucepan over medium heat and sprinkle the corn flour over it. Stir well to make a roux, or thick paste. Gradually add the vegetable stock, stirring well after each addition, to make a smooth sauce. Add the yeast extract, stir well, and remove the sauce from the heat.
Pour this sauce over the layered potatoes, cover the casserole, and bake 45 minutes. Serve hot with steamed green and yellow vegetables.

Allow 1 hour

Servings: 4; Calories per serving, 125; Protein (g) 5; Total fat (g) 4; Saturated fat (g) 0.5; Percent calories from fat, 25%.

ROASTED VEGETARIAN LOAF

Apart from being easy, this loaf is versatile: you may serve it hot, cold, or reheated to meet any meal occasion. It is light, as loaves go, without any of the nuts or seeds that can sometimes make vegetable roasts hard going.

⅓ cup red lentils, washed and drained
2 packets No-Salt VegeBurger dry mix
⅔ cup rolled oats
1 teaspoon chili powder
1 teaspoon freshly ground black pepper
2 teaspoons dried parsley
¾ cups water

SAUCE
2 tablespoons tomato purée
½ cup plus 2 tablespoons water
2 teaspoons mixed sweet dry herbs, such as Herbes de
    Provence

Lightly oil a loaf pan and preheat the oven to 325°F.

Stir together the lentils, burger mix, oats, and seasonings in a mixing bowl. Add the water, stir well, and leave the mixture to sit for 10 minutes.

Make the sauce by mixing the tomato purée, water, and herbs in a small bowl.

Stir the loaf mixture once again, then press firmly into the loaf pan.

Bake for 10 to 15 minutes. Remove from the oven, and pour the sauce over the loaf. Cover the loaf with aluminum foil and return to the oven. Bake for another 40 minutes.

Leave the loaf on a cooling rack, uncovered, for 5 to 10 minutes, then turn it out onto a serving platter. Slice and serve hot, with vegetables, or cold, in sandwiches. Or, slice the cold loaf, lightly sauté each slice, and serve with baked beans and grilled tomatoes.

Allow 1¼ hours.

Servings: 4; Calories per serving, 200; Protein (g) 15; Total fat (g) 5; Saturated fat (g) 0.1; Percent calories from fat, 23%.

SIMPLE VEGETABLE KEBABS

These kebabs are quick and easy to make, exceptionally pretty, and can be served to accompany any number of other dishes. They are perfect at a party or picnic or as a late-night supper.

2 medium onions, quartered
1 medium red pepper, coarsely chopped
1 medium green pepper, coarsely chopped
4 ounces button mushrooms, cleaned, and large ones halved
2 medium zucchini, quartered and cut into chunks
½ cup pitted olives, drained
1 large orange, peeled, divided into segments, and each
    segment halved

Preheat a broiler. On each of 8 skewers, thread a piece of onion, red pepper, green pepper, a mushroom, zucchini chunk, olive, and orange chunk. Repeat the procedure.

Lay the kebabs across a baking pan for support.

Broil the kebabs for 2 to 3 minutes, turn or rotate them, and broil them for another 2 minutes.

Serve immediately—2 kebabs per person—with rice or salad and a sauce of your choice, such as tomato or peanut sauce.

Allow 25 minutes.

Servings: 4; Calories per serving, 96; Protein (g) 2.5; Total fat (g) 3.5; Saturated fat (g) 0.5; Percent calories from fat, 28%.

VEGETARIAN SHEPHERD'S PIE

Tradition without trauma. A delicious example of how textured vegetable protein (TVP) can be used to make traditional dishes vegetarian. This dish gets finished in one sitting, even when you thought you weren't very hungry.

⅓ cup red lentils, rinsed and drained
½ cup soy mince (TVP) (see pages 272–73)
2 teaspoons freshly ground black pepper
1 tablespoon mixed sweet dry herbs, such as
    Herbes de Provence
1 tablespoon yeast extract
2¼ cups water
1 pound potatoes, peeled and quartered
1 tablespoon olive oil
3 to 5 cloves garlic, finely chopped
2 medium onions, finely chopped
8 ounces carrots, peeled and sliced
8 ounces brussels sprouts, trimmed and halved
¾ cup soy milk
1 tablespoon margarine

Preheat the oven to 350°F. Lightly oil a deep casserole dish.

Stir together the lentils, soy mince, pepper, and herbs in a large mixing bowl.

Dissolve the yeast extract in the water. Pour this over the lentil and soy mixture and stir well. Set aside.

Cook the potatoes in a vegetable steamer until tender.

Heat the oil in a frying pan and sauté the garlic and onion until tender. Add the carrots and brussels sprouts and stir frequently for 5 to 7 minutes more. Now stir this sauté into the lentil mixture in the mixing bowl. Turn the mixture into a deep casserole dish.

Mash the cooked potatoes with the milk and margarine and spread the mash over the mixture in the casserole. Draw a fork across the top of the mash to give it texture.

Cover the dish and bake for 30 minutes. Remove the cover and bake for 10 minutes more to brown the top. Serve hot with steamed vegetables.

Allow 1¼ hours.

Servings: 4; Calories per serving, 288; Protein (g) 16; Total fat (g) 4.8; Saturated fat (g) 1; Percent calories from fat, 15%.

CHILI CON BEANY

This dish is so tasty you'll wonder what all the con carne *fuss was about. It is quick enough for a spur-of-the-moment winter supper, but it also benefits from time, improving in flavor (and spiciness) when it's transported to a picnic or party, for instance.*

1 tablespoon olive oil
5 cloves garlic, finely chopped
1 medium onion, finely chopped
½ cup soy mince (TVP) (see pages 272–73)
2 cups water
½ cup plus 2 tablespoons tomato purée
1 14-ounce can chopped tomatoes
1 tablespoon soy sauce
1 teaspoon chili powder
1 (1-pound) can kidney beans
2 tablespoons cider vinegar

Heat the oil in a deep saucepan and place over high heat. Add the garlic and onion and sauté for 3 to 5 minutes, until tender. Add the soy mince to the sauté and stir for another 2 to 3 minutes.

Mix the water, tomato purée, and chopped tomatoes in a bowl and stir into the sauté. Reduce the heat and add the soy sauce, chili powder, and beans. Stir well, then cover the pan, reduce the heat, and simmer for 20 minutes.

Five minutes before serving, add the vinegar and stir once again. Serve in bowls with a plate of corn chips and a side salad.

Allow 40 minutes.

Servings: 4; Calories per serving, 225; Protein (g) 15; Total fat (g) 4.5; Saturated fat (g) 0.6; Percent calories from fat, 17%.

GREEK-STYLE SPINACH AND CHICKPEA SAUTÉ

I don't think I could ever love anyone who didn't love chickpeas. This is a variation of a classic Greek dish which, in its simplicity, captures the full flavors and nutritional benefits of its ingredients. For a quicker dish, canned chickpeas and frozen spinach may be substituted, though you may then need to adjust the seasoning.

1 cup dried chickpeas
2 pounds fresh spinach, washed and trimmed
1 tablespoon olive oil
5 cloves garlic, finely chopped
2 medium onions, finely chopped
2 teaspoons freshly ground black pepper
1 teaspoon ground cumin
3 teaspoons soy sauce or tandoori paste
½ cup plus 2 tablespoons water

Wash the chickpeas and soak them in cold water all day or overnight. Cook them over medium heat until tender, or pressure-cook according to the manufacturer's instructions.

Coarsely chop the spinach and allow to drain.

Heat the oil in a deep pan and place over medium heat. Add the garlic and onion and sauté until tender, stirring frequently. Add the pepper and cumin and sauté for another 3 minutes. Add the cooked chickpeas to the sauté, and cook, stirring often, for 5 minutes. Mix the soy sauce with the water and add to the sauté.

Now place the spinach on top of the chickpea mixture, cover the pan, and leave over a medium-low heat for 15 minutes. Do not remove the cover.

At the end of this time, stir the spinach into the chickpeas and cover again for another 5 minutes. Serve immediately by itself, or over rice or noodles.

Allow 35 minutes, plus extra time for the chickpeas to soak and cook.

Servings: 4; Calories per serving, 181; Protein (g) 14; Total fat (g) 2.7; Saturated fat (g) 0.3; Percent calories from fat, 12%.

HUNGARIAN GOULASH

Another traditionally "meaty" dish well served by the use of TVP chunks. Don't hurry this dish; it should be very thick, and the soy chunks, very tender.

        1 tablespoon olive oil
        5 to 7 cloves garlic, finely chopped
        1 large onion, finely chopped
        2 cups soy chunks (TVP) (see pages 272–73)
        5 medium potatoes, cubed
        2 large carrots, sliced
        2 tablespoons paprika
        1 teaspoon cayenne
        1 1-pound can chestnut purée
        4 cups water
        1 tablespoon soy sauce or yeast extract
        1 large green pepper, coarsely chopped
        plain vegan yogurt (optional)

Heat the oil in a large saucepan over a medium heat. Add the garlic and sauté for 2 to 3 minutes, until it begins to turn golden. Add the onion and sauté for another 2 to 3 minutes. Add the soy chunks and stir often so they don't absorb too much oil. Add the potatoes, carrots, paprika, cayenne, and chestnut purée. Add the water and yeast extract and stir well. Simmer, covered, over a medium heat for 30 to 40 minutes, stirring frequently.

Add the green pepper and simmer for another 5 minutes. Serve hot with a dollop of yogurt, if desired, over rice or noodles. Or serve the goulash in a bowl on its own, accompanied by slices of fresh bread.

Allow 1 hour

Servings: 4–6; Calories per serving, 380; Protein (g) 16; Total fat (g) 5; Saturated fat (g) 1; Percent calories from fat, 12%.

CREAM OF SPINACH SOUP

Look, no cow's milk! An utterly irresistible soup.

1 pound fresh spinach, washed and trimmed
2 teaspoons yeast extract
¼ cup water
3 cloves garlic, finely chopped
2 medium onions, finely chopped
2 teaspoons ground black pepper
2 cups vegetable stock or water
1 tablespoon olive oil
2 teaspoons caraway seeds
1 tablespoon corn flour
2 cups soy milk
1 teaspoon ground coriander

Cut the spinach into wide strips. Drain in a colander until needed.

Dissolve the yeast extract in the water and bring to a rapid simmer in a deep saucepan over medium heat. Add the garlic and onion and "sauté" until the onions are just tender, about 2 minutes.

Add the black pepper and stock and bring to a slow boil. Now add the drained spinach, reduce the heat, cover the pan, and simmer gently, stirring occasionally, for about 10 minutes.

Meanwhile, in a small saucepan, heat the oil and lightly sauté the caraway seeds over a low heat. Sprinkle the corn flour over the sauté and stir thoroughly to make a roux, or smooth paste. Keep the pan over the heat as you add the soy milk, a little at a time, stirring after each addition. Add the coriander and stir until smooth. Add the white sauce to the soup and stir until well blended. Cook the soup for another 5 to 10 minutes, stirring often. Serve hot.

Allow 45 minutes.

Servings: 4; Calories per serving, 135; Protein (g) 13; Total fat (g) 6.5; Saturated fat (g) 0.1; Percent calories from fat, 39%.

GREEN BEANS AND CARROTS IN SPICY TOMATO SAUCE

This is a very colorful and spicy dish that looks and tastes like it takes hours to prepare. Just perfect to serve unexpected guests.

1 tablespoon plus 1 teaspoon olive oil
1 whole bulb garlic, separated and finely chopped
1 large onion, finely chopped
1 pound carrots, thinly sliced
1 (14-ounce) can peeled tomatoes
1 teaspoon dried oregano
1 teaspoon dried basil
1 to 3 teaspoons freshly ground black pepper
2 (14-ounce) cans green beans

Divide the oil evenly between 2 saucepans and place both over medium heat. Add half the chopped garlic to each saucepan and sauté for 2 to 3 minutes, until the garlic begins to turn slightly golden. Add half the onions to each saucepan and continue the sauté for another 2 to 3 minutes, stirring both sautés frequently.

Add the carrots to one saucepan, stir well, cover, and reduce the heat. Cook the carrot sauté until the carrots are just tender, about 15 minutes. In the meantime, add the tomatoes, herbs, and pepper to the other sauté, stir well, cover, and reduce the heat. Simmer for 15 minutes, then remove from the heat.

Add the tomato sauce and the beans to the carrot sauté. Stir, cover, and simmer gently for a final 5 minutes, stirring occasionally.

Serve hot over rice, pasta, toast, or baked potato.

Allow 40 minutes.

Servings: 4; Calories per serving, 164; Protein (g) 5; Total fat (g) 5; Saturated fat (g) 1; Percent calories from fat, 26%.

SCRAMBLED TOFU

This quick dish is wonderfully pretty and makes the best Sunday morning breakfast you could dream of. It can be served as a main course with a selection of vegetables, or over toast as a snack and is a healthy alternative to omelettes and scrambled eggs.

    1 tablespoon olive oil
    1 small onion, finely chopped
    1 teaspoon ground turmeric
    1 medium carrot, thinly sliced
    1 medium zucchini, sliced
    2 ounces mushrooms, quartered
    1 (10½-ounce) package tofu, drained
    1 teaspoon freshly ground black pepper
    1 tablespoon finely chopped fresh parsley
    4 slices whole wheat bread, toasted

Heat the oil in a frying pan over medium heat and sauté the onion until tender. Add the turmeric and stir well to blend. Now add the carrot, zucchini, and mushrooms and sauté for another 10 minutes.

Crumble the tofu into the sauté and add the black pepper. Cook over a medium heat, stirring, for about 5 minutes. Add the chopped parsley, and cook for 1 minute. Place 1 slice of toast on each warmed plate and spoon the scrambled tofu over it. Delicious with a dash of soy sauce and accompanied by grilled tomatoes. Try this dish over rice or baked potatoes instead of toast, too.

Allow 20 minutes.

Servings: 2; Calories per serving, 320; Protein (g) 18; Total fat (g) 13; Saturated fat (g) 2; Percent calories from fat, 36%.

TEMPEH MARINADE

Tempeh (pronounced "tem-pay") is a fermented soybean cake. Like cheese, yogurt, and ginger beer, it is made with a cultured starter. It is highly digestible, smells like fresh mushrooms, and tastes remarkably similar to chicken. You can pan-fry it and top it with a sauce, dice and deep-fry it like french fries, add it to a stir-fry, or roast it. It's a significant source of vitamin B_{12}. You'll find it in the freezer at most health food stores. This unusual dish builds on the subtle, slightly nutty flavor of tempeh to create a rich, fragrant tempeh morsel. Use it as a protein-rich cornerstone to your meal.

    8 ounces (1 block) tempeh, defrosted
    ¾ cup cider vinegar
    ¼ cup olive oil
    ¼ cup soy sauce
    1 teaspoon mustard seed, slightly crushed
    12 whole cloves
    12 whole peppercorns, partly crushed
    6 cloves garlic, finely chopped
    2 small onions, finely chopped
    1¼ cups rice, rinsed and drained
    1 pound broccoli, trimmed and cut into florets

> 1 pound carrots, sliced
> 2 medium onions, quartered

Cut the tempeh into 1-inch cubes and place in a casserole dish.

Mix the vinegar, oil, soy sauce, mustard seed, cloves, peppercorns, and garlic in a small bowl or pitcher. Stir well and pour over the tempeh pieces. Cover the casserole and marinate the tempeh for 4 to 18 hours.

Bake, covered, at 325°F for 30 minutes. Remove the cover and bake for another 10 minutes. If a drier, crispier top is desired, remove the cover earlier in the baking time.

Meanwhile, cover the rice in twice its volume of water. Bring to a boil, cover, and cook over medium heat. Steam the broccoli and carrots until tender.

Place the pieces of onion in a shallow baking dish and broil them under a preheated broiler for 5 to 7 minutes, turning once or twice. Spoon the rice onto warmed plates. Top with the tempeh and its marinade, the roasted onions, and steamed vegetables. Add a dash of soy sauce if desired.

Allow 1 hour, plus time to marinate.

Servings: 4; Calories per serving, 519; Protein (g) 20; Total fat (g) 17; Saturated fat (g) 2; Percent calories from fat, 29%.

TOFU MARINADE

Tofu is very high in protein, low in saturated fats, and entirely cholesterol-free. It's used in east Asia in the same ways you would use eggs or meat. Tofu plays a tasty supporting role to almost anything in pies, dips, fritters, and sauces, complementing the main ingredients. Or you can use tofu as your star—in a tofu burger, tofu salad, tofu fried rice, chili con tofu. It is also extremely good barbecued. This simple dish is a gourmet delight that turns plain tofu into an exquisite appetizer or side dish.

1 (10½-ounce) package tofu, drained and cubed

1 cup cider vinegar

1 tablespoon soy sauce

1 teaspoon whole allspice, roughly crushed

1 teaspoon peppercorns, roughly crushed

6 whole cloves

1 cardamom seed

1 clove garlic, thinly sliced (optional)

1 thin slice fresh ginger (optional)

CRUDITÉS

1 medium carrot, cut into sticks

2 stalks celery, cut into sticks

½ cucumber, sliced

1 apple, cored and sliced

8 lettuce leaves, washed and drained

Arrange the tofu cubes in a deep bowl or dish; a single layer is preferable. Mix the remaining ingredients together in a pitcher and pour over the tofu. The cubes should be covered by the marinade. Cover the dish and marinate the tofu 6 to 24 hours in the fridge. Agitate the dish occasionally during this time, if possible.

Carefully remove the tofu cubes from the marinade and arrange on a large plate with the crudités.

You may reuse the marinade immediately, if you wish. (Do not use more than twice.)

Allow 20 minutes, plus marination time.

Servings: 4; Calories per serving, 123; Protein (g) 9; Total fat (g) 4; Saturated fat (g) 1; Percent calories from fat, 23%.

VEGETABLE MARINADE

Make this on Sunday evening and snack on it until Thursday lunch!
This dish improves by keeping it in the fridge and, provided you stir it
each day and serve it with a clean spoon, it will keep for 3 to 4 days,
if you can let it alone for that long. Very pretty, and easy to transport
to school or work.

MARINADE
1½ cups cups cider vinegar
¼ cup vegetable oil
2 teaspoons coarsely ground black pepper
1 teaspoon coarsely ground mustard seed
1 teaspoon coarsely ground caraway or fennel seed
Zest and juice of 1 lemon

1 medium cauliflower, cut into florets
1 pound broccoli, coarsely chopped
1 (1-pound) can kidney beans, drained
1 bunch scallions thinly sliced
5 cloves garlic, finely chopped

Put the marinade ingredients into a large, nonreactive saucepan and
place over a medium heat. Bring to a gentle simmer.

Add the remaining ingredients, stir well, and cover the pan. Cook
over medium heat for 15 minutes, stirring twice in that time.

Remove the pan from the heat and allow to cool without removing
the cover. Place in the fridge once the marinade has cooled to room
temperature. Serve as a starter, light lunch, or accompaniment to
other dishes.

Allow 45 minutes, plus time to cool and chill.

Servings: 4; Calories per serving, 300; Protein (g) 13; Total fat (g) 14; Saturated fat (g) 2; Percent calories from fat, 38%.

CHOCOLATE AND ALMOND CAKE

Now for a couple of desserts—if you've got room, that is. This one is a hit wherever it goes. It is light and slightly crumbly, and very pretty.

3 cups whole wheat flour
⅔ cup oatmeal flakes
½ cup dark brown sugar
2 teaspoons baking powder
¾ cup slivered almonds
⅔ cup carob or semisweet chocolate chips
¼ cup olive oil
1⅞ cups water
1 teaspoon almond extract

Preheat the oven to 350°F. Lightly oil a 6-inch round cake pan.

Mix together the whole wheat flour, oatmeal flakes, brown sugar, and baking powder in a large bowl, stirring until well blended. Add the almonds and chocolate chips and stir well.

Stir together the oil, water, and almond extract in a pitcher and pour into the center of the dry mixture. Stir to blend well. Pour the batter immediately into the cake pan.

Bake for 35 to 40 minutes. Cool on a wire rack.

Allow 50 minutes.

Servings: 8; Calories per serving, 300; Protein (g) 6.5; Total fat (g) 15; Saturated fat (g) 1.7; Percent calories from fat, 39%.

FAMILY FRUIT AND NUT CAKE

This is a tasty, substantial cake with lots of texture. It is simple to make, perfect for the kids to throw together. Serve it with soy pudding, soy ice cream, or on its own.

1 cup raisins or currants
¼ cup brown sugar
2 tablespoons olive oil
1¼ cups apple juice
2 cups whole wheat flour
⅔ cup rolled oats
2 teaspoons baking powder
1 teaspoon ground ginger
⅓ cup citrus peel
½ cup slivered almonds

Preheat the oven to 375°F. Lightly oil a 9-inch cake pan.

Stir together the currants, brown sugar, olive oil, and apple juice in a small mixing bowl and blend well. Set aside to soak.

Mix together the remaining ingredients in a large mixing bowl and stir well. Stir the raisin mixture into the dry mixture to make a thick batter. Turn the batter into the cake pan, and bake for 40 minutes.

Let the cake cool in the pan for 10 minutes, turn it onto a wire rack, and cool completely before serving.

Allow 1 hour.

Servings: 8; Calories per serving, 215; Protein (g) 5; Total fat (g) 8; Saturated fat (g) 1; Percent calories from fat, 30%.

6

YOUR QUESTIONS ANSWERED

Whenever I give a workshop or do a radio phone-in, I can guarantee that some of the following questions will crop up. So here they are, The Questions That Will Not Die, together with the answers. I hope this selection will help you, your family, and your friends to experience an easy transition to the new way of living!

"Does it take longer to prepare vegetarian meals?"

Only if you want it to! The example most often given to illustrate the convenience of a meat-based diet goes something like this: "I can come home from a long, tiring day and take a chop from the fridge and slap it under the broiler. It's ready to eat by the time the potatoes and peas have cooked—*and* I've slipped into something more comfortable."

Well, for those who wish to keep this particular schedule, you can prepare exactly the same meal using a vegetable burger, or grill instead of broil, and nothing else will change. However, you'd be missing a lot of the fun and flavor of eating without meat. In the same period of time, about thirty minutes, you can make

- Pasta topped with tomato, vegetable, or meat-free Bolognese sauce, accompanied by a green salad
- Stir-fried vegetables over basmati rice topped with a peanut sauce

- A robust chef's salad followed by onion soup
- Tempeh or vegetable burgers in sesame buns with the full compliment of garnishes, a side salad, and a baked potato
- Scrambled tofu on toast with grilled tomatoes and mushrooms, followed by fresh fruit salad topped with yogurt.

The list could go on and on. And if you are willing to spend just fifteen minutes longer over your meal, you can anticipate luscious homemade pizzas, a variety of vegetable quiches, curries, casseroles, and even tantalizing Mexican meals, such as tacos or tostadas with bean paste filling and spicy tomato sauce. Of course, most of these can be prepared even more quickly using those handy appliances of the modern kitchen, the pressure cooker, microwave, and food processor. And vegetarian cooking is quicker, still, if some of the meals make partial use of canned or frozen foods; the choice is yours. Certainly fresh is better if you can manage it, but speed and convenience are often paramount, and thank goodness for handy foods at those times.

Just a few words about beans: Many people suffer from fear of beans on three accounts. First, that a vegetarian diet relies almost entirely on them. Second, that they have drastic and dire effects on the digestive system. And third, that they take hours and hours to cook. On all three counts, the correct response is "not true," if you follow a few basic tips.

First, beans are a marvelous source of protein, fiber, iron, the B vitamins and, when sprouted, vitamin C. With such a healthy nutritional profile, who wouldn't be tempted to include them in every meal? It is important to remember, however, that beans can either look like beans, or they can be transformed into one of the many delicious and nutritious bean products that supply the food value but not the same "beany" experience. Among these are soy milk, tofu, TVP (textured vegetable protein), tempeh, soy yogurt and ice cream, marinated tofu, and soy cheeses of every description.

Second, it is true, beans can be a "musical" food if you don't follow the golden rules of cooking them:

- Let them soak overnight. Do it last thing before turning in, and you'll be able to use them anytime in the next day or so.

Isn't this a terrible hassle? Not really; it's the very small price we pay for what is practically the ultimate in convenience foods. What other foodstuff would be perfectly happy to wait around in your kitchen for months on end, and still be in great nutritional shape when you eventually decide to use it? Certainly not meat!

- Don't cook them in the soaking water, and never cook them without rinsing them.
- Make sure to cook the beans thoroughly (self-service salad bars often fail to do so). Here's the secret: Use the tongue test. Put one bean in your mouth, and try to squash it against the roof of your mouth, using normal pressure from your tongue. If you can't squash it, it isn't well cooked. Anything less may create gas and digestive discomfort.

Third, cooking beans in an open pot can indeed take hours, which is why I'd suggest you should use a pressure cooker. You can cook most beans in a pressure cooker in less than thirty minutes. Buy one made of stainless steel.

"My six-year-old won't eat meat; what should I do?"

Celebrate, quickly learn a few new meatless recipes (see next page for some cookbook suggestions) and then join her. Most children are naturally vegetarian, especially so if they have realized that the meat on their plates is actually dead animal. Because they empathize so strongly with animals (and we encourage them to do so with our gifts of teddy bears and tales of cute animals with human characteristics), they cannot easily bear the transition from "friend" to "food." By supporting your child in her choice, you are enabling her to live with one less hypocrisy in her life. You are also giving her a chance to avoid the horrific catalogue of diseases that accompanies a meat-based diet. Children come to us to be with us and learn from us, but also to change us. Accept your child's decision gladly for the changes and improvements it will inevitably make to your diet, your health, and your whole life.

"What are the best vegetarian cookbooks?"

Try *The Farm Vegetarian Cookbook*, edited by Louise Hagler and Dorothy R. Bates from the Book Publishing Co. (If it is not in your local bookstore, it is readily available from popular on-line "stores"— new or used!) This excellent cookbook is full of vegan recipes that use the soybean and its various products in wholesome and imaginative ways. It describes in simple terms how to make soy milk, tofu, soy yogurt, ice cream, and tempeh, and gives you recipes that are so tasty and aromatic you'll have the whole block knocking on your door.

"My doctor's told me I must eat meat. What should I do?"

Get a new doctor.

"Isn't vegetarian food more expensive?"

No, it's inevitably cheaper. In order to understand why this should be so, you have to grasp the underlying economics of the meat industry. A meat animal is treated as nothing more or less than a machine—a machine that the industry uses to convert vegetable protein into animal protein. As a machine, it is deplorably inefficient. For every pound of meat protein that is produced as a steak, twenty pounds of vegetable protein have to be put into it (twenty pounds that *could* have gone to feed human mouths). It is a disgraceful, obscene waste of food. Figure 6.1 shows you just what an inefficient "machine" food animals are.[1]

As you can see, beef animals are extraordinarily wasteful converters of vegetable protein, only managing to convert a miserly 6 percent of it into meat protein. This is the reason behind the desperate use of chemicals (and genetic engineering techniques) in animal rearing—it's an attempt by the farmer to improve on a process that is notoriously inefficient.

So when someone buys a steak, he's actually paying not just for the meat, but also for a vast amount of wasted vegetable food that the cow has consumed and excreted. This means that consumers are actually paying to create all the pollution problems associated with that

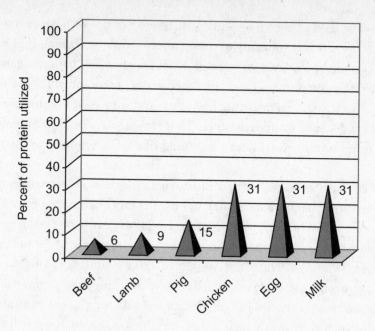

Figure 6.1. How much vegetable protein animals convert to meat protein.

excreta, too. For example, here's just one problem that most people don't know about: the global cattle population emits 100 million tons of methane gas each year.[2] Concentrations of methane in the air have been rising at the rate of 1 percent per year since 1950—four times the rate of increase of carbon dioxide. Scientists fear that soon, methane may be the prime greenhouse gas, responsible for global warming.

But let's return to the faulty economics of meat production, because this is where the story gets very intriguing. Although the meat industry constantly stresses the "naturalness" of meat, they go to great pains to conceal the fact that they themselves are violating one of the most fundamental laws of nature; the law that explains why large, fierce animals are rare, and why smaller, vegetable-feeding ones are much more numerous.

In the wild, food chains exist whereby one level of the chain consumes something on a lower level of the chain. Close to the bottom of the chain, there are lots and lots of animals feeding on a profusion of plant foods (for example, rabbits feeding on grass). At the top of the chain, there are just a few carnivorous animals who feed on the lower levels (foxes feeding on rabbits). Thus, the foxes are indirectly eating the lowest level of the chain—grass. If things get out of balance, and the fox population suddenly expands, there won't be enough rabbits to go round. So the foxes starve until things get back into balance again.

Therefore, if humans were designed to be predominantly carnivores, there would be relatively few of us, and we would live at a considerable distance from each other. That way, there would be enough flesh to go round. Now, does that sound like the way most of us live today?

Of course it doesn't. But that's just where the meat industry tries to buck nature. The more meat they sell us, the more cattle they have to breed, feed, and bleed. There are now 1.3 billion cattle on the face of our planet, consuming its food resources at a truly incredible rate. As biologist Dr. David Hamilton Wright of Emory University observes, "An alien ecologist observing Earth might conclude that cattle is the dominant animal species in our biosphere."[3] As long as we continue to eat at such a perilously high position in the food chain, there will be more and more cattle, creating bigger and bigger problems for our ravaged planet.

Says the president of the Greenhouse Crisis Foundation, Jeremy Rifkin:

In all of the ongoing public debates around the global environmental crisis a curious silence surrounds the issue of cattle, one of the most destructive environmental threats of the modern era. Cattle grazing is a primary cause of the spreading desertification process that is now enveloping whole continents. Cattle ranching is responsible for the destruction of much of the earth's remaining tropical rain forests. Cattle raising is indirectly responsible for the rapid depletion of fresh water on the planet, with some reservoirs and aquifers now at their lowest levels since the end of the last Ice Age. Cattle are a chief source of organic pollution; cow dung is poisoning the freshwater lakes, rivers, and the streams of the world. Growing herds of cattle are exerting unprecedented pressure on the carrying capacity of natural ecosystems, edging entire species of wildlife to the brink of extinction. Cattle are a growing source of global warming, and their increasing numbers now threaten the very chemical dynamics of the biosphere. Most

Americans and Europeans are simply unaware of the devastation wrought by the world's cattle. Now numbering over a billion, these ancient ungulates roam the countryside, trampling the soil, stripping the vegetation bare, laying waste to large tracts of the earth's biomass.[4]

Unfortunately, most of us don't realize that the meat industry is playing this grotesque game with nature. But it is, and consumers are paying for it. I hope you can now see that the original question raises some extremely profound, yet little-known, issues.

And now, to answer that question directly: The cheapest way to eat vegetarian food is to buy fruits and vegetables in season and use them, with a few grains and legumes, to design your menu. This approach can allow you to provide truly hearty meals for two to four persons every day of the week for something like $1.50 per meal. Of course, they're nothing fancy, nor are they five courses, but such meals are wholesome, tasty, nutritious, and, of course, cheap.

Next cheapest is to buy the same fruit and veggies but to add a few special things from the supermarket (tofu, soy milk, pastas, nuts, vegetable burgers) and ethnic grocers (Asian, Chinese, Jamaican) to liven up your cooking repertoire. A revolution has been taking place over the past few years that has meant foods such as herbs, spices, soy- and meat-replacement products are stocked in most of the major supermarket chains, and at reasonable prices.

"If everyone was vegetarian, what would happen to all the farm animals?"

That's a silly question.

"No, I'm serious! What would happen to them?"

I pull my hair out when people ask me this in all seriousness. It reveals such an astounding depth of ignorance about the wretched lives of today's food animals. And implicit in it lies the logic of the lunatic asylum. It suggests:

1. We have a duty to eat animals, because if we didn't eat them they wouldn't be born.
2. If they weren't born, they wouldn't get a chance to experience life, even though that existence is wretched and painful.
3. It is a greater evil to deny the possibility of existence to a potential animal than it is to inflict real suffering on a real, live animal.

The simple answer is this: if everyone was vegetarian, fewer and fewer food animals would be born. Eventually, we would have just a few cows, a few pigs, and so on—all valued as beautiful creatures in their own right, rather than as lumps of flesh to be consumed.

"Which kitchen utensils should I buy?"

These are the ones I find most useful:

- Pressure cooker. A must for beans and pulses.
- Cast-iron pans. Enamel are fine, too, but not aluminum or copper.
- Wok. Good for really fast stir-frying of vegetables using minimal oil. With care it can even be used without any oil if you watch over it and sprinkle water on when necessary.
- Garlic press. It releases the flavor better than chopping.
- A food processor. It allows you to make delicious raw salads, including such tasty vegetables as beets, turnip, rutabaga, and carrot, in a flash.
- Steamer. Never boil the nutrients in vegetables away again!
- Mortar and pestle. For grinding spices.

"I've heard that plants scream when you dig them up, isn't that just as cruel as eating meat?"

No. Unlike animals, plants don't have a central nervous system, and they can't feel pain. This crackpot idea is trotted out by meat eaters with guilty consciences. They figure that if they can only convince themselves that chickpeas suffer as much as chickens, there's really no difference between meat eating and vegetarianism, so they might just as well carry on eating flesh. Nevertheless, it's a little piece of lunacy that regularly comes up, so I tried to find out where it originated. As far as I can discover, it first arose when that expert self-publicist, L. Ron Hubbard (that's right, the founder of Scientology), came to England.

"It was not long before television and Fleet Street reporters were beating a path to Saint Hill manor [his chosen home near East Grinstead, Sussex] demanding to interview Hubbard about his novel theories," wrote Russell Miller in his biography of Hubbard. "Always pleased to help the gentlemen of the press, he was memorably photographed looking compassionately at a tomato jabbed by probes attached to an E-meter—a picture that eventually found its way into *Newsweek* magazine, causing a good deal of harmless merriment at his expense. Alan Whicker, a well-known British television interviewer, did his best to make Hubbard look like a crank, but Hubbard contrived to come across as a rather likeable and confident personality. When Whicker moved in for the kill, sarcastically inquiring if rose pruning should be stopped lest it cause pain and anxiety, Hubbard neatly side-stepped the question and drew a parallel with an essential life-preserving medical operation on a human being. He might have wacky ideas, Whicker discovered, but he was certainly no fool."[5]

So it seems as if that particularly deranged notion is all part of L. Ron's rich legacy to humankind.

"How can I lose weight on a vegetarian diet?"

In my experience, people who change to the vegetarian way of living automatically start to "normalize" their body weight. And it's true that you see very few overweight vegetarians. So don't bother about trying to lose weight if you've recently gone meat-free, you may find that your body will naturally stabilize at an optimum weight, and it's certainly more difficult to overeat without all those calories from saturated fat in meat.

Meanwhile, give a little thought to the whole question of *why* we overeat. Did you know that humans are the only species on the face of the planet to have a chronic weight problem? No other animal has so much excess body fat as we do, and no other animal so regularly commits suicide by overeating. One very successful evolutionary strategy our bodies have developed is the ability to store food energy in the form of fat all over our bodies. Humans actually have more fat cells (known as adipocytes) in proportion to their body mass than almost *any other creature*—only hedgehogs and whales have a greater proportion of fat in their bodies! Even animals that we traditionally think of as fatties, such as pigs, seals, bears, and camels, all have less fat than we do!

This evolutionary adaptation is an outstanding success story, which has allowed us to cope with the uncertainty of a highly variable food supply. Today, of course, some of us have access to far more food than we know what to do with. However, our old survival instincts tell us to go on eating, just in case.

People who sell us foodstuffs know very well how to exploit these deep-rooted, unconscious instincts of ours. Take, for instance, the routine use of the word "NEW" on food products of all types. Have you ever wondered why this word is repeated so incessantly? The answer again lies in an old and once-useful behavior pattern that we and other successful omnivores have evolved. Omnivores are animals that have adapted to eat a highly varied diet. Their successful survival strategy is to continually search out *new* types of food, so that if one staple in the diet fails for any reason, there is always another food source ready to replace it. A great idea! But in nature, the urge to experiment with new food is counterbalanced by the desire to be cautious. You can see both of these clever survival mechanisms demonstrated in the behavior patterns of that other hugely successful omnivore feeder—the common rat.

Rats, just like humans, are always ready to experiment with anything new. When a rat finds something unusual to eat (and like us, they are on the lookout all the time), he will carefully nibble a small amount, then leave it strictly alone for a day or so. If the animal suffers no ill effects in the meantime, he will return to the new food and start to include it in his diet. However, if the rat feels sick or ill after eating that small sample, he will *never* return to that food again. This is a highly successful feeding strategy, which is still present deep inside all of us. Here's the proof: Think back to a time when you felt sick shortly after eating a particularly distinctive type of food. It doesn't really matter whether your sick feeling was actually *caused* by the food you remember eating; what matters is that you now *associate* that food with the unpleasant feelings afterwards, and in all probability, you will never eat that particular food again. It's in ways like this that our old survival mechanisms try to keep us away from food that may be dangerous for us. However, it's the other side of this mechanism—the strong desire that we all have to try out anything marked "NEW"—that gets us into so much trouble these days, simply because there's *so much* temptation all around us. It is this desire to constantly look for—and experiment with—new foodstuffs that makes us so vulnerable to all those advertising come-ons.

When you go vegetarian, you're reclaiming control over what you eat—it's an act of personal liberation. For probably the first time in your life, you are consciously deciding what feeding strategy you will adopt. Now this, all by itself, gives you power, and takes away power from those food industries that seek to limit your food choices, and exploit your instinctive feeding strategies for their own purposes. Again, this makes it far less likely that you will continue to be overweight.

Here are two ridiculously simple but highly effective ways of losing weight: First, try a mainly raw food diet. It's almost impossible to overeat on raw food. Second, don't eat after sundown (you should drink, of course, but not alcohol). This, also, allows your body to normalize itself. Obviously, if you have diabetes or another metabolic disease, or are pregnant, don't diet without first discussing it with your doctor.

"Is it OK to wear leather?"

Only if you think it's OK to eat meat. Bear in mind that 25 to 50 percent of slaughterhouse profits come from the leather industry.[6] Leather alternatives are increasingly available in the shops, and the more you ask for them, the more there will be.

"Hitler was a vegetarian, wasn't he?"

I used to think that this was a silly question, but so many people kept asking it that I'm now prepared to give it a serious answer. This is inevitably a loaded question: the clear implication is that Hitler and vegetarians share some kind of weird moral ground. Here's how a certain Robert Milch put it, in a testy letter to the *New York Times*: "Adolf Hitler was a vegetarian all his life and wrote extensively on the subject. If vegetarians choose not to eat meat, they ought to acknowledge that it is a personal quirk and not preach at the rest of us so self-righteously."[7]

Sometimes, the specter of Hitler is evoked in other ways. Most vegetarians are also opposed to vivisection, and vivisectors have on occasion found it useful to exhume the old Nazi to use as a weapon against those who oppose their cruel trade. In a recent British television program, one of those trendy, jeans-wearing scientists whom the media find so irresistible put forward an argument that vegetarians everywhere will find deeply offensive.[8] According to the vivisector, vegetarian Hitler banned animal experiments because he preferred to use Jews, Gypsies, and other "defectives" instead. This, apparently, is supposed to prove that vegetarians and others opposed to vivisection are racist Nazis. In the anti-Nazi magazine *Searchlight*, writer Colin Meider took him severely to task for such abhorrent and incoherent reasoning:

"It is not only profoundly unscientific, it is especially rich coming from a man whose own profession devised and carried out the program of human mutilation and slaughter. It was scientists and doctors who executed the Nazi program of racial hygiene whereby all 'inferior' humans were at first sterilized and then exterminated. . . . In 1932 the German Medical Association was already discussing eugenics in the service of the state. No other profession supported it on such a scale."[9]

But was Hitler a vegetarian? And in any case, does it matter? It certainly matters to our critics, who seem to believe that the entire vegetarian ethos can be demolished on the basis of it. "The bigger the lie, the easier it is to deceive people," said Hitler's head of propaganda, Josef Goebbels. He might well have been talking about the modern-day myth of Hitler's vegetarianism. Historian and author of *Judaism and Vegetarianism*, Richard H. Schwartz, makes this reply:

"Because Hitler suffered from excessive flatulence he occasionally went on a vegetarian diet. But his primary diet included meat. In 'The Life and Death of Adolf Hitler,' Robert Payne mentions Hitler's fondness for Bavarian sausages. Other biographers, including Albert Speer, point out that he also ate ham, liver, and game. Hitler banned vegetarian organizations in Germany and the occupied countries, though vegetarian diets would have helped solve Germany's World War II food shortage."[10]

This hardly sounds like a card-carrying member of the Vegetarian Society. Adds Jewish historian Ralph Meyer, writing in *The Jewish Vegetarian*:

"How can someone be a strict vegetarian and take injections of pulverized bull testicles, as Hitler did? How can someone be a strict vegetarian who ordered his enemies 'hung up like carcasses of meat,' who urged the Hitler youth to become 'like beasts of prey,' who said 'it is not by the principles of humanity that man lives but brute force . . . close your eyes to pity . . . act brutally.' Surely a person who worshipped brutality and literally shrieked for blood is the antithesis of a vegetarian."[11]

Ultimately, I don't believe we have to brawl over the amount of sausage that Hitler ate, nor his prodigious appetite for stuffed squab (baby pigeon), which was, according to chef Dione Lucas, "a great favorite with Mr. Hitler." And she should know—she cooked it for him.[12]

"What are hot dogs made from?"

Many people are rather nauseated when they find out what goes into burgers, but hot dogs have, so far, escaped much scrutiny. That is about to change! A good friend of mine had the opportunity to tour a factory where these especially loathsome comestibles were made, and in the process somehow seemed to acquire a copy of the recipe (I put it down to chaos theory). It passed to me in due course, and I reprint it here, with no further comment, since nothing I could say would be more revolting than the recipe itself:

Fish
Chicken feet
Chicken carcasses
Chicken heads
Lungs plus trachea
Udder
Liver
Fresh blood
Wheat flour
Salt
PP530
Water
Phosphate
Carageenan

"Should I buy vegetarian cheeses?"

Many cheeses contain rennet, an enzyme taken from the stomachs of slaughtered baby calves, a small amount of which helps to coagulate milk into cheese. Not all cheese includes animal rennet, but if you want to be sure, buy a specially marked cheese from a health food store, or a growing number of supermarkets. Vegetable rennet is sometimes called "rennin," to distinguish it from the animal-derived type. In my view, the rennet controversy tends to be exaggerated by some vegetarians. If you're buying dairy products, you are economically contributing to the meat industry, in any case. There's a growing range of completely animal-free cheeses on the market (try your local health food store), which I would urge you to investigate. Personally, I ate a vegetarian diet for many years before I went vegan, and I found that dairy products simply became less and less important in my diet, until one day I realized that I'd made the transition.

"How can I get enough vitamin D?"

Although vegetarians who consume dairy products get some in milk, most people—vegetarian, vegan or meat eating—get most vitamin D from the action of sunlight on their skin. In fact, food sources of vitamin D are relatively unimportant. Comments the expert on vegan nutrition Dr. Gill Langley, "Bright sunshine is not necessary: even the 'skyshine' on a cloudy day will stimulate the formation of some vitamin D_2 in the skin, while a short summer holiday in the open air will increase serum levels of vitamin D two- or three-fold."[13] In recent years, there have been moves to reclassify this substance as a steroid hormone rather than as a vitamin.[14] In addition there have been scientific suggestions that, when taken by nondeficient people, low level ingestion of calciferol (the name for this group of substances) may accelerate the aging of arteries, kidneys, and bones.[15]

"Should I eat fish or take fish oil?"

In recent years, it has become accepted wisdom among a wide variety of people—doctors, health-food shoppers, and even among some vegetarians—that fish, and particularly fish oil, is healthy. There's certainly no disputing that fish oil can make you very healthy, indeed, if, that is, you happen to manufacture fish oil capsules! For several years, they've been the fastest-moving items in health food stores. According to these manufacturers, fish oil can treat asthma, prevent cancer, lower your cholesterol level, and banish arthritis. But what is the evidence?

Fish oil is indeed a significant source of the omega-3 essential fatty acids. There are two important groups of essential fatty acids: omega-6 acids, found in abundance in corn, soy, safflower, and other vegetable oils; and omega-3 acids, found in fatty fish. Each group has distinct—and often antagonistic—physiological effects.

But, contrary to popular opinion, fish is not the *only* source of omega-3 acids. Flaxseed (linseed) oil actually contains about twice as much omega-3 essential fatty acids as is found in fish oil. According to nutritionist Ann Louise Gittleman, M.S., coauthor of *Beyond Pritikin*, flaxseed oil's greatest attribute is its ranking as the vegetable source highest in omega-3 fatty acids. "Fish is the best-known source of the omega-3's," she says, "but flaxseed oil contains 55 to 60 percent omega-3—about twice as much as is found in fish oil."[16] Flaxseed is also rich in omega-6 fatty acids. It is a highly polyunsaturated oil, capable of providing the raw material necessary for the production of prostaglandins in the human body. Prostaglandins are vital, hormone-like compounds that regulate every function in the body at the molecular level. Without enough prostaglandins, our bodies cannot properly use the food we eat. Note that foods containing omega-3 oils go bad easily because the unsaturated fatty acids attract oxygen and become oxidized or turn rancid.

Fish oil has been touted as the ultimate cure for heart disease. Some studies have indeed shown that large doses of fish oil can lower triglycerides (blood fats). But when continued over a longer period of time—six months or so—the initial triglyceride-lowering effect of fish off in patients with high levels almost disappears.[17]

Another study casts doubt on the benefits of fish oil for heart patients who have had angioplasty, a medical treatment for narrowed arteries. Because fish oil makes your blood thinner, it was thought that it could help keep clogged arteries open, and three small studies first hinted that it could. However, a larger study from Harvard Medical School and Beth Israel Hospital shows that people taking fish oil actually had a higher rate of recurrent narrowing of the arteries and more heart attacks than people taking olive oil![18]

It has now passed into folklore that Eskimos have much less heart disease than other Westerners, and that this reduction in heart disease is due to the fish oil they consume. Actually, if you study almost any native population, you'll find they have much less heart disease than we do. In March 1990, the American Journal of Public Health published a review of scientific work on this subject. The author of the review wrote:

"Several studies have reported that Arctic populations, which typically consume large amounts of fatty fish, have a low rate of atherosclerosis and cardiovascular disease. But a thorough examination of the methods used in these projects reveals that the evidence may not have been reliable. Two studies that reported causes of death used data from a modest number of autopsies that were performed without standard procedures by inadequately trained personnel."[19]

In fact, there have been persistent questions asked in scientific journals about the accuracy of the "Eskimo" evidence. One medical critic has already pointed out the original study was seriously flawed, because far fewer deaths from cardiovascular disease were recorded than actually took place.[20]

The same research that was supposed to demonstrate that fish oil could reduce deaths from heart disease also revealed that Eskimos were dying in greater numbers from cerebrovascular hemorrhages—hemorrhagic strokes. Since fish oil is known to thin the blood, this is a perfectly possible consequence. But this finding has received very little publicity.

A recent study conducted to assess the benefits of fish oil on young people with raised levels of fats in their blood ended up providing just how dramatic this blood-thinning effect can be. Of eleven patients, eight of them had nosebleeds while taking the oil. "It is concluded," wrote the scientists, "that the dose of fish oil necessary to reduce blood lipid levels may be associated with an extremely high risk of bleeding problems in adolescents."[21]

Can fish oil help in arthritis? Again, the evidence is far less conclusive than the publicity indicates. A 1985 study found that people who took one specific omega 3 (known as EPA) reported less morning stiffness when compared to another group of people who didn't take the oil.[22] But there were no improvements in other areas, such as grip strength, exercise ability, fatigue, or swelling. Note that the people on fish oil didn't actually get any better, it was just that the people *not* taking fish oil got worse.

As far as cholesterol is concerned, the results are very mixed, indeed. Some studies have shown that large doses of fish oil can lower cholesterol levels dramatically. But other studies have shown just the opposite—that it can, in fact, raise them, and in particular raise the level of "bad" LDL cholesterol.[23]

"Can my cat and dog go vegetarian?"

Yes, both animals can be fed a vegetarian diet. Indeed, the flesh of animals who fall into one of the categories of the four D's—dead, dying, diseased, or disabled—is what often goes into pet food. Many of these animals have died of infections, dehydration, or exposure to extreme heat or cold. In all but a few states, it is legal to remove unusable parts from chickens and sell them to pet food manufacturers. If you are concerned about your companion animal's health and about the cruelties of the meat industry, it's a good idea to stop buying meat-based pet food. Note that cats need food fortified with an amino acid called taurine, found in the muscles of animals. Synthetic taurine has been developed, and vegetarian cats should be fed it as a supplement. Below is a list of companies that sell vegan dog and/or cat food:

Boss Bars
P.O. Box 517,
Patagonia, AZ 85624
888-207-9114; fax: 888-207-9114
(100% certified organic dog biscuits, four flavors, including wheat- and corn-free)

Evolution
815 S. Robert St.,
St. Paul, MN 55107
612-228-0467, 612-227-2414, 612-228-0632
(Dog and cat kibble and canned food, ferret kibble, fish food)

F&O Pet Products
1740 NE 86th St. Suite 205,
Seattle, WA 98115
Website: www.vegancats.safeshopper.com
(Wide variety of vegetarian dog and cat products, including "starter packs")

Harbingers of a New Age
717 E. Missoula Ave.,
Troy, MT 59935
406-295-4944
(Vegecat, Vegekit, and Vegedog supplements; recipes for homemade vegan dog, cat, and kitten food; digestive enzymes, and acidifying nutritional yeast)

Natural Life Pet Products
1601 W. McKay,
Frontenac, KS 66763
800-367-2391; fax: 316-231-0071
(Canned and kibble dog food)

Nature's Recipe
341 Bonnie Circle
Corona, CA 91720
800-843-4008; fax: 909-278-9727
(Canned and kibble dog food. Call for closest distributor.)

Pet Guard
P.O. Box 728,
Orange Park, FL 32067-0728
800-874-3221, fax: 904-264-0802
(Canned dog food and biscuits, digestive enzymes)

Wow-Bow Distributors
13-B Lucon Dr.,
Deer Park, NY 11729
516-254-6064; fax: 516-254-6036
(Canned and kibble dog food and biscuits, nutritional supplements)

Wysong Corporation
1880 N. Eastman Rd.,
Midland, MI 48642
800-748-0188; fax: 517-631-8801
(Dog and cat kibble)

If you decide to prepare your own vegetarian dog or cat food, please read *Vegetarian Cats and Dogs* or *Vegetarian Dogs* by Verona Reibow and Jonathan Dune (P.O. Box 7056, Halcyon, CA 93421; 805-481-8581) to ensure that you understand the nutritional needs of dogs and cats.

"Which organizations should I join?"

It depends on what you want. Some organizations campaign effectively on behalf of animals, and achieve some real successes; others merely seem to generate much in-fighting and waste huge amounts of energy and resources. Most have Websites these days, so you should be able to find what you're looking for reasonably quickly.

UNITED STATES

The American Vegan Society
P.O. Box 369, Malaga, NJ 08328-0908
856-694-2887; Fax: 856-694-2288

Boston Vegetarian Society
P.O. Box 381071, Cambridge, MA 02238;
617-424-8846
E-mail: bvs@ivu.org Website: www.bostonveg.org

CARE (Compassion for Animals and Respect for the Environment)
P.O. Box 847, West Chester, PA 19381
215-242-0465; fax: 610-524-1637
E-mail: care@libertynet.org Website: www.libertynet.org/care

Club Veg
P.O. Box 625 WVS, Binghamton, NY 13905
607-655-2993
E-mail: Clubveg@aol.com Website: www.clubveg.org

Christian Vegetarian Association
U.S.: P.O. Box 201791, Cleveland, OH, 44120
phone/fax 216-283-6702 Canada: 30 Mary's Point Road,
Harvey, New Brunswick, Canada E4H 2N1
506-386-2498; fax 506-882-1013
Website: www.veg.faithweb.com

Food for Life Global
P.O. Box 59037, Potomac, MD 20859
703-204-1689; fax: 801-730-1372
E-mail: priya@ffl.org Website: www.ffl.org

Hampton Roads Vegetarian and Living Foods Community
60 Maxwell La., Newport News, VA 23606
757-930-1189
E-mail: hrv@ivu.org Website: www.ivu.org/hrv

Illinois and Midwest Vegetarian Entertainment Group
P.O. Box 7044, Elgin, IL 60121-7044
E-mail: iamveg@ivu.org Website: www.ivu.org/iamveg

Jewish Vegetarians of North America
6938 Reliance Rd. Federalsburg, MD 21632
410-754-5550
E-mail: imossman@skipjack.bluecrab.org

North American Vegetarian Society
P.O. Box 72, Dolgeville, NY, 13329
518-568-7970 fax: 518-568-7979
Website: www.navs-online.org

Pittsburgh Vegetarian Society
P.O. Box 44276, Pittsburgh, PA 15205-2004
412-734-5554

Springfield Vegetarian Association
325 S. Illinois St., Springfield, IL 62704
217-787-0014; fax: 217-793-9220
E-mail: hershey@famvid.com

Triangle Vegetarian Society
P.O. Box 3364
Chapel Hill, NC 27515-3364
919-489-3340
E-mail: tvs@ivu.org Website: www.trianglevegsociety.org

Vegans in Motion
2593 Columbia, Berkley, MI 48072 Phone/fax: 248-591-9543
E-mail: VIM@all4vegan.net Website: www.all4vegan.net/vim.htm

Vegetarian Resource Center
P.O. Box 38-1068, Cambridge, MA 02238-1068
617-625-3790; fax: 815-346-1306
E-mail: vrc@ivu.org

336 YOU DON'T NEED MEAT

The Vegetarian Resource Group
P.O. Box 1463, Baltimore, MD 21203
E-mail: vrg@vrg.org Website: www.vrg.org

Vegetarian Society of Colorado
P.O. Box 6773, Denver, CO, 80206-6773
303-777-4828
E-mail: info@vsc.org Website: www.vsc.org

Vegetarian Society of the District of Columbia
P.O. Box 4921, Washington, DC, 20008-4921
Voice mail: 202-362-VEGY
E-mail: vsdc@vsdc.org Website: www.vsdc.org

Vegetarian Society of Hawaii
P.O. Box 23208, Honolulu, HI 96823-3208
808-944-vegi (808-944-8344)
E-mail: info@vsh.org Website: www.vsh.org

Vegetarian Society of Houston
P.O. Box 541998, Houston, TX 77254-1998
713-880-1055; fax: 281-652-3277
E-mail: Vegsochouston@aol.com
Website: www.delos.net/vegsochou

Vegetarian Society of Richmond
P.O. Box 71342, Richmond VA 23255
804-344-4356
E-mail: vsr@ivu.org Website: www.ivu.org/vsr

Vegetarian Society of Yakima
E-mail: vsy@ivu.org Website: www.ivu.org/vsy

Vermont Vegetarian Society
P.O. Box 1797, North Ferrisburg, VT 05473-1797
E-mail: vvs@ivu.org Website: www.ivu.org/vvs

Very Vegetarian Society of Winston-Salem
620 Bellview St., Winston-Salem, NC, 27103-35
336-765-2614

CANADA

Ottawa Vegetarian Society
P.O. Box 4477, STN. E, Ottawa, Ontario, Canada K1S 5B4
819-776-6095
E-mail: ATIDMA@aol.com Website: www.flora.org/ovs

Toronto Vegetarian Association
2300 Yonge St., Suite 1101, P.O. Box 2307, Toronto, Ontario, Canada
M4P 1E4
416-544-9800; fax: 416-544-9094
E-mail: tva@veg.on.ca Wesbsite: www.veg.on.ca

Winnipeg Vegetarian Association
P.O. Box 2721, Winnipeg, Manitoba, R3C 4B3
204-889-5789; fax: 204-947-6514 (c/o Manitoba Eco-Network)
E-mail: wva@ivu.org

ALSO CONSIDER

The Humane Society of the United States
2100 L St, NW, Washington, DC 20037
Website: www.hsus.org

People for the Ethical Treatment of Animals
501 Front St., Norfolk, VA 23510
757-622-PETA (757-622-7382) fax: 757-622-0457
E-mail: info@peta-online.org Website: www.peta.com

"I'm a Christian, and the Bible says I can eat meat."

Well, the Bible says a great many things, and with selective quotation, you can prove almost anything. Nineteenth-century American slave owners frequently justified themselves with pious Biblical quotations. Many books have been written about this subject, but I'd like to make three points here. First, if we loved the animals today in the way humans loved them in the Garden of Eden, we would not eat them. It is only after Adam and Eve had been expelled from the Garden of Eden, after Noah and his family emerged from the Ark in the wake of the great flood, that people started killing for food. Other cultures have essentially similar tales of a fall from a once-perfect state of universal kinship. The Cherokee Indians have a tribal myth that says that humans once lived in perfect harmony with all their fellow creatures and plants, and all of them could speak to each other. In China, the Taoist Chuang Tsu wrote in the fourth century B.C. of a past "age of virtue," when all humankind lived a common, co-operative life with the birds and the beasts. And in Greece, the philosopher Empedocles wrote of a "golden age, an age of love" when "no altar was wet with the shameful slaughter of bulls," and he maintained that the primal sin was man's slaughter of animals. The Old Testament tells us that the world that God created was, initially, perfect. It is quite clear that in this perfect state, it was not intended that humans eat the flesh of other creatures: "Behold I have given you every herb yielding seed, which is upon the face of the earth, and every tree, in which is the fruit of a tree yielding seed; to you it shall be for meat." Clearly, our task is to strive for that state of perfection once again, and a good starting point is to stop slaughtering our fellow creatures.

Second, as Rev. Dr. Andrew Linzey puts it, "The Christian argument for vegetarianism is simple: since animals belong to God, have value to God and live for God, then their needless destruction is sinful."[24] Andrew Brown, religious affairs correspondent for a British newspaper, rather brilliantly describes this "needless destruction" in the following passage:

"They [factory-farmed animals] are martyred in the cause of mediocrity, confined and tortured to make our diets blander. Not even the weariest and most jaded epicure has ever crowned a lifetime of increasingly decadent sensuality by reaching, as his final perverted thrill, for a handful of chicken McNuggets. This is of course pleasingly moralistic: the fruits of sin turn to fast food in our mouths, as they should."[25]

And thirdly, I would urge you to consider what is, for many people, the kernel of Christianity, expressed in Christ's Sermon on the Mount. I won't indulge in selective quotation from it here; read the whole of it (Matthew, Chapter 5) and then consider these words written by Richard Whitehead:

"Let us take two images and place them side by side. The first is of a young preacher, healing the sick, washing his disciples feet preaching gentleness and humility and going to the cross without so much as raising a hand against his persecutors. The second is of an industry which systematically and mercilessly slaughters millions of animals which it has compelled to spend their brief lives in cramped, dingy, smelly sheds, and stuffed full of every chemical under the sun in order to produce meat to the maximum economic efficiency, a product which it spends millions of pounds persuading the public to buy. Clearly the two images are not simply incompatible; they are diametrically opposed. Can we really envisage Jesus being anything *but* a vegetarian if he were to be born into our society?"[26]

Well, there we are. I don't imagine for a moment that I've answered all the questions that you may have, although I hope some of the most common ones have been put to rest. What's really important now is that you feel confident enough to go ahead and live the new lifestyle for yourself, finding out things along the way. You'll enjoy it!

Finally, I have a request to make of you. Now that you know the truth about all this, you have a responsibility to pass it on to someone else. This is the best way, and perhaps the only way, that things will ever really change.

NOTES

1: EVERYTHING YOU'RE NOT SUPPOSED TO KNOW

1. de Tocqueville, A., *Journeys to England and Ireland*, ed. J. P. Mayer (1958), 105–6.
2. Spencer, C., *The Heretics Feast*, (Fourth Estate, 1993).
3. Phillips, R. L., Lemon, F. R., Beeson, W. L., Kuzma, J. W., "Coronary Heart Disease Mortality Among Seventh-Day Adventists with Differing Dietary Habits: A Preliminary Report." *American Journal of Clinical Nutrition* 31, (Oct. 1978) S191–S198.
4. *Dorland's Medical Dictionary*, 26th edition, (Fort Worth, Tex.: W. B. Saunders Co., 1985).
5. Snowdon, D. A., Phillips, R. L., Fraser, G. E., "Meat Consumption and Fatal Ischemic Heart Disease." *Preventive Medicine* 13: 5 (Sept. 1984), 490–500.
6. Hirayama, T., "Mortality in Japanese with Life-styles Similar to Seventh-Day Adventists: Strategy for Risk Reduction by Life-style Modification." *National Cancer Institute Monograph* 69 (Dec. 1985), 143–153.
7. Frentzel-Beyme, R., Claude, J., Eilber, U., "Mortality Among German Vegetarians: first Results After Five Years of Follow-up," *Nutrition and Cancer* 11: (2) (1988), 17–26.
8. Burr, M. L., Butland, B. K., "Heart Disease in British Vegetarians," *American Journal of Clinical Nutrition*. 48: 3 Suppl (Sept. 1988), 830–832.
9. *The New York Times*, 8 May 1990.
10. Coleman, V., *The Health Scandal* (Sidgwick & Jackson, 1988).
11. Medawar, C., "The Wrong Kind of Medicine?" Consumers Association, 1984.
12. Collier, J., *The Health Conspiracy* (Century, 1989).
13. Campbell, T. C., "A Study on Diet, Nutrition and Disease in the People's Republic of China, Part I." *Boletín de la Asociación Médica de Puerto Rico* 82: 3 (Mar 1990), 132–134.

14. Turpeineu, O., "Effect of Cholesterol-Lowering Diet on Mortality from Coronary Heart Disease and Other Causes." *Circulation* 59: 1 (Jan. 1979), 1–7.

15. Collens, W. S., "Atherosclerotic Disease: An Anthropologic Theory." *Medical Counterpoint* 1 (Dec. 1969); 53–57.

16. More information from www.pcrm.org.

17. More information from www.drmcdougall.com.

18. More information from www.ornish.com.

19. More information from www.vegsource.com/klaper.

20. More information from www.vegsource.com/harris.

21. More information from www.drfuhrman.com.

22. More information from www.newveg.av.org/health/kradjian.htm.

23. *The Guardian*, 23 November 1988.

24. *Meat Trades Journal*, 28 June 1984.

25. *Meat Trades Journal*, 20 March 1986.

26. *The Guardian*, 30 November 1984.

27. *Meat Trades Journal*, 25 June 1987.

28. *Meat Trades Journal*, 25 August 1988.

29. *Newsweek*, 27 June 1988.

30. *U.S. News & World Report* 103: 23 (7 December 1987), 57.

31. UPI newswire, 22 April 1988.

32. UPI newswire, 16 June 1988.

33. *Newsweek*, 27 June 1988.

34. *Advertising Standards Authority*, November 1991.

35. *Marketing*, 13 June 1991.

36. Lyman, H. F., *Mad Cowboy* (New York: Scribner 1998).

37. The judgment can be read at www.ca5.uscourts.gov/opinions/pub/98/98-10391-CVO.HTM.

38. Meat and Food History. Background papers on meat related topics. Meat and Livestock Commission, 1992.

39. *Meat Messenger*, Meat and Livestock Commission, 12 (Summer 1992).

40. *Academic American Encyclopedia*, 1992.

41. Morris, D., *The Naked Ape*, (Jonathan Cape).

42. Fornaciari, G., Mallegni, F., "Paleonutritional Studies on Skeletal Remains of Ancient Populations from the Mediterranean Area: An Attempt to Interpretation." *Anthropologischer Anzeiger* 45: 4 (Dec. 1987), 361–370.

43. *Meat in the News*, Meat and Livestock Commission, February 1992.

44. Konner, E., "Paleolithic Nutrition: A Consideration of Its Nature and Current Implications." *New England Journal of Medicine* 312: 5, 283–289.

45. Zihlman, A., in *Woman the Gatherer*, Dahlberg, F., ed., (New Haven, Conn.: Yale University Press, 1981).

46. Truswell & Hanson, "Medical Research Amongst the !Kung," in *Kalahari Hunter-Gatherers*, Lee, DeVore ed., (Cambridge Mass: Harvard University Press, 1976).

47. Coon, C. S., *The Hunting Peoples* (Jonathan Cape, 1972).

48. Benney, N., *Reclaim the Earth* (The Women's Press).

49. Howard, J., *Darwin* (Oxford: Oxford University Press, 1982).

50. Zihlman, A., in *Woman the Gatherer*, Dahlberg, F. ed., (New Haven, Conn.: Yale University Press, 1981).

51. *Meat in the News*, Meat and Livestock Commission, February 1992.

52. Associated Press, 8 September 1992.

53. Budker, P., *Whales and Whaling* (Harrap, 1958).

54. Spengler, O., *Der Mensch und die Technike* (Munich 1931).

2: APOCALYPSE COW!

1. Interestingly, this scenario may not be as unlikely as it sounds. An article in *War and Peace Digest* 2: 3 (Aug, 1992) states, "On June 19, 1992, the United States conducted an underground nuclear bomb test in Nevada. Another test was conducted only four days afterwards. Three days later, a series of heavy earthquakes as high as 7.6 on the Richter scale rocked the Mojave desert 176 miles to the south. They were the biggest earthquakes to hit California this century. Only 22 hours later, an 'unrelated' earthquake of 5.6 struck less than 20 miles from the Nevada test site itself. It was the biggest earthquake ever recorded near the test site and caused one-million dollars of damage to buildings in an area designated for permanent disposal of highly radioactive nuclear wastes only fifteen miles from the epicenter of the earthquake."

2. *Unfit for Human Consumption*, Lacey, R. (Souvenir Press, 1991).

3. Nebehay, S., Reuters online service, 22 December 2000.

4. *The Guardian*, 8 January 2000.

5. Fiennes, T. W., R.N., *Zoonoses and the Origins and Ecology of Human Disease* (Orlando Fla.: Academic Press, 1978).

6. Ibid.

7. Ibid.

8. Ibid.

9. Cannon, G., *The Politics of Food* (Century, 1987).

10. Prusiner, S. B., "Molecular Biology of Prisons Causing Infectious and Genetic Encephalopathies of Humans as Well as Scrapie of Sheep and BSE of Cattle." *Developments in Biological Standardization* 75 (1991), 55–74.

11. Carp, R. I., Kascsak, R. J., Wisniewski, H. M., Merz, P. A., Rubenstein, R., Bendheim, P., Bolton, D., "The Nature of the Unconventional Slow Infection Agents Remains a Puzzle." *Alzheimer's Disease and Associated Disorders* 3: 1–2 (Spring–Summer 1989), 79–99.

12. Wells, G.A.H., et al, "A Novel Progressive Spongiform Encephalopathy in Cattle." *Veterinary Record*, 31 October 1987, 419.

13. Parry, H. B., *Scrapie Disease in Sheep* (Orlando, Fla.: Academic Press, 1983).

14. Anon., "On the disease called goggles in sheep; by a gentleman in Wiltshire." *Bath Papers* (1788), 1 42–44.

15. Jones, T. C., Hunt, R. D., *Veterinary Pathology* (Lea & Feibiger, 1983).

16. "Bovine Spongiform Encephalopathy." *The Veterinary Record*, 23 June 1990, 626–627.

17. Morgan, K. L. "Bovine spongiform Encephalopathy: Time to Take Scrapie Seriously," *The Veterinary Record* 122: 18 (30 April 1988), 445–446.

18. Lantos, P. L., "From Slow Virus to Prion: A Review of Transmissible Spongiform Encephalopathies." *Histopathology* 20: 1 (January 1992).

19. Quoted in *Developments in Biological Standardization* 75 (1991), 56.

20. Seale, J. R., "Kuru, AIDS and Aberrant Social Behaviour." 80: 4 (April 1987), 200–2.

21. Hornabrook, R. W., ed., *Essays on Kuru*, Institute of Human Biology Papua New Guinea Monograph Series 3 (1976).

22. Ibid.

23. Ibid.

24. Calculated from Ministry of Agriculture data and data in *Developments in Biological Standardization* 75 (1991).

25. Bastian, F. O., "Creutzfeldt-Jakob disease and other transmissible spongiform encephalopathies." *Mosby Year Book* (1991).

26. Ibid.

27. Ibid.

28. *The Independent*, 14 June 1992.

29. *The Sunday Telegraph*, 21 August 1988.

30. Morgan, K. L., "Bovine Spongiform Encephalopathy: Time to Take Scrapie Seriously." *The Veterinary Record* 122: 18. (30 April 1988), 445–446.

31. From data cited in "Beef and Bovine Spongiform Encephalopathy: The Risk Persists." *Nutrition* and *Health*. Dealler, S., Lacey, R. 7: 3 (1991), 117–133.

32. "CheckOut '92," Channel Four Television, 8 July 1992.

33. *The Guardian*, 7 July 1992.

34. "CheckOut '92," Channel Four Television, 8 July 1992.

35. Ibid.

36. Agriculture Committee Fifth Report 89–90: "Bovine Spongiform Encephalopathy (BSE) Report" and Proceedings of the Committee. HCP 449 89/90.

37. Memorandum submitted by Professor Ivor H. Mills. Agriculture Committee Fifth Report 89–90: "Bovine Spongiform Encephalopathy (BSE)," Report and Proceedings of the Committee. HCP 449 89/90.

38. Mills, I. H. letter to *The Times*, 15 May 1990.

39. Agriculture Committee Fifth Report 89–90: "Bovine Spongiform Encephalopathy (BSE) Report" and Proceedings of the Committee. HCP 449 89/90.

40. *The Guardian*, 13 December 1985.

41. *The Guardian*, 8 August 1986.

42. Agriculture Committee Fifth Report 89–90: "Bovine Spongiform Encephalopathy (BSE) Report" and Proceedings of the Committee. HCP 449 89/90.

43. BBC Television, 1989.

44. *Meat Trades Journal*, 28 August 1986.

45. Ibid.

46. *Country File*, BBC Television, July 1989.

47. Agriculture Committee Fifth Report 89–90: "Bovine Spongiform Encepha-
     lopathy (BSE) Report" and Proceedings of the Committee. HCP 449 89/90.

48. Lacey, R. W., Dealler, S. F., "The BSE Time-Bomb? The Causes, the Risks and
     the Solutions to the BSE Epidemic." *The Ecologist* 21: 3 (1991) 117–122.

49. Agriculture Committee Fifth Report 89–90: "Bovine Spongiform Encepha-
     lopathy (BSE) Report" and Proceedings of the Committee. HCP 449 89/90.

50. Wells, G.A.H. et al, "A novel progessive spongiform encephalopathy in cat-
     tle." *The Veterinary Record*, 31 October 1987.

51. *The Times*, 29 December 1987.

52. *Sunday Telegraph*, 24 April 1988.

53. *Meat Trades Journal*, 5 April 1990.

54. Agriculture Committee Fifth Report 89–90: "Bovine Spongiform Encepha-
     lopathy (BSE) Report" and Proceedings of the Committee. HCP 449 89/90.

55. Kew, B., *The Pocketbook of Animal Facts and Figures* (Green Print, 1991).

56. "Disease Update: Bovine Spongiform Encephalopathy." *The Veterinary
     Record* 122: 20 (14 May, 1988), 477–478.

57. Morgan, K. L., "Bovine Spongiform Encephalopathy: Time to Take Scrapie
     Seriously." *The Veterinary Record* 122: 18 (30 April, 1988), 445–446.

58. "Disease Update: Bovine Spongiform Encephalopathy." *The Veterinary
     Record* 122: 20 (14 May, 1988), 477–478.

59. Lacey, R., *Unfit for Human Consumption* (Souvenir Press, 1991).

60. *The Times*, 9 June 1988.

61. *Meat Trades Journal*, 9 June 1988.

62. *Meat Trades Journal*, 4 August 1988.

63. *Sunday Telegraph*, 21 August 1988.

64. Associated Press newswire, 2 September 1988.

65. Wilesmith, J. W., Wells, G. A., Cranwell, M. P., Ryan, J. B. "Bovine Spongi-
     form Encephalopathy: Epidemiological Studies." *The Veterinary Record* 123:
     25 (17 December 1988), 638–644.

66. *The Independent*, 14 May 1990.

67. Ibid.

68. King Lear, V, iii, 20.

69. *The Times*, 30 January 1989.

70. Granada Television, 1990.

71. *The Guardian*, 11 February 1989.

72. *The Guardian*, 15 February 1989.

73. *The Times*, 16 February 1989.

74. "Report on the Working Party on Bovine Spongiform Encephalopathy." 1989
     HMSO.

75. Agriculture Committee Fifth Report 89–90: "Bovine Spongiform Encepha-
     lopathy (BSE) Report" and Proceedings of the Committee. HCP 449 89/90.

76. Ibid.

77. *Hansard*, 27 February 1989.

78. Ibid.

79. *The Times*, 1 March 1989.

80. From data cited in Dealler, S., Lacey, R., "Beef and Bovine Spongiform Encephalopathy: The Risk Persists." *Nutrition and Health.* 7: 3 (1991), 117–133.

81. *Hansard*, 13 March 1989.

82. *Hansard*, 9 March 1989.

83. *Hansard*, 16 March 1989.

84. BBC Television, 1989.

85. *Meat Trades Journal*, 27 April 1989.

86. *Daily Telegraph*, 26 May 1989.

87. Cited in Agriculture Committee Fifth Report 89–90: "Bovine Spongiform Encephalopathy (BSE) Report" and Proceedings of the Committee. HCP 449 89/90.

88. Ibid.

89. *The Sunday Times*, 9 July 1989.

90. Lacey, R., *Unfit for Human Consumption* (Souvenir Press, 1991).

91. *The Independent*, 4 January 1990.

92. Dawson, M., Wells, G.A.H., Parker B.N.J., "Preliminary Evidence of the Experimental Transmissibility of Bovine Spongiform Encephalopathy to Cattle." *The Veterinary Record* 126: 5 (3 February 1990) 112–113.

93. Granada Television, 1990.

94. *The Independent*, 14 April 1990.

95. Agriculture Committee Fifth Report 89–90: "Bovine Spongiform Encephalopathy (BSE) Report" and Proceedings of the Committee. HCP 449 89/90.

96. Ibid.

97. *Daily Mail*, 11 May 1990.

98. *The Independent*, 11 May 1990.

99. *Evening Standard*, 25 May 1990.

100. *The Times*, 15 May 1990.

101. Ibid.

102. *The Independent*, 16 May 1990.

103. *The Independent*, 18 May 1990.

104. Agriculture Committee Fifth Report 89–90: "Bovine Spongiform Encephalopathy (BSE) Report" and Proceedings of the Committee. HCP 449 89/90.

105. *The Shorter Oxford English Dictionary*, 3rd edition.

106. Herzberg L., Herzberg B. N., Gibbs, C. J., Jr, Sullivan, W., Amyx H., Gajdusek, D. C., Letter: "Creutzfeldt-Jakob Disease: Hypothesis for High Incidence in Libyan Jews in Israel." *Science* 186: 4166 (29 November 1974), 848.

107. Kahana, E., Alter, M., Braham, J., Sofer, D., "Creutzfeldt-Jakob Disease: Focus among Libyan Jews in Israel." *Science* 183: 120 (11 January 1974), 90–91.

108. *Science* 186: 4166 (29 November 1974), 848.

109. Goldberg, H., Alter, M., Kahana, E., "The Libyan Jewish Focus of Creutzfeldt-Jakob Disease: A Search for the Mode of Natural Transmission," in eds. Prusiner & Hadlow, *Slow Transmissible Diseases of the Nervous System* (Orlando, Fla.: Academic Press, 1979).

110. Neugut, R. H., Neugut, A. I., Kahana, E., Stein, Z., Alter, M., "Creutzfeldt-Jakob Disease: Familial Clustering Among Libyan-Born Israelis." *Neurology* 29:2 (February 1979), 225–231.

111. Palsson, P., Sigurdsson, B., in *Proceedings of the 8th Nordiska Veterinary Congress*, Helsinki, 1958.

112. Bobowick, A., Brody, J., Matthews, J. M., Roos, R., Gajdusek, D. *American Journal of Epidemiology* 98:381 (1973).

113. Malmgren, R. et al., "The epidemiology of Creutzfeldt-Jakob disease," in Prusiner & Hadlow, eds., *Slow Transmissible Diseases of the Nervous System* (Orlando, Fla.: Academic Press, 1979).

114. National Center for Health Statistics, *Eighth Revision International Classifications of Diseases* (Washington, D.C.: U.S. Govt. Printing Office).

115. *The Lancet* 336 (1990) 21–22.

116. Masters, C. L., et al, "Creutzfeldt-Jakob Disease: Patterns of Worldwide Occurance," in *Slow Transmissible Diseases of the Nervous System*, Prusiner & Hadlow eds. (Orlando, Fla.: Academic Press 1979).

117. Davanipour, Z., Alter, M., Sobel, E., Callahan, M., "Sheep Consumption: A Possible Source of Spongiform Encephalopathy in Humans." *Neuroepidemiology* 4: 4 (1985), 240–249.

118. Chatelain, J., Cathala, F., Brown P., Raharison, S., Court, L., Gajdusek, D.C., "Epidemiologic Comparisons Between Creutzfeldt-Jakob Disease and Scrapie in France During the 12-Year Period 1968–1979." *Journal of Neurological Science* 51:3 (September 1981), 329–337.

119. Cathala, F., Brown P., Raharison, S., Chatelain, J., Lecanuet, P., Castaigne, P., Gibbs, C. J. Jr., Gajdusek, D. C., "Maladie de Creutzfeldt-Jakob en France: Contribution a une recherche epidemiologique." *Revue Neurologique* 138:1 (1982), 39–51.

120. Brown, P., Cathala, F., Raubertas, R. F., Gajdusek, D. C., Castaigne, P., "The Epidemiology of Creutzfeldt-Jakob Disease: Conclusion of a 15-Year Investigation in France and Review of the World Literature." *Neurology* 37: 6 (June 1987) 895–904.

121. *The Economist*, 28 July 1990.

122. Korczyn, A. D., "Creutzfeldt-Jakob Disease Among Libyan Jews." *European Journal of Epidemiology* 7:5 (September 1991), 490–493.

123. Goldfarb, L. G., Korczyn, A. D., Brown, P., Chapman, J., Gajdusek, D. C., "Mutation in Codon 200 of Scrapie Amyloid Precursor Gene Linked to Creutzfeldt-Jakob Disease in Sephardic Jews of Libyan and Non-Libyan Origin." *The Lancet* 336: 8715 (September 1990), 637–638.

124. Gajdusek, D. C., "The transmissible Amyloidoses: Genetical Control of Spontaneous Generation of Infectious Amyloid Proteins by Nucleation of Configurational Change in Host Precursors: Kuru-CJD-GSS-Scrapie-BSE." *Journal of Epidemiology* 7:5 (September 1991), 567–577.

125. *Scientific American* (August 1990).

126. Gajdusek, D. C., "The Transmissible Amyloidoses: Genetical Control of Spon-

taneous Generation of Infectious Amyloid Proteins by Nucleation of Configurational Change in Host Precursors: Kuru-CJD-GSS-Scrapie-BSE." *European Journal of Epidemiology* 7:5 (September 1991), 567–577.

127. Goldfarb, L. G., Mitrova, E., Brown, P., Toh, B. K., Gajdusek, D. C., "Mutation in Codon 200 of Scrapie Amyloid Protein Gene in Two Clusters of Creutzfeldt-Jakob Disease in Slovakia." *The Lancet* 336:8713 (25 August 1990), 514–515.

128. Mitrova, E., Huncaga, S., Hocman, G., Nyitrayova, O., Tatara, M., "Clusters of CJD in Slovakia: The First Laboratory Evidence of Scrapie." *European Journal of Epidemiology* 7:5 (September 1991), 520–523.

129. Mitrova E., Brown, P., Hroncova, D., Tatara, M., Zilak, J., "Focal Accumulation of CJD in Slovakia: Retrospective Investigation of a New Rural Family Cluster." *European Journal of Epidemiology* 7:5 (September 1991), 487–489.

130. Ibid.

131. Mitrova, E., Huncaga, S., Hocman, G., Nyitrayova, O., Tatara, M., "Clusters of CJD in Slovakia: The First laboratory Evidence of Scrapie." *European Journal of Epidemiology* 7:5 (September 1991), 520–523.

132. "Some New Aspects of CJD Epidemiology in Slovakia." Mitrova, E., *European Journal of Epidemiology* 7:5 (September 1991), 439–449.

133. Mitrova E., Huncaga S., Hocman, G., Nyitrayova, O., Tatara, M., " 'Clusters' of CJD in Slovakia: The First Laboratory Evidence of Scrapie." *European Journal of Epidemiology* 7:5 (September 1991), 520–523.

134. *Meat Trades Journal*, 9 January 1992.

135. *Meat Trades Journal*, 12 March 1992.

136. *The Independent*, 5 March 1992.

137. *The Daily Telegraph*, 21 March 1996.

138. *The New York Times*, 25 July 2000.

139. Walker, K. D., Hueston, W. D., Hurd, H. S., Wilesmith, J. W., "Comparison of Bovine Spongiform Encephalopathy Risk Factors in the United States and Great Britain." *Journal of the American Veterinary Medical Association.* 199 (1991) 1554–1561.

140. "Mad Cow Disease Must be found in US Cows in Low Levels, Says Research," *Food Chemical News*, 3 June 1996.

141. "Stringent Steps Taken by US on Cow Illness," *The New York Times*, 14 January 2001.

142. *USA Today*, 6 February 2001.

143. *The New York Times*, 8 February 2001.

144. *British Journal of Psychiatry* 158 (1991), 457–470.

145. *Newsweek*, 4 August 1996, 58–59.

146. *PR Watch* 3:1 (1996), 1–8.

147. *American Journal of Medical Genetics* 60 (1995), 12–18.

148. *Neuroepidemiology* (1993) 12(1): 28–36

149. Physicians Committee for Responsible Medicine 24 January 2001.

3: PIG TALES

1. Singer, P., *Practical Ethics* (Cambridge U.K.: Cambridge University Press, 1979).
2. Singer, I. B., *The Séance and Other Stories*, 1968.
3. The Simon Wiesenthal Center.
4. The Humane Society of the United States.
5. Eisnitz, Gail, *Slaughterhouse: The Shocking Story of Greed, Neglect, and In humane Treatment Inside the U.S. Meat Industry*, Prometheus Books, 1997.
6. Katme, Dr. A. M., letter to *The Guardian*, 20 August 1985.
7. Edmunds, M., "What is Ritual Slaughter?" *She*, July 1985.
8. Berkovits, letter to *The Independent*, 15 March 1989.
9. *New Scientist*, 7 April 1988.
10. *Birmingham Evening Mail*, 3 July 1985.
11. Pick, P. L. ed., *Tree of Life* (A. S. Barnes & Co, 1977).
12. Adcock, D.V.M. and Finelli, M., "Against Nature: The Sensitive Pig versus the Hostile Environment of the Modern Pig Farm." *HSUS News*, Spring 1996.
13. Brophy, B., quoted in "Unlived Life—a Manifesto Against Factory Farming." in Wynne-Tyson, J. ed., *The Extended Circle*. (Centaur Press, 1985).
14. Bly, R., *Iron John* (Reading, MA: Addison-Wesley Publishing Co., 1990).

4: A MANUAL OF VEGETARIAN HEALTH

1. www.beef.org/nutrition/index.htm
2. *Meat in the News*, February 1992.
3. See, for example, "Beef/Meat-Containing vs. Vegetarian Diets & Health," Series No. FS/N 023 2000, National Cattlemen's Beef Association and Cattlemen's Beef Board; and "Facts For Your File: Adolescent Vegetarianism," 1999, National Cattlemen's Beef Association.
4. Scrimshaw, N. S., "Iron deficiency." *Scientific American* 265:4 (October 1991), 46–47.
5. Barber, S. A., Bull, N. L., Buss, D. H., "Low Iron Intakes Among Young Women in Britain." *British Medical Journal*, 290:9 (March 1985), 743–744.
6. "Dietary Reference Values for Food Energy and Nutrients for the United Kingdom," Department of Health, 1991.
7. Sanders, T. A., Ellis, F. R., Dickerson, J. W. "Haematological Studies on Vegans." *British Journal of Nutrition*, 40:1 (July 1978), 9–15.
8. Havala, S., R.D. and Dwyer, D.SC., R.D. "Position of the American Dietetic Association: Vegetarian Diets-Technical Support Paper." *Journal of the American Dietetic Association* 88:3 (March 1988), 352–355.
9. Carlson, E., Kipps, M.; Lockie, A., Thomson, J. J., "A Comparative Evaluation of Vegan, Vegetarian and Omnivore Diets." *Journal of Plant Foods* 6, (1985), 89–100.
10. Rana, S. K., Sanders, T. A. "Taurine Concentrations in the Diet, Plasma, Urine and Breast Milk of Vegans Compared with Omnivores." *British Journal of Nutrition* 56:1 (1986), 17–27.

11. Sanders, T. A., Key, T. J., "Blood Pressure, Plasma Renin Activity and Aldosterone Concentrations in Vegans and Omnivore Controls." *Human Nutrition–Applied Nutrition*, 41:3 (June 1987), 204–211.

12. Levin, N., Rattan, J., Gilat, T., "Mineral Intake and Blood Levels in Vegetarians." *Israel Journal of Medical Sciences*, 22:2 (February 1986), 105–108.

13. Van Staveren, W. A., Dhuyvetter, J. H., Bons, A., Zeelen, M., Hautvast, J. G., "Food Consumption and Height/Weight Status of Dutch Preschool Children on Alternative Diets." *Journal of American Dietetic Association* 85:12 (December 1985), 1579–1584.

14. Abdulla, M., Andersson, I., Asp, N. G., Berthelsen, K., Birkhed, D., Dencker, I., Johansson, C. G., Jagerstad, M., Kolar, K., Nair, B. M., Nilsson-Ehle P., Norden, A., Rassner, S., Akesson, B., Ockerman, P. A., "Nutrient Intake and Health Status of Vegans: Chemical Analyses of Diets Using the Duplicate Portion Sampling Technique." *American Journal of Clinical Nutrition*, 34:11 (November 1981), 2464–2477.

15. "Anderson, B. M., Gibson, R. S., Sabry, J. H., "The Iron and Zinc Status of Long-Term Vegetarian Women." *American Journal of Clinical Nutrition*, 34:6 (June 1981), 1042–1048.

16. Hunt, J. R., Hoverson, B. S., Gallagher, S. K., Johnson, L. K., "Low or High Meat Consumption: Effects on Triglycerides, HDL Cholesterol and Indices of Iron Nutriture in Postmenopausal Women." Proceedings of the American Dietetic Association, 76th Annual General Meeting, 25–28 October 1993.

17. MEDLINE® database produced by the U.S. National Library of Medicine.

18. Seshadri, S., Shah, A., Bhade, S., "Haematologic Response of Anaemic Preschool Children to Ascorbic Acid Supplementation." *Human Nutrition–Applied Nutrition* 39: 2 (April 1985) 151–154.

19. Emery, T., *Iron And Your Health: Facts and Fallacies.* (Boston: CRC Press 1991).

20. "Good Medicine," Winter 1993, Physicians Committee for Responsible Medicine, Washington, D.C.

21. Salonen, J. T., Nyyssonen, K., Korpela H., Tuomilehto, J., Seppanen, R., Salonen, R., "High Stored Iron Levels are Associated with Excess Risk of Myocardial Infarction in Eastern Finnish Men." *Circulation* 86: 3 (September 1992), 803–811.

22. Narins, D. in *Biochemistry of Nonheme Iron*, Bezkorovainy, A. (New York: Ed. Plenum, 1980).

23. The Associated Press Newswire, 18 February 1993.

24. Oski, F. A., "Is Bovine Milk a Health Hazard?" *Pediatrics*, 75, 182–86.

25. "Control of Nutritional Anemia with Special Reference to Iron Deficiency." WHO Technical Report Series, 1985, 580.

26. Anyon, C., "A cause of iron-deficiency anaemia in infants." *New Zealand Medical Journal*, 74, 24–25.

27. UPI Newswire, 8 October 1993.

28. Thrash & Thrash, *Nutrition for Vegetarians*, 1982.

29. *Vegetarian Times* 184:6 (December 1992), 56.

30. "Dietary Reference Values for Food Energy and Nutrients for the United Kingdom." Department of Health, 1991.

31. Beilin, L. J., "Strategies and Difficulties in Dietary Intervention in Myocardial Infarction Patients." *Clinical and Experimentalist Hypertension,* [A] 14: 1–2 (1992), 213–221.

32. Barnard, N., *Food for life* (New York: Harmony Books, 1993).

33. *The University of California, Berkeley Wellness Letter* 6:8 (May 1990), p. 1.

34. Adam, O. Z., "Ernahrung als adjuvante Therapie bei chronischer Polyarthritis." *Rheumotology,* 52: 5 (September–October 1993) 275–280.

35. Skoldstam, L., "Fasting and Vegan Diet in Rheumatoid Arthritis." *Scandinavian Journal of Rheumatology* 15 (1986), 219–223.

36. Panush, R. S., Stroud, R. M., Webster, E. M., "Food-Induced (Allergic) Arthritis: Inflammatory Arthritis Exacerbated by Milk." *Arthritis and Rheumatism,* 29: 2 (February 1986) p. 220–226.

37. Kjeldsen-Kragh, J., Haugen, M., Borchgrevink, C. F., Laerum, E., Eek, M., Mowinkel, P., Hovi, K., Forre, O., "Controlled Trial of Fasting and One-Year Vegetarian Diet in Rheumatoid Arthritis." *The Lancet* 338: 8772 (12 October 1991) 899–902.

38. *The Independent,* 7 January 1992.

39. *The Guardian,* 1 March 1986.

40. Childers, N., and Russo, G. M., "The Nightshades and Health." (Somerville, N.J.: Horticulture Publications, 1973).

41. Sorbel, D., Klein, A., *Arthritis: What Works* (New York: St. Martin's Press).

42. The work of Dr. Alan Ebringer, Department of Rheumatology, Middlesex Hospital, and immunologist at King's College, London.

43. Shatin, R., M.D., reported in *Bestways,* 17: 9, (September 1989), 42.

44. Bingham, R., Bellew, B. A., and Bellew, J. G., "Yucca Plant Saponin in the Management of Arthritis." *Journal Applied Nutrition* 27 (1975), 45–50.

45. The Associated Press Newswire, 12 August 1993.

46. The Associated Press Newswire, 2 October 1992.

47. *Panorama,* BBC1 Television, 14 February 1994.

48. Sabbah, A., "L'allergie alimentaire dans l'asthme de l'enfant." *Allergie et Immunologie* 22: 8 (October 1990) 325–331.

49. Lindahl, O., Lindwall, L., Spangberg, A., Stenram, A., Ockerman, P. A., "Vegan Regimen with Reduced Medication in the Treatment of Bronchial Asthma." *Journal of Asthma,* 22: 1 (1985), 45–55.

50. Dahlen, S. E., Hansson, G., Hedqvist, P. et al., "Allergen Challenge of Lung Tissue from Asthmatics Elicits Bronchial Contraction That Correlates with the Release of Leukotrienes C_4, D_4, E_4." *Proceedings of the National Academy of Sciences* 1983: 80, 1712–1716.

51. Arm, J. P., Lee, T. H., "The use of fish oil in bronchial asthma." *Allergy Proceedings,* 10: 3 (May–June 1989), 185–187.

52. Kirsch, C. M., Payan, D. G., Wong, M. Y., Dohlman, J. G., Blake, V. A., Petri,

M. A., Offenberger, J., Goetzl, E. J., Gold, W. M., "Effect of Eicosapentaenoic Acid in Asthma." *Clinical Allergy* 18: 2 (March 1988), 177–187.

53. Picado, C., Castillo, J. A., Schinca, N., Pujades, M., Ordinas, A., Coronas, A., Agusti-Vidal, A., "Effects of a Fish Oil Enriched Diet on Aspirin Intolerant Asthmatic Patients: a Pilot Study." *Thorax* 43: 2 (Feb 1998), 93–97.

54. Reynolds, R. D., Natta, C. L. "Depressed Plasma Pyridoxal Phosphate Concentrations in Adult Asthmatics." *American Journal of Clinical Nutritionists* 41 (1985) 684–688.

55. Pauling, L. *How to Live Longer and Feel Better.* (New York: Avon Books, 1987).

56. Ogilvy, C. S., Douglas, J. D., Tabatabai, M., Dubois, M., "Ascorbic Acid Reverses Bronchconstriction Caused by Methacholine Aerosol in Man." *Physiologist* 21, (1978), 86.

57. Anah, C. O., Jarike, L. N., Baig, H. A., "High Dose Ascorbic Acid in Nigerian Asthmatics." *Tropical and Geographical Medicine,* 32 (1980) 132–137.

58. Bricklin, M., *Practical Encyclopedia of Natural Healing* (Emmaus, Penn.: Rodale Press, 1983).

59. Allen, D. H., Delohery, J., Baker, G., "Monosodium L-Glutamate–Induced Asthma." *Journal of Allergy and Clinical Immunology,* 80: 4 (October 1987), 530–537.

60. The Associated Press Newswire, 19 June 1992.

61. Anibarro, B., Martin, E. M., Martinez, A. F., Pascual, M. C., Ojeda, C., "Egg Protein Sensitization in Patients with Bird Feather Allergy." *JA Allergy* 46: 8 (November 1991), 614–618.

62. Singh, V., Wisniewski, A., Britton, J., Tattersfield, A., "Effect of Yoga Breathing Exercises (Pranayama) on Airway Reactivity in Subjects with Asthma." *The Lancet* 335: 8702 (9 June 1990), 1381.

63. *The Lancet,* 24 August 1990.

64. National Cancer Institute; The Associated Press newswire, 25 September 1992; Brady, J., ed., *Women with Cancer Confront an Epidemic.* (Cleis Press, 1992).

65. Higson, J., Muir, C. S., "Environmental Carcinogenesis." *Journal of the National Cancer Institute* 63 (1979), 1291–1298.

66. Tyler, A., "Political Cripples." *New Statesman & Society,* 12 June 1992.

67. Letter to *New Statesman & Society,* 26 June 1992.

68. *The Independent,* 17 April 1992.

69. Personal communication, March 1992.

70. Doll, R., and Peto, R., *The Causes of Cancer* (Oxford, UK: Oxford Medical Publications, 1981).

71. *Scientific American,* January 1892.

72. Abernethy, J., *Surgical Observations on Tumours.* (1804). Cited in *The Heretic's Feast,* Spencer, C. (Fourth Estate, 1993).

73. Gregor, O., Toman, R., Prusova, F., "Gastrointestinal Cancer and Nutrition." *Gut* 10: 12 (1969), 1031–1034.

74. Wynder, E. L., Shigematsu, T., "Environmental Factors of Cancer of the Colon and Rectum." *Cancer* 20:9 (1967), 1528.

75. Phillips, R. L., "Role of Life-style and Dietary Habits in Risk of Cancer among Seventh-Day Adventists." *Cancer Research* 35 (1975), 3513–3522.

76. Ibid.

77. Phillips, R. L., Snowdon, D. A., "Association of Meat and Coffee Use with Cancers of the Large Bowel, Breast and Prostate among Seventh-Day Adventists: Preliminary Results." *Cancer Research* 43 (1983), 2403–2408.

78. Howell, M. A., "Diet as an Etiological Factor in the Development of Cancers of the Colon and Rectum." *Journal of Chronic Diseases* 28 (1975), 67–80.

79. Palgi, A., "Association between Dietary Changes and Mortality Rates: Israel 1949–1977: A Trend-Free Regression Model." *American Journal of Clinical Nutrition* 34 (1981), 1569–1583.

80. Lubin, J. H., Burns, P. E., Blot, W. J., Ziegler, R. G., Lees, A. W., Fraumeni, J. F., "Dietary Factors and Breast Cancer Risk." *International Journal of Cancer* 28 (1981), 685–689.

81. Kolonel, L. N., Hankin, J. H., Lee, J., Chu, S. Y., Nomura, A.M.Y., Hines, M. W., "Nutrient Intakes in Relation to Cancer Incidence in Hawaii." *British Journal of Cancer* 44 (1981), 332.

82. Correa, P., "Epidemiological Correlations Between Diet and Cancer Frequency." *Cancer Research* 41, 3685–3690.

83. Willett, W. C., Stampfer, M. J., Colditz, G. A., Rosner, B. A., Speizer, F. E., "Relation of Meat, Fat, and Fiber Intake to the Risk of Colon Cancer in a Prospective Study among Women." *New England Journal of Medicine* 323: 24 (13 December 1990), 1664–1672.

84. *The Independent*, 14 December 1990.

85. Manousos, O., Day, N. E., Trichopoulos, D., Gerovassilis, F., Tzonou, A., "Diet and Colo-Rectal Cancer: A Case-Control Study in Greece." *International Journal of Cancer* 32 (1983), 1–5.

86. Lijinsky, W., and Shubik, P., "Benzo(a)pyrene and Other Polynuclear Hydrocarbons in Charcoal-Broiled Meat." *Science* 145, 53–55.

87. UPI Newswire, 10 May 1986.

88. Committee on Nitrate Accumulation, National Academy of Sciences: "Accumulation of Nitrate 1972."

89. Physician's Committee for Responsible Medicine, March 1992.

90. "National Pork Producers Council Recommends Hog Farmers Suspend Use of Sulphamethazine," UPI Newswire, 29 January 1988.

91. Korpela, J. T., Adlercreutz, H, Turunen, M.J.S, "Fecal Free and Conjugated Bile Acids and Neutral Sterols in Vegetarians, Omnivores, and Patients with Colorectal Cancer," *Scandinavian Journal of Gastroenterology* 23: 3 (April 1988), 277–283.

92. Malter, M., Schriever, G., Eilber, U., "Natural Killer Cells, Vitamins, and Other Blood Components of Vegetarian and Omnivorous Men." *Nutrition and Cancer* 12: 3 (1989), 271–278.

93. van Kaam, A. H., Koopman-Esseboom, C., Sulkers, E. J., Sauer, P. J., van der Paauw, C. G., Tuinstra, L. G., "Polychloorbifenylen (PCB's) in moedermelk,

vetweefsel, plasma en navelstrengbloed, gehalten en correlaties." *Nederlands Tijdschrift Voor Geneeskunde* 135:31 (3 August 1991), 1399–1403.

94. Hall, R. H., "A New Threat to Public Health: Organochlorines and Food." *Nutrition and Health* 8:1 (1992), 33–43.

95. "Can Vitamins Help Prevent Cancer?" *Consumer Reports*, 48:5 (May 1983), 243–245.

96. Troll, W., "Prevention of Cancer by Agents That Suppress Oxygen Radical Formation." *Free Radical Research Communications* 12–13: Part 2 (1991), 751–757.

97. *Academic American Encyclopedia.*

98. Thrash, A. M., and Thrash, C. L., *The Animal Connection.* (Yuchi Pines Institute, 1983).

99. Gardner, M. B., "Viruses as Environmental Carcinogens: An Agricultural Perspective." *Basic Life Science* 21 (1982), 171–188.

100. Johnson, E. S., Fischman, H. R., Matanoski, G. M., Diamond, E., "Cancer Mortality among White Males in the Meat industry." *Journal of Occupational Medicine* 28:1 (January 1986), 23–32.

101. Diglio, C. A., Ferrer, J. F., "Induction of Syncytia by the Bovine C-Type Leukaemia Virus." *Cancer Research*, 36, 1056–1067.

102. Rifkin, J., *Beyond Beef.* (New York: Dutton, 1992).

103. *New Scientist*, 7 January 1989.

104. McClure, H. M., Keeling, M. E., Custer, R. P., Marshak, R. R., Abt, D. A., Ferrer, J. F., "Erythroleukaemia in Two Infant Chimpanzees Fed Milk from Cows Naturally Infected with the Bovine C-Type Virus." *Cancer Research* 34, 2745–2757.

105. Lemon, H. M., "Food-Born Viruses and Malignant Hemopoietic Diseases." *Bacteriological Review* 28, 490–492.

106. Aleksandrowicz, J., "Leukaemia in Humans and Animals in the Light of Epidemiological Studies with Reference to Problems of Its Prevention." *Acta Medica Polona* 9, 217–230.

107. Muszynski, B., "Wplyw biaLaczek bydLa na powstawanie chorob nowotworo, wych u ludzi na podstawie materiaLow zebranych w powiecie zlotowskim." *Przegl Lek* 25:9, 660–661.

108. Linos, A., Kyle, R. A., Elveback, L. R., Kurland, L. T., "Leukemia in Olmsted county, Minnesota, 1965–1974." *Mayo Clinic Proceedings* 53, 714–718.

109. Donham, K. J., Berg, J. W., Sawin, R. S., "Epidemiologic Relationships of the Bovine Population and Human Leukemia in Iowa." *American Journal of Epidemiology* 112 (1980), 80–92.

110. Blair, A., Hayes, H. M., "Cancer and Other Causes of Death among US Veterinarians 1966–1977." *International Journal of Cancer* 25, 181–185.

111. Lenfant-Pejovic, M. H., Mlika-Cabanne, N., Bouchardy, C., Auquier, A., "Risk Factors for Male Breast Cancer: A Franco-Swiss Case-Control Study." *International Journal of Cancer* 45:4 (15 April 1990), 661–665.

112. Magnani, C., Pastore, G., Luzzatto, L., Carli, M., Lubrano, P., Terracini, B.,

"Risk Factors for Soft Tissue Sarcomas in Childhood: A Case-Control Study." *Tumori* 75:4 (31 August 1989), 396–400.

113. *Vibrant Life*, 8:3 (May–June 1992), 20.

114. Physicians' Health Study, begun 1982, Dr. Charles Hennekens, Harvard Medical School and Brigham & Women's Hospital, Boston National Cancer Institute, Cancer Research Laboratory, Bethesda, Maryland, USA, Regina Ziegler, Ph.D., Environmental Epidemiology Department.

115. "Can vitamins help prevent cancer?" *Consumer Reports* 48:5 (May 1983), 243–245.

116. *Redbook*, 172:6, (April 1989), 96.

117. "Good Diet 'Curbs Cancer Risk,' " *The Independent*, 3 October 1989.

118. Gerhard Schrauzer, Ph.D., of the University of California, cited in *Better Nutrition* 51:11 (November 1989) 14.

119. *Redbook* 172:6, (April 1989), 96.

120. Spallholz, J. E., Stewart, J. R., "Advances in the Role of Minerals in Immunobiology." *Biological Trace Element Research* 19:3 (March 1989), 129–151.

121. Knekt, P., et al., "Selenium Deficiency and Increased Risk of Lung Cancer." Abstract of paper read at the Fourth International Symposium on Selenium in Biology and Medicine, Tubingen, West Germany, July 1988.

122. Reinhold, U., et al. "Selenium Deficiency and Lethal Skin Cancer." Abstract of paper read at the Fourth International Symposium on Selenium in Biology and Medicine, Tubingen, West Germany, July 1988.

123. Garland, C., and Garland, F., *The Calcium Connection* (New York: Simon & Schuster, 1989). C. Garland is director of the Cancer Center Epidemiology Program, University of California, San Diego.

124. American Cancer Society, "Nutritional Guidelines?" *Health* 16, (June 1984), 9.

125. "Can Vitamins Help Cancer?" *Consumer Reports* 48:5 (May 1983), 243–245.

126. National Advisory Committee on Nutrition Education, "Proposals for Nutritional Guidelines for Health Education in Britain," The Health Education Council, September 1983.

127. Burkitt, D. P., Walker, A.R.P., Painter, N. S., "Effect of Dietary Fibre on Stools and Transit Times, and Its Role in the Causation of Disease." *The Lancet*, 30 December 1972.

128. "Dietary Reference Values for Food Energy and Nutrients for the United Kingdom," Department of Health, 1991.

129. Handler, S., "Dietary Fiber: Can It Prevent Certain Colonic Diseases?" *Postgraduate Medicine* 73:2 (Feb. 1983), 301–307.

130. *Cosmopolitan* 207:4 (October 1989), 98.

131. Davies, G. J., Crowder, M., Dickerson, J. W., "Dietary Fibre Intakes of Individuals with Different Eating Patterns." *Human Nutrition–Applied Nutrition* 39 (2) (Apr. 1985) 139–48.

132. Goldin, B. R., Adlercreutz, H., Gorbach, S. L., Warram, J. H., Dwyer, J. T., Swenson, L., Woods, M. N., "Estrogen Excretion Patterns and Plasma Levels

in Vegetarian and Omnivorous Women." *New England Journal of Medicine* 307:25 (16 December 1982) 1542–1547.

133.   Abdulla, M., Aly, K. O., Andersson, I., Asp, N. G., Birkhed, D., Denker, I., Johansson, C. G., Jagerstad, M., Kolar, K., Nair, B. M., et al, "Nutrient Intake and Health Status of Lactovegetarians: Chemical Analyses of Diets Using the Duplicate Portion Sampling Technique." *American Journal of Clinical Nutrition* 40:2 (Aug 1984), 325–338.

134.   Levin, N., Rattan, J., Gilat, T., "Mineral Intake and Blood Levels in Vegetarians." *Israel Journal of Medical Sciences* 22:2 (Feb. 1986), 105–108.

135.   Slavin, J. L., "Dietary Fiber: Classification, Chemical Analyses, and Food Sources." *Journal of the American Dietetic Association* 87:9 (September 1987), 1164–1171.

136.   Rattan, J., Levin, N., Graff, E., Weizer, N., Gilat, T. "A High-Fiber Diet Does Not Cause Mineral and Nutrient Deficiencies." *Journal of Clinical Gastroenterology* 3:4 (December 1981), 389–393.

137.   Kelsay, J. L., Frazier, C. W., Prather, E. S., Canary, J. J., Clark, W. M., Powell, A. S., "Impact of Variation in Carbohydrate Intake on Mineral Utilization by Vegetarians." *American Journal of Clinical Nutrition* 48:3 Suppl. (September 1988), 875–879.

138.   Langley, G., "Vegan Nutrition: A Survey of Research." Vegan Society, 1988.

139.   "Introducing Diabetes," British Diabetic Association.

140.   "Diabetes in the United Kingdom, 1988," British Diabetic Association.

141.   Diabetes Epidemiology Research International, "Preventing Insulin Dependent Diabetes Mellitus: The environmental challenge." *British Medical Journal (Clinical Research)*, 295: 6596 (22 August 1987), 479–481.

142.   Anderson, J. W. "Plant Fiber and Blood Pressure" *Annals of Internal Medicine* 1983:98, 842–846.

143.   American Diabetes Association, "Nutritional Recommendations and Principles for Individuals With Diabetes Mellitus: 1986." *Diabetes Care* 10: 1 (January–February 1987).

144.   Snowdon, D. A., Phillips, R. L., "Does a Vegetarian Diet Reduce the Occurrence of Diabetes?" *American Journal of Public Health* 75 (1985), 507–512.

145.   Krieb, R. and Beebe, C., "Food Choices Can Affect Your Risks for Diabetes Complications." *Diabetes in the News* 6:5 (September–October 1989), 12.

146.   Scott, F. W., "Cow Milk and Insulin-Dependent Diabetes Mellitus: Is There a Relationship?" *American Journal of Clinical Nutrition* 51:3 (March 1990), 489.

147.   Tuomilehto, J. et al, Department of Epidemiology, National Public Health Institute, Helsinki, Finland, "Coffee Consumption as Trigger for Insulin Dependent Diabetes Mellitus in Childhood." *British Medical Journal*, 300:6725 (10 March 1990), 642–643.

148.   *Better Nutrition for Today's Living*, 52:6 (June 1990), 22–23.

149.   Putzier, E., "[Dermatomycoses and an Antifungal Diet] Haurmykosen und Antipilzdiat" *Wiener Medizinische Wochenschrift* (Austria) 139:15–16 (31 August 1989), 379–380.

150. Sir James Black, quoted in *The Independent*, 22 October 1988.

151. Black, Sir J., and J. J., Voorhees, M.D. in *Archives of Dermatology* and *Better Nutrition for Today's Living*, 52:6 (June 1990), 22–23.

152. Rudin, D. O., M.D., "The Omega-3 Phenomenon." *Better Nutrition for Today's Living* 52:6 (June 1990), 22–23.

153. Fry, L. et al, "The Mechanism of Folate Deficiency in Psoriasis." *British Journal of Dermatology* 84 (1971), 539–544.

154. Chandra, R. K., Puri S., Hamed, Azza, "Influence of Maternal Diet During Lactation and Use of Formula Feeds on Development of Atopic Eczema in High Risk Infants." *British Medical Journal*, 298:6693 (22 July 1989), 228.

155. Poilolainen, K. et al, National Public Health Institute, Helsinki, as reported in *The Independent*, 23 March 1990.

156. Bruckstein, A. H., "Nonsurgical Management of Cholelithiasis." *The Archives of Internal Medicine* 150:5 (May 1990), 960.

157. Pixley, F., Wilson, D. McPherson, K., Mann, J., "Effect of Vegetarianism on Development of Gallstones in Women." *British Medical Journal*, 291 (6 July 1985).

158. Pixley F., Mann, J., "Dietary Factors in the Aetiology of Gall Stones: A case Control Study." *Gut* 29:11 (November 1988), 1511–1515.

159. *The Edell Health Letter*, 8:6 (June 1989), 1.

160. *Prevention* 41:5 (May 1989), 66.

161. Roberts, W. C., "We Think We Are One, We Act As If We Are One, But We Are Not One." *American Journal of Cardiology* 66:10 (1 October 1990), 896.

162. Hirayama, T., "Mortality in Japanese with Life-styles Similar to Seventh-Day Adventists: Strategy for Risk Reduction by Life-style Modification." *National Cancer Institute Monograph* 69 (December 1985) 143–153.

163. Thorogood, M., Carter, R., Benfield L., McPherson, K., Mann, J. I., "Plasma Lipids and Lipoprotein Cholesterol Concentrations in People with Different Diets in Britain." *British Medical Journal*, (Clinical Research Edition) 295:6594 (8 August 1987), 351–353.

164. Frentzel-Beyme, R., Claude, J., Eilber, U. "Mortality Among German Vegetarians: First Results After Five Years of Follow-Up." *Nutrition and Cancer* 11:2 (1988), 117–126.

165. Fonnebo, V. J., "Mortality in Norwegian Seventh-Day Adventists 1962–1986." *Journal of Clinical Epidemiology* 45:2 (February 1992), 157–167.

166. Arntzenius, A. C., Kromhout, D., Barth, J. D., Reiber, J. H., Bruschke, A. V., Buis, B., van Gent, C. M., Kempen-Voogd, N., Strikwerda, S., van der Velde, E. A., "Diet, Lipoproteins, and the Progression of Coronary Atherosclerosis: The Leiden Intervention Trial." *New England Journal of Medicine* 312:13 (28 March 1985), 805–811.

167. *Time*, 29 October 1990.

168. Ornish, D., Brown, S. E., Scherwitz, L. W., Billings, J. H., Armstrong, W. T., Ports, T. A., McLanahan, S. M., Kirkeeide, R. L., Brand, R. J., Gould, K. L.,

"Can Lifestyle Changes Reverse Coronary Heart Disease? The Lifestyle Heart Trial." *The Lancet*: 336: 8708 (21 July 1990), 129–133.

169. *Time*, 29 October 1990.

170. Associated Press Newswire, 13 November 1990.

171. Watts, G. F., Lewis, B., Brunt, J. N., Lewis, E. S., Coltart, D. J., Smith, L. D., Mann, J. I., Swan, A. V., "Effects on Coronary Artery Disease of Lipid-Lowering Diet, or Diet Plus Cholestyramine, in the St. Thomas' Atherosclerosis Regression Study (STARS)." *The Lancet* 339: 8793 (7 March 1992), 563–569.

172. Gould, K. L., Ornish, D., Kirkeeide, R., Brown, S., Stuart, Y., Buchi, M., Billings, J., Armstrong, W., Ports, T., Scherwitz, L., "Improved Stenosis Geometry by Quantitative Coronary Arteriography after Vigorous Risk Factor Modification." *American Journal of Cardiology* 69:9 (1 April 1992), 845–853.

173. "Proposals for Nutritional Guidelines for Health Education in Britain," The Health Education Council, National Advisory Committee on Nutrition Education, September 1983.

174. Donaldson, A. N., "The Relation of Protein Foods to Hypertension." *Californian and Western Medicine* 1926:24, 328.

175. Armstrong, B., Van Merwyk, A. J., Coates, H., "Blood Pressure in Seventh-Day Adventist Vegetarians." *American Journal of Epidemiology* 105:5 (1977), 444–449.

176. Haines, A. P., Chakrabarti, R., Fisher, D., Meade, T. W., North, W.R.S., Stirling, Y., "Haemostatic Variables in Vegetarians and Non-vegetarians." *Thrombosis Research 19*, (1980), 139–148.

177. Sacks, F. M., Castelli, W. P., Donner, A., Kass, E. H., "Plasma Lipids and Lipoproteins in Vegetarians and Controls." *New England Journal of Medicine* 292: (1975), 1148–1151.

178. Anderson, J. W., "Plant Fiber and Blood Pressure." *Annals of Internal Medicine* 98, (1983) 842–846.

179. Margetts, B. M., Beilin, L. J., Vandongen, R., Armstrong, B. K., "Vegetarian Diet in Mild Hypertension: A Randomised Controlled Trial." *British Medical Journal (Clinical Research Edition)* (6 Dec 1986).

180. Margetts, B. M., Beilin, L. J., Armstrong, B. K., Vandongen, R., "A Randomized Control Trial of a Vegetarian Diet in the Treatment of Mild Hypertension." *Clinical & Experimental Pharmacology & Physiology*, 12 (1985), 263–266

181. Lindahl, O., Lindwall, L., Spångberg, Å., Stenram, Å., Öckerman, P. A., "A Vegan Regime with Reduced Medication in the Treatment of Hypertension." *British Journal of Nutrition* 52, (1984), 11–20.

182. Beilin, L. J., "Vegetarian Approach to Hypertension." *Canadian Journal of Physiology and Pharmacology* 64:6 (Jun 1986), 852–855.

183. *Los Angeles Times*, 18 July 1989.

184. *HeartCorps* 2:3, (Dec. 1989), 67.

185. Witteman, J. C. M., Willett, W. C., Stampfer, M. J., Colditz, G. A., Kok, F. J., Sacks, F. M., Speizer, F. E., Rosner, B., Hennekens, C. H., "Relation of Mod-

erate Alcohol Consumption and Risk of Systemic Hypertension in Women."
American Journal of Cardiology, 65:9 (1 March 1990). 633.

186.   *Journal of the American Medical Association*, 11 April 1990.

187.   Seedat, Y. K., "Nutritional aspects of hypertension." *South African Medical Journal* 75:4 (18 February 1989), 175–177.

188.   *Better Nutrition*, 52: 7 (July 1990), 14

189.   Uza, G., Vlaicu, R., "Serum Calcium and Salt Restriction in the Diet of Patients with Essential Arterial Hypertension." Institute of Hygiene and Public Health Medical Clinic no. 1, Cluj-Napoca, Romania. *Med Interne* 27:2 (April–June 1989), 93–97.

190.   *Medical World News*, 31:4, (26 February 1990), 22.

191.   "Selenium and High Blood Pressure," *The Cleveland Clinic*, March, 1976.

192.   McDougall, J., *Vegetarian Times*, 142, (June 1989), 60.

193.   *American Journal of Medicine* 220 (1950), 421.

194.   Swank, R. L., "Multiple Sclerosis: Twenty Years on Low Fat Diet." *Archives of Neurology* 23:5 (November 1970), 460–474.

195.   Swank, R. L., and Pullen, M. H., *The Multiple Sclerosis Diet Book* (Garden City, N.Y.: Doubleday, 1977).

196.   *The Edell Health Letter* 8: 5 (May 1989), 6; Hall, C., "Low-fat Diet May Cut Deaths From MS," *The Independent*, 6 July 1990, Swank, R. L., Dugan, B. B., "Effect of Low Saturated Fat Diet in Early and Late Cases of Multiple Sclerosis." *The Lancet*, 336:8706 (7 July 1990), 37.

197.   *The Lancet*, 336: 8706 (7 July 1990), 25.

198.   McDougall, J., *Vegetarian Times* 142 (June 1989), 60

199.   "Newsletter of the National Osteoporosis Society No. 1."

200.   National Osteoporosis Society, "Leaflet no. 2."

201.   *The Independent*, 23 October 1990.

202.   Ibid.

203.   John Studd, consultant gynaecologist, Kings College & Dulwich Hospitals, vice chairman of the National Osteoporosis Society.

204.   Lufkin, E. G., Ory, S. J., "Estrogen Replacement Therapy for the Prevention of Osteoporosis." *American Family Physician* 40:3 (September 1989), 205.

205.   Mack, T. M., Pike, M. C., Henderson, B. E, et al, "Estrogens and Endometrial Cancer in a Retirement Community." *New England Journal of Medicine* 294 (1976), 1262–1267.

206.   Cust M. P., Gangar, K. F., Hillard, T. C., Whitehead, M. I., "A Risk-Benefit Assessment of Estrogen Therapy in Postmenopausal Women." *Drug Safety* 5:5 (September–October), 345–358, Hulka, B. S., "Hormone-Replacement Therapy and the Risk of Breast Cancer." *A Cancer Journal for Clinicians* (Sept.–Oct. 1990) 40(5) 289–96.

207.   Quoted in *Bestways* 18:2 (February 1990), 26.

208.   "Osteoporosis: Bone Up on the Facts," *Better Nutrition*, 1990.

209.   Ibid.

210.   Data for 2% fat milk from U.S. Department of Agriculture "Handbook no. 8."

211. Data for cheddar cheese from U.S. Department of Agriculture "Handbook no. 8."

212. *The New York Times*, 8 May 1990.

213. Mazess, R. B., Mather, W., "Bone Mineral Content of North Alaskan Eskimos." *American Journal of Clinical Nutrition* 27:9 (September 1974), 916–925.

214. *Vegetarian Times* 43, 22.

215. Hegsted, M., Schuette, S. A., "Urinary Calcium and Calcium Balance in Young Men as Affected by Level of Protein and Phosphorus Intake." *Journal of Nutrition* 111 (1981) 553–562.

216. Johnson, N. E., Alcantara, E. N., Linkswiler, H., "Effect of Level of Protein Intake on Urinary and Fecal Calcium and Calcium Retention of Young Adult Males." *Journal of Nutrition* (1970), 100:1425

217. Breslau, N. A., Brinkley, L., Hill, K. D., Pak, C. Y., "Relationship of Animal Protein-Rich Diet to Kidney Stone Formation and Calcium Metabolism." *Journal of Endocrinology and Metabolism* 66:1 (January 1988), 140–146.

218. Scharffenberg, J. A., *Problems with Meat*. (Woodbridge Press Publishing Company, 1979).

219. Nielsen, F. H., Hunt, C. D., Mullen, L. M., Hunt, J. R., "Effect of Dietary Boron on Mineral, Estrogen, and Testosterone Metabolism in Postmenopausal Women." *FASEB Journal* 1:5 (November 1987), 394–397

220. UPI Newswire, 4 November 1987.

221. *Bestways* 18:3 (March 1990), 14

222. Marsh, A. G., Sanchez, T. V., Michelsen, O., Chaffee, F. L., Fagal, S. M., "Vegetarian lifestyle and bone mineral density." *American Journal of Clinical Nutrition* 48:3 Suppl (September 1988), p 837–841.

223. Lufkin, E. G., Ory, S. J., "Estrogen Replacement Therapy for the Prevention of Osteoporosis." *American Family Physician* 40:3 (Sept. 1989), 205.

224. Heaney, R. P., Recker, R. R., "Effects of Nitrogen Phosphorus, and Caffeine on Calcium Balance in Women." *Journal of Laboratory and Clinical Medicine* 99:1 (Jan. 1982), 46–55.

225. "What Everyone Needs to Know about Osteoporosis," The National Osteoporosis Society.

226. White, J. E., "Osteoporosis Strategies For Prevention." Family Nurse Practitioner Program, University of Pittsburgh School of Nursing. *Nurse Practitioner* 11:9 (1986), 36–46, 50.

227. *Meat Messenger* 12, 1992.

228. Erlichman, J., "Britain's Foul Abattoirs Anger Europe," *The Guardian*, 8 March 1989.

229. Cox, P., *Why You Don't Need Meat*, (Thorsons, 1986).

230. Mason, D., Vines, G., "Eggs and the Fragile Food Chain." *New Scientist*, 17 December 1988.

231. "Give Salmonella the Elbow." *New Scientist*, 17 Sept. 1987, Erlichman, J., *Gluttons for Punishment* (New York: Penguin Books, 1986).

232. *The Independent*, 31 July 1992.
233. "The Top 10 Most Censored Stories of 1989," Project Censored, Sonoma State University.
234. Associated Press Newswire, 18 September 1992.
235. *Meat Trades Journal*, 13 February 1986.
236. *The Observer*, 23 July 1989.
237. *Sunday Correspondent*, 4 November 1990.
238. *The Sunday Telegraph*, 16 July 1989.
239. *The Independent*, 12 June 1991.
240. Miller, J. A., "Diseases for our Future: Global Ecology and Emerging Issues." *BioScience*, 39:8 (Sept. 1989), 509.
241. Kilbourne, E. D., "New Viral Diseases: A Real and Potential Problem without Boundaries." *Journal of the American Medical Association* 26:1 (4 July 1990), 68.
242. *Newsday*, 30 May 1989.
243. *Black's Veterinary Dictionary* (A & C Black, 1988).
244. *Veterinary Medicine*, 7th Edition (Baillière Tindall, 1989).
245. *The Wall Street Journal*, 31 May 1991.
246. Gonda, M. A., Braun, M. J., Carter, S. G., Kost, T. A., Bess, J. W., Jr., Arthur, L. O., Van der Maaten, M. J., "Characterization and Molecular Cloning of a Bovine Lentivirus Related to Human Immunodeficiency Virus." *Nature* 330:6146 (November 26–December 2, 1987), 388–391.
247. Grote, J., "Bovine Visna Virus and the Origin of HIV." *Journal of the Royal Society of Medicine* 82:6 (1989), 380.
248. Benz, E. W., Moses, H. L., "Small Virus-like Particles Detected in Bovine Sera by Electron Microscopy." *Journal of the National Cancer Institute* (1974) 52:1931.
249. Lucas, M. H., Roberts, D. H., "Bovine Visna Virus and the Origin of HIV." *Journal of the Royal Society of Medicine* 82 (May 1989), 317.
250. Thomas, S., Pruett, S., St. Cyr-Coats, K., "BIV and BLV Infection of Mississippi Dairy Cattle: A Seroepidemiological Survey." *AIDS Weekly* (22 June 1992), 15.
251. *The New York Times*, 1 June 1991.
252. Kilbourne, E. D., "New Viral Diseases: A Real and Potential Problem without Boundaries" *Journal of the American Medical Association* 264:1 (4 July 1990), 68; Lederberg, J., "Pandemic as a Natural Evolutionary Phenomenon." *Journal of Social Research* 55 (1988), 344–359.

5: HOW TO GO VEGETARIAN

1. The names of interviewees in this chapter have been changed to fictional ones, any similarity to the names of living people is pure coincidence. The case histories are, however, entirely real and are told by the interviewees in their own words.

2. Klaper, M., from "Pregnancy, Children and the Vegan Diet." *Gentle World*, 1987.

3. Regan, T., *The Case for Animal Rights*. (Berkeley, Calif.: University of California Press, 1983).

4. Recipes analyzed by Nutri-Calc Plus using USDA data, supplemented with McCance & Widdowson, and manufacturers' analyses.

6: YOUR QUESTIONS ANSWERED

1. From data in Wilson, P. N., "Biological Ceilings and Economic Efficiencies for the Production of Animal Protein A.D. 2000." *Chemistry & Industry*, 6 July 1968.

2. Pearce, F., "Methane: The Hidden Greenhouse Gas." *New Scientist*, 1989.

3. Foundation on Economic Trends, Washington, D.C., 1992.

4. Beyond Beef Campaign, Washington, D.C. 1992.

5. Miller, R., *Bare-Faced Messiah*. (Michal Joseph, 1987).

6. Howlett, L., "Cruelty-Free Shopper." (Bloomsbury, 1989).

7. *The New York Times*, 2 September 1991.

8. "Open Space—Flying Fur," BBC2 Television, 1991.

9. *Searchlight* June 1991. See also: Proctor, R., *Racial Hygiene: Medicine Under the Nazis* (Cambridge, Mass.: Harvard, 1988).

10. *The New York Times*, 21 September 1991.

11. *The Jewish Vegetarian*, December 1989.

12. *The New York Times*, 21 September 1991, citing *The Gourmet Cooking School Cookbook* (1964).

13. Langley, G., "Vegan Nutrition." Vegan Society, 1988.

14. Norman, A. W., *Vitamin D: The Calcium Homeostatic Steroid Hormone*. (Orlando, Fla.: Academic Press, 1979).

15. Moon, J., "Factors Affecting Arterial Calcification Associated with Atherosclerosis." *Atherosclerosis* 16:199, 26.

16. *Better Nutrition* 52:2 (February 1990), 24.

17. *Nutrition Research Newsletter* 8:5 (May 1989), 56.

18. Reis, G. J., Boucher, T. M., Sipperly, M. E., Silverman, D. I., McCabe, C. H., Baim, D. S., Sacks, F. M., Grossman, W., Pasternak, R. C., "Randomised Trial of Fish Oil for Prevention of Restenosis After Coronary Angioplasty." *The Lancet* 2:8656 (22 July 1989), 177–181.

19. Middaugh, J. P., "Cardiovascular Deaths Among Alaskan Natives, 1980–86." *The American Journal of Public Health* 80:3 (March 1990), 282.

20. Cliff, W. J., "Coronary Heart Disease: Animal Fat on Trial." *Pathology* 19 (1987), 325–328.

21. Clarke, J.T.R., Cullen-Dean, G., Regelink, E., Chan, L., Rose, V., "Increased Incidence of Epistaxis in Adolescents with Familial Hypercholesterolemia Treated with Fish Oil." *Journal of Pediatrics* 116:1 (January 1990) 116:1, 139.

22. *Men's Health* 5:7 (July 1989), 4.

23. Lamperl, K. D., et al., "Effects on Serum Lipids and Blood Coagulation in Dialysis Patients." *American Journal of Disease* (February 1988) 11: 170–175.

24. Linzey, A., *Christianity and the Rights of Animals* (New York: Crossroads Publishing Company).

25. *The Independent*, 7 July 1990.

26. Personal correspondence, January 1988.

INDEX